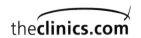
theclinics.com

CLINICS IN PODIATRIC MEDICINE AND SURGERY OF NORTH AMERICA

The Management of Lower Extremity Trauma and Complications

GUEST EDITORS
Thomas Zgonis, DPM
Demetrios G. Polyzois, MD

CONSULTING EDITOR
Vincent J. Mandracchia, DPM, MS

April 2006 • Volume 23 • Number 2

SAUNDERS

An Imprint of Elsevier, Inc.
PHILADELPHIA   LONDON   TORONTO   MONTREAL   SYDNEY   TOKYO

W.B. SAUNDERS COMPANY
A Division of Elsevier Inc.

1600 John F. Kennedy Blvd., Suite 1800, Philadelphia, PA 19103-2899

http://www.theclinics.com

CLINICS IN PODIATRIC MEDICINE
AND SURGERY   Volume 23, Number 2
April 2006   ISSN 0891-8422
Editor: Alexandra Gavenda   ISBN 1-4160-3523-0

The ideas and opinions expressed in *Clinics in Podiatric Medicine and Surgery* do not necessarily reflect those of the Publisher. The Publisher does not assume any responsibility for any injury and/or damage to persons or property arising out of or related to any use of the material contained in this periodical. The reader is advised to check the appropriate medical literature and the product information currently provided by the manufacturer of each drug to be administered to verify the dosage, the method and duration of administration, or contraindications. It is the responsibility of the treating physician or other health care professional, relying on independent experience and knowledge of the patient, to determine drug dosages and the best treatment for the patient. Mention of any product in this issue should not be construed as endorsement by the contributors, editors, or the Publisher of the product or manufacturers' claims.

Reprints. For copies of 100 or more of articles in this publication, please contact the Commercial Reprints Department, Elsevier Inc., 360 Park Avenue South, New York, New York 10010-1710 Tel.: (212) 633-3813, Fax: (212) 462-1935, e-mail: reprints@elsevier.com

Clinics in Podiatric Medicine and Surgery (ISSN 0891-8422) is published quarterly by W.B. Saunders, 360 Park Avenue South, New York, NY 10010-1710. Months of publication are January, April, July, and October. Business and Editorial Offices: 1600 John F. Kennedy Blvd., Suite 1800, Philadelphia, PA 19103-2899. Accounting and circulation offices: 6277 Sea Harbor Drive, Orlando, FL 32887-4800. Periodicals postage paid at New York, NY, and additional mailing offices. Subscription prices are $175.00 per year for US individuals, $280.00 per year for US institutions, $90.00 per year for US students and residents, $210.00 per year for Canadian individuals, $340.00 per year for Canadian institutions, $235.00 for international individuals, $340.00 for international institutions and $120.00 per year for Canadian and foreign students/residents. To receive student/resident rate, orders must be accompanied by name of affiliated institution, date of term, and the *signature* of program/residency coordinator on institution letterhead. Orders will be billed at individual rate until proof of status is received. Foreign air speed delivery is included in all *Clinics* subscription prices. All prices are subject to change without notice. POSTMASTER: Send address changes to *Clinics in Podiatric Medicine and Surgery*, Elsevier Periodicals Customer Service, 6277 Sea Harbor Drive, Orlando, FL 32887-4800. **Customer Service: 1-800-654-2452 (US). From outside of the US, call 1-407-345-1000.**

Clinics in Podiatric Medicine and Surgery is covered in *Index Medicus* and *EMBASE/ Excerpta Medica*.

Printed in the United States of America.

CONSULTING EDITOR

VINCENT J. MANDRACCHIA, DPM, MS, Section Chief, Podiatric Surgery, Department of Surgery, Broadlawns Medical Center; Clinical Professor, Department of Podiatric Medicine and Surgery, College of Podiatric Medicine and Surgery, Des Moines University–Osteopathic Medicine Center, Des Moines, Iowa

GUEST EDITORS

THOMAS ZGONIS, DPM, FACFAS, Assistant Professor, Division of Podiatry, Department of Orthopaedics, University of Texas Health Science Center at San Antonio, San Antonio, Texas; Director, Fellowship Training Programs, and Diplomate, American Board of Podiatric Surgery

DEMETRIOS G. POLYZOIS, MD, Director, Department of Orthopaedic Surgery, Metropolitan Hospital, Athens, Greece; President, Hellenic College of Orthopaedic Surgeons

CONTRIBUTORS

PAOLA ACQUARO, MD, Casa di Cura "Villa dei Gerani", Dott. A. Ricevuto srl, Sant'erice, Trapani, Italy

ANGELOS AYAZI, MD, Chief of Traumatology, IASO General Hospital, Athens, Greece

ALEXANDROS E. BERIS, MD, Professor, Department of Orthopaedics and Traumatology, University of Ioannina Medical School, Ioannina, Greece

ANDREAS GKIOKAS, MD, Director, Department of Orthopaedic Surgery and Traumatology, P and A Kyriakou Children's Hospital, Athens, Greece

THEODOROS B. GRIVAS, MD, Orthopaedic Surgeon, Director of the Orthopaedic Department, Thriasio General Hospital, Athens, Greece

JENNIFER B. HALLIGAN, DPM, Resident, Podiatric Surgery and Traumatology, Section of Podiatric Surgery, Department of Surgery, Broadlawns Medical Center, Des Moines, Iowa

GEORGIOS E. KOUFOPOULOS, MD, Orthopaedic Resident, Thriasio General Hospital, Athens, Greece

DENISE M. MANDI, DPM, Director of Externship Training and Faculty Member, Section of Podiatric Surgery, Department of Surgery, Broadlawns Medical Center; Clinical Assistant Professor, College of Podiatric Medicine and Surgery, Des Moines University, Des Moines, Iowa

VINCENT J. MANDRACCHIA, DPM, MS, Section Chief, Podiatric Surgery, Department of Surgery, Broadlawns Medical Center; Clinical Professor, Department of Podiatric Medicine and Surgery, College of Podiatric Medicine and Surgery, Des Moines University–Osteopathic Medicine Center, Des Moines, Iowa

LUIS E. MARIN, DPM, FACFAS, Residency Director, Palmetto General Hospital, Hialeah, Florida

W. ASHTON NICKLES, DPM, Resident, Podiatric Surgery/Traumatology, Section of Podiatric Surgery, Department of Surgery, Broadlawns Medical Center, Des Moines, Iowa

IOANNIS PAPAKOSTAS, MD, Attending Orthopaedic Surgeon, KAT Hospital, University of Athens Medical School, Athens, Greece

ENRICO PARINO, MD, Center for Foot Surgery, Casa di Cura Fornaca di Sessant, Torino, Italy

PIER CARLO PISANI, MD, Center for Foot Surgery, Casa di Cura Fornaca di Sessant, Torino, Italy

DEMETRIOS G. POLYZOIS, MD, Director, Department of Orthopaedic Surgery, Metropolitan Hospital, Athens, Greece; President, Hellenic College of Orthopaedic Surgeons

VASILIOS D. POLYZOIS, MD, PhD, Chief, Department of Orthopaedic Traumatology, KAT Hospital, University of Athens Medical School, Athens, Greece

THOMAS S. ROUKIS, DPM, FACFAS, Chief, Limb Preservation Service; Director, Diabetic Research Fellowship; Department of Vascular Surgery MCHJ-SOP, Madigan Army Medical Center, Tacoma, Washington

PANAYOTIS N. SOUCACOS, MD, Professor and Director, 1st Department of Orthopaedics and Traumatology, University of Athens Medical School, Athens, Greece

EMMANOUIL D. STAMATIS, MD, Attending Orthopaedic Surgeon, 401 General Army Hospital, Athens, Greece

PATRIS A. TONEY, DPM, MPH, Resident, Podiatric Surgery and Traumatology, Section of Podiatric Surgery, Department of Surgery, Broadlawns Medical Center, Des Moines, Iowa

ELIAS VASILIADIS, MD, Attending Orthopaedic Surgeon, Thriasio General Hospital, Athens, Greece

DANE K. WUKICH, MD, Assistant Professor, Department of Orthopaedic Surgery; Chief, Division of Orthopaedic Foot and Ankle Surgery, University of Pittsburgh School of Medicine, Pittsburgh, Pennsylvania

THOMAS ZGONIS, DPM, FACFAS, Assistant Professor, Division of Podiatry, Department of Orthopaedics, University of Texas Health Science Center at San Antonio, San Antonio, Texas; Director, Fellowship Training Programs, and Diplomate, American Board of Podiatric Surgery

CONTENTS

reported in the literature with a fairly high incidence of posttraumatic osteoarthritis of the subtalar joint, symptomatic hindfoot stiffness (especially when fixed in varus), wound dehiscence, and potential for the development of osteomyelitis caused by the extensive soft tissue trauma inherent with these injuries. For these reasons, closed treatment techniques using minimally invasive reduction procedures with application of ring-type fine-wire external fixation have recently gained popularity.

FORTHCOMING ISSUES

July 2006
Diagnosis and Treatment of Peripheral Nerve Entrapments and Neuropathy
Babak Baravarian, DPM, *Guest Editor*

October 2006
Implants in Foot and Ankle Surgery: Pros and Cons
Jesse B. Burks, DPM, MS, *Guest Editor*

January 2007
Residency Training
George F. Wallace, DPM, MBA, *Guest Editor*

RECENT ISSUES

January 2006
Pediatric Foot and Ankle Disorders
Jonathan M. Labovitz, DPM, *Guest Editor*

October 2005
Orthobiologics
Glenn M. Weintraub, DPM, *Guest Editor*

July 2005
Pedal Amputations
George F. Wallace, DPM, MBA, *Guest Editor*

THE CLINICS ARE NOW AVAILABLE ONLINE!

http://www.theclinics.com

ELSEVIER
SAUNDERS

Clin Podiatr Med Surg
23 (2006) xi–xii

CLINICS IN
PODIATRIC
MEDICINE AND
SURGERY

Foreword

The Management of Lower Extremity Trauma and Complications

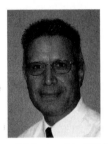

Vincent J. Mandracchia, DPM, MS
Consulting Editor

Life is what happens while you are busy making other plans

—John Lennon

How many times has it happened to you? You are busy making plans, and wham! Life either happens or passes you by—or, more importantly, makes the plans for you. This occurs in our personal and professional lives, and I have personally experienced this phenomenon in my professional life. Upon completion of residency training, my plans turned to private practice and plans for a podiatric generalist lifestyle. At that particular time, handling foot and especially ankle trauma was low on the priority list. After all, trauma was the purview of the orthopedic surgeon and not something that, although intriguing and exciting, most, if any, podiatric surgeons handled. But once again, life happened, regardless of other plans. Necessity is, after all, truly the mother of invention, and the supply-and-demand theory demanded of podiatrists that they expertly handle foot and ankle trauma.

I know first hand how true this is, working as a salaried podiatrist for a county hospital with a large, uninsured population. When confronted by the emergency department physician about the need to treat an ankle fracture, with no orthopedic

0891-8422/06/$ – see front matter © 2006 Elsevier Inc. All rights reserved.
doi:10.1016/j.cpm.2006.01.014

podiatric.theclinics.com

coverage available, it was necessary for us to "step up to the plate." That was 14 years ago, and man, things have changed. Without a doubt, podiatry has found a clearly defined place in the treatment of the most basic to the most complicated foot and ankle trauma. In fact, at our hospital, podiatry is first call for all lower-extremity trauma. Once again, life has happened, and plans have changed.

The podiatric colleges now offer specific foot and ankle trauma courses preparing students to handle lower extremity trauma in their residencies. National and state meetings of the College of Foot and Ankle Surgeons offer basic and advanced training for the trauma podiatrist. In short, treating trauma has become an unavoidable fact and a way of life for podiatrists.

This issue of the *Clinics in Podiatric Medicine and Surgery* is dedicated to management of lower extremity trauma and complications. Drs. Thomas Zgonis and Demetrios Polyzois have done an excellent job in gathering an international cast of authors to cover these topics. I thank them for their dedication to the dissemination of knowledge that is so important to our professional future.

As always, I encourage readers to use this issue as a reference and guide in their day-to-day experiences dealing with the patient who has foot and ankle trauma.

Vincent J. Mandracchia, DPM, MS
Broadlawns Medical Center
1801 Hickman Road
Des Moines, IA 50314, USA
E-mail address: vmandracchia@broadlawns.org

ELSEVIER
SAUNDERS

Clin Podiatr Med Surg
23 (2006) xiii–xiv

CLINICS IN
PODIATRIC
MEDICINE AND
SURGERY

Preface

The Management of Lower Extremity Trauma and Complications

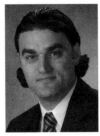 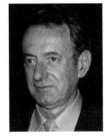

Thomas Zgonis, DPM   Demetrios G. Polyzois, MD
Guest Editors

One of the most difficult and challenging problems for the reconstructive and trauma surgeon is dealing with the extensive lower extremity injuries and complications. During my reconstructive foot and ankle surgery fellowship, I had the honor and privilege of spending some time at the Traumatology Center–Thriasio Hospital, Athens, Greece, under the direct supervision and guidance of my co-Editor, Dr. Demetrios Polyzois.

Dr. Polyzois is an internationally recognized lecturer in the methods and application of the Ilizarov apparatus and has authored numerous articles and book chapters in the field of lower extremity reconstructive surgery. Currently, he is the Director of the Department of Orthopaedic Surgery–Metropolitan Hospital, Athens, Greece, and has been elected as the President of the Hellenic College of Orthopaedic Surgeons. I have been grateful to know him as a personal colleague, friend, and mentor.

In this issue, a great international faculty has been selected to share some of their ideas and techniques of dealing with the most challenging trauma cases and complications. As you read through these articles, keep in mind the variety and different opinions of each surgeon dealing with the lower extremity trauma. I hope this issue serves as a guide to those interested on the field of traumatology and helps expand the possible therapies that are offered to their patients.

doi:10.1016/j.cpm.2005.12.001   *podiatric.theclinics.com*

I would like to thank Dr. Polyzois, all of the American and European invited authors, and, finally, my wife, Kristen, for her support and understanding throughout this intensive project. Thank you for allowing me to be a moderator of this great international invited faculty.

Thomas Zgonis, DPM
Division of Podiatry
Department of Orthopaedics
University of Texas Health Science Center at San Antonio
7773 Floyd Curl Drive, Mail Code 7776
San Antonio, TX 78229, USA
E-mail address: zgonis@uthscsa.edu

Demetrios G. Polyzois, MD
Department of Orthopaedic Surgery
Metropolitan Hospital
9 Eth. Makariou & El. Venizelou 1, N. Faliro
18547 Athens, Greece
E-mail address: dpolyzois@yahoo.com

ELSEVIER
SAUNDERS

Clin Podiatr Med Surg
23 (2006) 241–255

CLINICS IN
PODIATRIC
MEDICINE AND
SURGERY

Pediatric Fractures of the Foot and Ankle

Vasilios D. Polyzois, MD, PhD[a],*, Elias Vasiliadis, MD[b],
Thomas Zgonis, DPM[c], Angelos Ayazi, MD[d],
Andreas Gkiokas, MD[e], Alexandros E. Beris, MD[f]

[a]Department of Orthopaedic Traumatology, KAT Hospital, University of Athens Medical School,
Athens, Greece
[b]Orthopaedics Department, Thriasio General Hospital, Athens, Greece
[c]Division of Podiatry, Department of Orthopaedics, University of Texas Health Science Center at
San Antonio, 7773 Floyd Curl Drive, San Antonio, TX 78229, USA
[d]Traumatology Department, IASO General Hospital, Athens, Greece
[e]Department of Orthopaedic Surgery and Traumatology, P and A Kyriakou Children's Hospital,
Athens, Greece
[f]Department of Orthopaedics and Traumatology, University of Ioannina Medical School,
PO Box 1186, 451 10 Ioannina, Greece

Distal tibial physeal injuries are second in frequency only to distal radial physeal injuries [1]. They usually occur during sports activities and are more common in boys than in girls [2]. The prevalence is higher between the ages of 8 and 15 years [2], accounting for 10% to 40% of all injuries to skeletally immature patients [3–6]. In 1898 Poland [7] reported that in children ligaments are stronger than physeal cartilage, so that forces that result in ligament damage in adults cause fractures of the physes in children.

Distal tibial physis appears at 6 to 24 months of age and begins to ossify asymmetrically around the age of 14 years. Closure usually takes approximately 18 months and occurs first in the central part of the physis, extending next to the medial side and finally laterally. Tillaux and triplane fractures, which are known as transitional fractures [8–12], occur during that period. The anterior tibiofibular ligament plays an important role in the pathomechanics of transitional ankle fractures.

There are numerous accessory ossification centers around the ankle. Those accessory bones are common and may be injured.

* Corresponding author.
E-mail address: bpolyzois@yahoo.com (V.D. Polyzois).

0891-8422/06/$ – see front matter © 2006 Elsevier Inc. All rights reserved.
doi:10.1016/j.cpm.2006.01.010   *podiatric.theclinics.com*

The pediatric foot is characterized by a gradual maturation to an adult configuration. Ossification centers appear and fuse progressively, providing the child's foot with unique plasticity that prevents major injuries. Pediatric foot fractures are uncommon, especially in the early childhood, but become more frequent as the child matures.

Distal tibial fractures

Classification

Many classification systems have been proposed in the literature [13–21].

The Salter-Harris classification for physeal injuries is the most common anatomic system and is appropriate for every region of the skeleton (Table 1).

The Dias and Tachdjian mechanism-of-injury classification is the most widely used for ankle fractures in children. It is a modification of Lauge-Hansen classification for ankle fractures in adults and is based on their review of 71 fractures [21]. Their classification consists of eight types (Table 2). In the first four types the first word refers to the position of the foot at the time of injury and the second word refers to the force that produces the injury. The fifth type, axial compression, describes the mechanism of injury but not the position of the foot. Juvenile Tillaux and triplane fractures are believed to be caused by external rotation.

Diagnosis

A high index of suspicion is required for nondisplaced or minimally displaced fractures, because there is no severe pain or swelling, and there is no deformity. A radiograph should be obtained for accurate diagnosis. In patients who have significantly displaced fractures, pain, swelling, and deformity are marked, and the diagnosis is easier. Vascular and neurologic status should always be recorded before radiographic evaluation. The position of the foot relative to the leg may provide important information about the mechanism of injury.

Table 1
Salter-Harris classification of physeal injuries

Type	Description
I	A transverse fracture through the hypertrophic or calcified zone of the plate
II	A fracture similar to type I, but towards the edge the fracture deviates away from the physis and splits off a triangular metaphyseal fragment of bone
III	A fracture that splits the epiphysis and then veers off transversely to one side or the other through the hypertrophic layer of the physis
IV	A fracture that splits the epiphysis but extends into the metaphysis
V	A longitudinal compression injury of the physis

Table 2
Dias and Tachdjian mechanism-of-injury classification of pediatric distal tibial fractures

Type	Mechanism
Supination-inversion	
Grade I	The adduction or inversion force avulses the distal fibular epiphysis (Salter-Harris type I or II fracture)
Grade II	Further inversion produces a tibial fracture, usually a Salter-Harris type III or IV or, rarely, a Salter-Harris type I or II injury
Supination-plantarflexion	The plantarflexion force displaces the epiphysis directly posteriorly, resulting in a Salter-Harris type I or II fracture
Supination–external rotation	
Grade I	The external rotation force results in a Salter-Harris type II fracture of the distal tibia; the distal fragment is displaced posteriorly
Grade II	With further external rotation, a spiral fracture of the fibula is produced, running from anteroinferior to posterosuperior
Pronation–eversion–external rotation	A Salter-Harris type I or II fracture of the distal tibia occurs simultaneously with a transverse fibular fracture; the distal tibial fragment is displaced laterally
Axial compression	A Salter-Harris type V injury of the distal tibial physis
Juvenile Tillaux fracture	A Salter-Harris type III fracture involving the anterolateral distal tibia; the portion of the physis not involved in the fracture is closed
Triplane fracture	A group of fractures that have in common the appearance of a Salter-Harris type III fracture on the anteroposterior radiograph and of a Salter-Harris type II fracture on the lateral radiograph
Other physeal injuries	All fractures that do not fit into any of the other seven types

Anteroposterior and lateral radiographs of the affected ankle are usually sufficient. An additional mortise view may be required for nondisplaced fractures. CT scans are useful in the evaluation of intra-articular fractures, especially juvenile Tillaux and triplane fractures. MRI is occasionally useful in the identification of osteochondral injuries [22]. MRI scans supply information about the possibility of growth disturbance and potential physeal bars [23,24].

Treatment

The most important factors that must be considered when treating distal physeal fractures in children are the anatomic type as defined by Salter-Harris classification and the mechanism of injury as described by Dias and Tachdjian classification.

Salter-Harris type I and II fractures

Nondisplaced Salter-Harris type I and II fractures of the distal tibia can be treated adequately by immobilization in a non–weight-bearing long cast for 3 weeks, followed by 3 weeks of immobilization in a short-leg walking cast.

Closed reduction under general anesthesia, adequate muscle relaxation, and image intensifier control should be attempted for most displaced Salter-Harris type I and II fractures. For unstable fractures smooth-wire fixation across the physis may be required.

Immobilization should be performed with an above-knee non–weight-bearing cast for 4 weeks followed by a short-leg walking cast for an additional 3 to 4 weeks.

The accepted residual displacement or angulation is relevant to the remaining period of growth. For patients who have less than 2 years of growth remaining, no more than 5° is acceptable in each plane. When more than 2 years of growth are remaining, up to 10° of valgus or 15° of plantar tilt may be corrected by remodeling procedures. No varus deformity is acceptable [25].

Periosteum interposition may cause incomplete reduction. Open reduction through an anteromedial incision and extraction of the periosteal flap is recommended [26]. Interposition of the neurovascular bundle has also been reported, resulting in circulatory embarrassment when closed reduction was attempted [27]. Open reduction is obviously required.

It is important to obtain follow-up radiographs every 6 months for 2 years until there is no evidence of physeal deformity.

Salter-Harris type III and IV fractures

For nondisplaced Salter-Harris types III and IV fractures, above-knee cast immobilization is sufficient. A thorough radiographic evaluation is required weekly for the first 3 weeks to detect any displacement after casting. Occasionally a CT scan may be required.

Displaced fractures are intra-articular and require a precise anatomic reduction. Articular incongruity frequently results in posttraumatic arthritis and in an increased risk of growth arrest [28].

Reduction by closed methods should be reserved for minimally displaced fractures (<1 mm of displacement), must be undertaken under general anesthesia, and must be followed by stabilization using percutaneous pins or screws (if the epiphysis is large enough), supplemented by a cast. Smooth pins should be inserted within the epiphysis, parallel to the physis, and should be checked by image intensifier.

Displaced fractures (>2 mm) require open reduction. An additional arthrotomy may be required to evaluate the reduction. Options for internal fixation include smooth Kirschner wires, small-fragment cortical and cancellous screws, 4-mm cannulated screws, and absorbable pins [17,29,30]. The selection of the fixation device is determined mainly by the size of the fragment. An associated unstable fracture of the distal fibula should be stabilized using percutaneous pins. Postoperatively an above-knee nonwalking cast is applied for 6 weeks. Patients should be followed until skeletal maturity (every 6–12 months) to detect any growth abnormality that may arise.

Salter-Harris type V fractures

Unfortunately the diagnosis of Salter-Harris type V fractures is made only on follow-up radiographs. No specific treatment recommendations are available in the literature.

Juvenile Tillaux fractures

Tillaux fractures are usually nondisplaced because the fibula prevents displacement. Immobilization with a below-knee cast with the foot internally rotated for 6 weeks is adequate.

If a displacement greater than 2 mm exists, closed or open reduction is required. Direct pressure is applied to the anterolateral aspect of the distal tibia with the foot kept internally rotated as a closed reduction is attempted. A percutaneously inserted pin can be used to manipulate the displaced fragment into anatomic position [31]. If closed reduction is not successful, open reduction is required through an anterolateral approach, and fixation is performed with a cannulated or cancellous screw. Because growth preservation is not a concern, the screw does not have to be intra-epiphyseal.

Triplane fractures

For nondisplaced or minimally displaced (< 2 mm) fractures, immobilization in a long-leg cast with the knee flexed 30° is sufficient. The foot is held in internal rotation if the fracture is lateral or in eversion if the fracture is medial. Evaluation with a CT scan is recommended after casting to verify that there is no displacement. At 4 weeks, the cast is changed to a below-knee walking cast for another 3 to 4 weeks.

For fractures that are displaced more than 2 mm, a closed reduction under general anesthesia is attempted first. Reduction maneuvers are determined by the fracture pattern. Lateral triplane fractures are reduced by rotating the foot internally, and medial triplane fractures are reduced by abduction. Reduction is checked by image intensifier; if the reduction is considered adequate, an above-knee cast is applied, or percutaneous screws are inserted for fixation, if necessary, avoiding the physis. If closed reduction is unsuccessful, open reduction is required through an anterolateral approach for lateral triplane fractures or through an anteromedial approach for medial triplane fractures. Additional incisions are frequently necessary for adequate exposure. A preoperative CT scan may be helpful for evaluating the position of the fracture fragments in the anteroposterior and lateral planes and for determining the appropriate skin incisions. Occasionally a fibular osteotomy is required if the fibula is not fractured.

Direct vision through anteromedial arthrotomy and image intensification is used to confirm accurate reduction. Stabilization is performed by using two 4-mm cancellous screws. The entry point and the direction of the screws depend on the fracture pattern.

Postoperatively a below-knee cast is applied for 6 to 8 weeks.

Isolated fractures of the fibula

Isolated fractures of the fibula are usually Salter-Harris type I or II fractures that are caused by a supination-inversion injury. The most common pattern is a minimally displaced fracture that can be treated with short-leg cast immobilization for 6 weeks. Displaced fibular fractures accompany Salter-Harris type III and IV distal tibial fractures; if they are unstable, they may require fixation with a smooth intramedullary or obliquely inserted pin.

External fixation in pediatric fractures around the ankle

There are few indications for external fixation in pediatric fractures. The healing potential of the pediatric skeleton limits the usefulness of the complex treatment modalities that are used in adults. Severe open fractures or complex intra-articular fractures are uncommon in children. Only about 20% of severe open ankle fractures resulting from high-velocity motor vehicular accidents or lawn-mower injuries occur in children.

Meticulous mechanical débridement, copious irrigation, tetanus toxoid, and intravenous antibiotics are the basic principles of treatment. Skin grafting is occasionally required if local coverage is not possible.

The bone fragments are fixed with smooth pins, and the articular surface and physis should be restored. Care should be taken to avoid crossing the physis whenever possible. The pins can be incorporated in an external fixator and fixed to the metaphysis. Ideally a ring fixator such as an Ilizarov apparatus can be used. Using the device, the surgeon can correct any malalignment and allow the patient early weight bearing. Wound problems can be managed in a secure and stable environment that allows the bone to heal.

Complications

Delayed union and nonunion

Delayed union and nonunion are uncommon in pediatric ankle fractures and only a few case reports have been reported in the literature [22].

Malunion

Axis deviation or rotational deformity can arise after incomplete reduction or loss of reduction after cast immobilization. The remodeling process is limited mainly by the remaining growth of the child. The accepted angulation in each plane should not exceed 15° for younger children or 10° for older ones. Rotation is not acceptable and should be restored initially, because it cannot be corrected by remodeling.

If a malunion occurs, a corrective supramalleolar osteotomy should be performed. The procedure is demanding, especially if there is a potential for growth; it is wiser to reserve it for skeletally mature patients.

Growth arrest

Fractures that produce a physeal bar may result in a deformity that progresses with continued growth. Whether open reduction and internal fixation decreases physeal bar formation is controversial [16,28,32–34]. Leg-length discrepancy is another complication that may arise from growth arrest.

Growth abnormalities can be predicted by Harris growth lines [35] or with bone-scanning techniques.

Excision of bony bars and corrective osteotomy for significant angular deformity are required. Physeal bars, angular deformity, and leg-length discrepancy should be evaluated simultaneously.

Arthritis

Intra-articular fractures have an increased risk of posttraumatic arthritis. Arthritis occurs late, usually 5 to 8 years after skeletal maturity. Open reduction when there is a displacement of more than 2 mm can prevent this complication.

Fractures of the talus

Fractures of the talus are uncommon in children. The mechanism of injury in most reported cases is a forced dorsiflexion [36,37], and the fracture usually involves the talar neck.

The talus has a unique anatomic configuration. It is divided into the body, the neck, and the head. The artery of the tarsal canal with its deltoid branch and the artery of the sinus tarsi are the main arterial sources supplying the talus and are vulnerable to injury, especially fractures of the talar neck, where most arterial branches enter the body.

Talar neck fractures

A high index of suspicion is required for diagnosis of nondisplaced fractures of the talar neck. More severe injuries are accompanied by marked clinical signs such as swelling, pain, and localized tenderness. Anteroposterior, lateral, and oblique radiographs are sufficient for radiographic evaluation of the talar fractures. Occasionally, specific views are required [38].

The principles of treatment of fractures of the talar neck in children are similar to those in adults. For nondisplaced fractures, immobilization in an above-knee cast is recommended for 6 weeks. Any displacement greater than 5 mm is an indication for either closed or open reduction [38].

Forced plantarflexion of the foot in conjunction with inversion or eversion of the hindfoot is the maneuver for closed reduction, always under general anesthesia. The stability of the reduction is checked by fluoroscopy and is demonstrated by the maintenance of the reduction when the foot is dorsiflexed. If the reduction is stable, the leg is immobilized in a long cast for 6 to 8 weeks. If the reduction is not stable, an open reduction is indicated. Through a limited dorsomedial approach the reduction is held with Kirschner wires either through the navicular and the head of the talus or through the head of the talus only. If the talus is large enough, screw fixation should be used. It has been reported that posterior-to-anterior fixation is biomechanically superior, but in children it is wiser to avoid extended approaches that may injury the supplying arteries.

Meticulous follow-up with a radiograph every month for the first 6 months after injury and for a total period of 2 to 3 years is recommended to monitor healing and the vascular status of the talus [39].

The most severe complication of fractures of the talus in children is avascular necrosis. The risk for avascular necrosis depends on the degree of displacement at the time of injury and the vascular injury. Displacement can be managed during treatment, but little can be done for arterial disruption. The presence of the Hawkins sign, a subchondral lucency in the dome of the talus on radiograph, is not a reliable indicator of viability of the talar body after fracture in children because the subchondral area is cartilaginous [40]. A bone scan or MRI should be used for diagnosis of avascular necrosis.

When an avascular necrosis is detected, a restriction in weight bearing is recommended, ideally until completion of reossification [38,41,42], although such prolonged protection is not feasible in most cases. The remodeling potential is greater in children, and management should be more conservative than in adults. Talectomy for management of avascular necrosis of the talus is rarely indicated.

Other fractures of the talus

Fractures of the body of the talus are uncommon in children. There is no well-established method of treatment for this age group in the literature.

Fractures of the lateral or the posterior process of the talus also seem to be rare in children. Os trigonum may be a source of confusion that requires careful inspection of the radiographs.

Osteochondral fractures of the talus

The use of CT, MRI, or arthroscopy in evaluation of ankle pathology revealed an increased prevalence of osteochondral fractures of the talus among young adolescents as well as in adults [43].

A torsional impaction is the main mechanism of injury that produces either a posteromedial or an anterolateral lesion [44]. Posteromedial lesions may have a vascular cause. Osteochondral fractures of the talus may accompany an ankle injury with rupture of the talofibular ligaments.

A useful classification system based on CT and MRI is that of Anderson and colleagues [45], which divides osteochondral fractures into four stages. In stage I there is a subchondral fracture without collapse that is recognizable only with MRI. In stage II there is incomplete separation of the fragment. In stage III the fragment is unattached but still nondisplaced. In stage IV it is unattached and displaced.

Diagnosis is confirmed with a bone scan, a CT scan, or MRI in a persistently painful posttraumatic ankle. Radiographs are insufficient to expose early-stage osteochondral fractures. MRI is superior for evaluating the subchondral bone but is not recommended when the lesion is evident on a radiograph. CT is helpful for staging the lesion and for preoperative planning.

Stage I and II lesions are managed by non–weight bearing for 6 weeks. More advanced lesions require surgical treatment, either arthroscopically or by open techniques. Drilling, fixation with absorbable pins, and excision of the fragment are options for surgical intervention that follow the same principles as in adults.

Fractures of the calcaneus

Reports of calcaneal fractures in children have increased in recent years. This increase seems to result from improved diagnosis of the nondisplaced or minimally displaced fractures that predominate in children.

The calcaneus is the first bone of the foot to ossify. There are some anatomic differences between the immature and mature talus and calcaneus. Joint depression injuries are less severe in children, because the lateral process of the talus is small, and the posterior facet is parallel to the ground rather than inclined, resulting in a smaller impaction force to the cartilaginous calcaneus.

The most widely used classification for calcaneal fractures is that of Essex-Lopresti [46–49]. Calcaneal fractures are divided into intra- and extra-articular fracture patterns.

Localized tenderness is a reliable indicator of a minimally displaced calcaneal fracture. More severe injuries are characterized by pain, swelling, and inability to walk.

Lateral, axial, and dorso-plantar views are recommended for the diagnosis of calcaneal fractures. A lateral view of the spine should be made if there is tenderness over the spine, because compression fractures of the spine can be related to fractures of the calcaneus in children as well as in adults [48]. Böhler's angle, which is normally smaller in young children, should be measured.

A bone scan is helpful in demonstrating unrecognized calcaneal fractures.

CT scanning for calcaneal fractures has been studied less extensively in children than in adults, but CT is recommended in fractures with significant comminution and in older adolescents [39].

Treatment of calcaneal fractures in children is conservative. Simple immobilization in a short-leg walking cast for 4 to 6 weeks is sufficient for non-displaced fractures. For displaced intra-articular fractures, a non–weight-bearing policy should be followed to prevent further displacement. It has been reported that joint depression fractures in children are followed by overgrowth of the inferior articular facet of the talus that accommodates the joint depression of the calcaneus precisely [50]. Operative treatment is rarely indicated for intra-articular fractures in children, because remodeling leads to satisfactory results.

Fracture of the anterior process is a challenge, because it cannot be seen on radiographs until about age 10 years. Open reduction for larger displaced anterior calcaneal fractures is controversial [51]. Avulsion fractures of the tuberosity of the calcaneus may need open reduction if they are severely displaced [52].

Midfoot and tarsometatarsal injuries

Midfoot and tarsometatarsal injuries are extremely rare in children. Only a few case reports are available in the literature. There is not a specific mechanism of injury or a classification system for children, and currently the principles of treatment are the same as for adults (Figs. 1–4).

Metatarsal fractures

Metatarsal shaft and neck

Metatarsal fractures are relatively common in children. A direct or an indirect force may be the mechanism of injury. A torque applied to the forefoot usually results in a fracture of the metatarsal neck fracture, and a direct blow results in a fracture of the shaft.

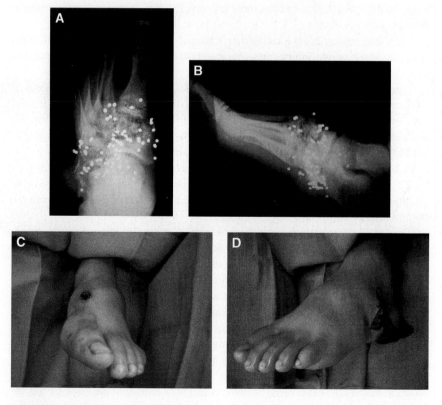

Fig. 1. Preoperative (*A*) anteroposterior and (*B*) lateral radiographs and (*C*, *D*) clinical presentation of a gunshot injury of the tarso-metatarsal joint in a 10- year-old boy.

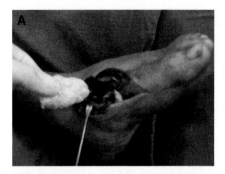

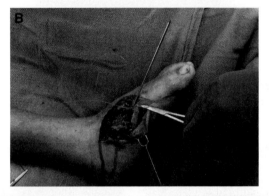

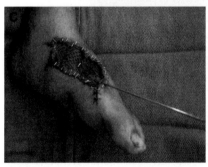 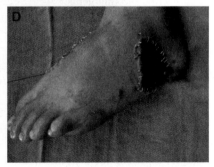

Fig. 2. Intraoperative pictures of (A) bone grafting, (B) abductor hallucis muscle flap, and (C, D) split-thickness skin grafting to the entrance and exit wounds.

Pain, swelling, ecchymosis, and localized tenderness are the principle symptoms. Metatarsal fractures can easily be diagnosed on anteroposterior, true lateral, and oblique radiographs.

Marked swelling and soft tissue injury should alert the physician to a possible compartment syndrome.

Initial management depends on the severity of injury. Stretched, taut skin accompanied by venous congestion in the toes and marked pain is an indication for fasciotomy. All nine compartments should be released.

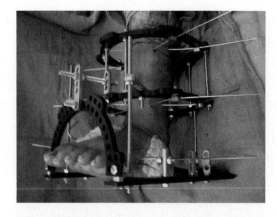

Fig. 3. Application of a circular multiplane external fixator for the tarso-metatarsal joint arthrodesis.

Most fractures of the metatarsals in children require immobilization in a short-leg walking cast for 3 to 6 weeks.

For the first and fifth metatarsals, reduction may be required. If the reduction is unstable, percutaneous Kirschner-wire fixation can be helpful. In most cases weight bearing adds to the beneficial result of remodeling. For the rare cases in which an open reduction through dorsal approach is required, a Kirschner wire is used to hold the fragments.

Complications generally are minimal, except for those already mentioned relating to the severity of the injury, circulatory compromise, or premature physeal closure.

Fractures of the base of the fifth metatarsal

Fractures of the base of the fifth metatarsal are common in children and are often been confused with an apophyseal growth center or the os vesalianum.

They occur after an avulsion injury of the base by the action of the peroneus brevis. A specific fracture pattern, the Jones fracture, must be differentiated from a fracture of the tuberosity, because the two differ considerably in prognosis and management.

Treatment consists of immobilization in a short-leg weight-bearing cast for 3 to 6 weeks. Removal of the cast is determined by the subsidence of swelling and tenderness rather than by radiographic appearance. Intramedullary screw fixation, with or without bone grafting, is rarely indicated in older children.

Stress fractures of the metatarsals

A skeletally maturing adolescent starting to participate in intensive training for sports may suffer a metatarsal stress fracture. Pain on weight bearing and localized tenderness are marked. A high index of suspicion is required. Bone

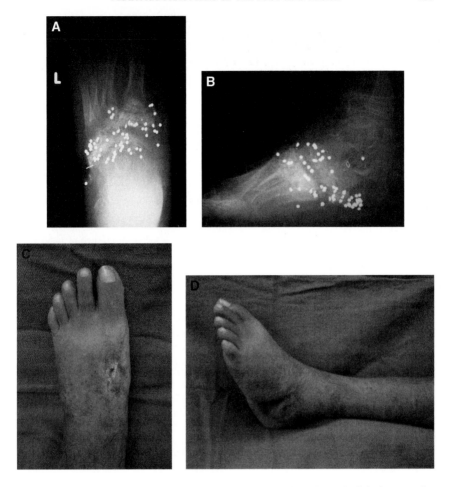

Fig. 4. Postoperative (*A*) anteroposterior and (*B*) lateral radiographs and (*C, D*) clinical presentation 3 months after the initial injury.

scans can elicit the lesion during the first 2 to 3 weeks, when radiographs are usually normal. Radiographs reveal periosteal callus formation 2 to 3 weeks after the onset of symptoms. A short period of immobilization, usually 3 weeks in a short-leg cast, followed by restriction of sports activities is recommended.

Fractures of the phalanges

Phalangeal fractures in children are extremely rare. The mechanism of injury is a direct blow, and the diagnosis is confirmed by radiographic examination. Treatment consists of immobilizing the injured toe by taping it to the adjacent one, which is serves as a splint. Reduction is required when there is rotational malalignment. The nail bed of the injured toe should be in the same plane as the other nail beds. Occasionally, a percutaneous Kirschner-wire fixation or open reduction may be indicated for a fracture of the proximal phalanx of the great toe in an older child. Three weeks of immobilization is sufficient, with a further 3 weeks of activity restriction.

References

[1] Peterson CA, Peterson HA. Analysis of the incidence of injuries to the epiphyseal growth plate. J Trauma 1972;12:275–81.
[2] Spiegel P, Cooperman D, Laros G. Epiphyseal fractures of the distal ends of the tibia and fibula. J Bone Joint Surg [Am] 1978;60:1046–50.
[3] Nilsson S, Roaas A. Soccer injuries in adolescents. Am J Sports Med 1978;6:358–61.
[4] Orava S, Saarela J. Exertion injuries to young athletes: a follow-up research of orthopaedic problems of young track and field athletes. Am J Sports Med 1978;6:68–74.
[5] Roser LA, Clawson DK. Football injuries in the very young athlete. Clin Orthop 1970;69: 219–23.
[6] Sullivan JA, Gross RH, Grana WA, et al. Evaluation of injuries in youth soccer. Am J Sports Med 1980;8:325–7.
[7] Poland J. Traumatic separation of the epiphysis. London: Smith, Elder & Co; 1898.
[8] Zaricznyj B, Shattuck LJ, Mast TA, et al. Sports-related injuries in school age children. Am J Sports Med 1980;8:318–24.
[9] Marmor L. An unusual fracture of the tibial epiphysis. Clin Orthop Relat Res 1970;73:132–5.
[10] Cooperman DR, Spiegel PG, Laros GS. Tibial fractures involving the ankle in children: the so-called triplane epiphyseal fracture. J Bone Joint Surg [Am] 1978;60:1040–6.
[11] Kaarholm J, Hansson LI, Laurin S. Computed tomography of intraarticular supination–eversion fractures of the ankle in adolescents. J Pediatr Orthop 1981;1:181–7.
[12] Denton JR, Fischer SJ. The medial triplane fracture: report of an unusual injury. J Trauma 1981;21:991–5.
[13] Aitken AP. The end results of the fractured distal tibial epiphysis. J Bone Joint Surg [Am] 1936; 18:685.
[14] Ashhurst APC, Bromer RS. Classification and mechanism of fractures of the leg bones involving the ankle. Arch Surg 1922;4:51.
[15] Bishop PA. Fractures and epiphyseal separation fractures of the ankle. AJR Am J Roentgenol 1932;28:49.
[16] Carothers CO, Crenshaw AH. Clinical significance of a classification of epiphyseal injuries at the ankle. Am J Surg 1955;89:879–89.
[17] Bucholz RW, Henry S, Henley MB. Fixation with bioabsorbable screws for the treatment of fractures of the ankle. J Bone Joint Surg [Am] 1994;76:319–24.
[18] Ogden JA. Skeletal injury in the child. Philadelphia: Lea & Febiger; 1982.
[19] Peterson HA. Physeal fractures: III. Classification. J Pediatr Orthop 1994;14:439.
[20] Salter RB. Injuries of the ankle in children. Orthop Clin North Am 1974;5:147–52.
[21] Lauge-Hansen N. Fractures of the ankle II. Arch Surg 1950;60:957–85.
[22] Kerr R, Forrester DM, Kingston S. Magnetic resonance imaging of foot and ankle trauma. Orthop Clin North Am 1990;21:591–601.
[23] Gabel GT, Peterson HA, Berquist TH. Premature partial physeal arrest: diagnosis by magnetic resonance imaging in two cases. Clin Orthop 1991;272:242–7.
[24] Havranek P, Lizler J. Magnetic resonance imaging in the evaluation of partial growth arrest after physeal injuries in children. J Bone Joint Surg [Am] 1991;73:1234–41.
[25] Cummings RJ. Fractures and dislocations of the foot. In: Rockwood Jr CA, Green DP, editors. Fractures in children. 4th edition. Philadelphia: JB Lippincott; 1996.

[26] Kling T. Fractures of the ankle and foot. In: Drennan J, editor. The child's foot and ankle. New York: Raven Press; 1992.

[27] Grace DL. Irreducible fracture-separations of the distal tibial epiphysis. J Bone Joint Surg [Br] 1983;65:160–2.

[28] Kling T, Bright R, Hensinger R. Distal tibial physeal fractures in children that may require open reduction. J Bone Joint Surg [Am] 1984;66:647–57.

[29] Benz G, Kallieris D, Seebock T, et al. bioresorbable pins and screws in paediatric traumatology. Eur J Pediatr Surg 1994;4:103–7.

[30] Bostman OM, Makela EA, Sodergard J, et al. Absorbable polyglycolide pins in internal fixation of fractures in children. J Pediatr Orthop 1993;13:242.

[31] Schlesinger I, Wedge JH. Percutaneous reduction and fixation of displaced juvenile tillaux fractures: a new surgical technique. J Pediatr Orthop 1993;13:389.

[32] Cass JR, Peterson HA. Salter-Harris type IV injuries of the distal tibial epiphyseal growth plate, with emphasis on those involving the medial malleolus. J Bone Joint Surg [Am] 1983;65: 1059–70.

[33] Crenshaw AH. Injuries of the distal tibial epiphysis. Clin Orthop 1965;41:98–107.

[34] Johnson Jr EW, Fahl JC. Fractures involving the distal epiphysis of the tibia and fibula in children. Am J Surg 1957;93:778–81.

[35] Hynes D, O'Brien T. Growth disturbance lines after injury of the distal tibial physis. J Bone Joint Surg [Br] 1988;70:231–3.

[36] Coltart WD. Aviator's astragalus. J Bone Joint Surg [Br] 1952;34:545–66.

[37] Mazel C, Rigault P, Padovani JP, et al. Fractures of the talus in children. Apropos of 23 cases. Rev Chir Orthop Reparatrice Appar Mot 1986;72(3):183–95.

[38] Canale ST, Kelly Jr FB. Fractures of the neck of the talus. Long-term evaluation of 71 cases. J Bone Joint Surg [Am] 1978;60:143–56.

[39] Gross RH. Fractures and dislocations of the foot. In: Rockwood Jr CA, Green DP, editors. Fractures in children. 4th edition. Philadelphia: JB Lippincott; 1996.

[40] Ogden JA. Skeletal injury in the child. Philadelphia: W.B. Saunders; 1990.

[41] Hawkins LG. Fractures of the lateral process of the talus. J Bone Joint Surg [Am] 1965;47: 1170–5.

[42] Hawkins LG. Fractures of the neck of the talus. J Bone Joint Surg [Am] 1970;52:991–1002.

[43] Canale ST, Belding RH. Osteochondral lesions of the talus. J Bone Joint Surg [Am] 1980; 62:97–102.

[44] Berndt AL, Harty M. Transchondral fractures (osteochondritis dissecans) of the talus. J Bone Joint Surg [Am] 1959;41:988–1020.

[45] Anderson IF, Crichton KJ, Grattan-Smith T, et al. Osteochondral fractures of the dome of the talus. J Bone Joint Surg [Am] 1989;71:1143–52.

[46] Essex-Lopresti P. The mechanism, reduction technique, and results in fractures of the os calcis. Br J Surg 1952;39:395–419.

[47] Rasmussen F, Schantz K. Radiologic aspects of calcaneal fractures in childhood and adolescence. Acta Radiol Diagn (Stockh) 1986;27(5):575–80.

[48] Scully TJ, Besterman G. Stress fracture—a preventable training injury. Mil Med 1982;147: 285–7.

[49] Wiley JJ, Profitt A. Fractures of the os calcis in children. Clin Orthop 1984;188:131–8.

[50] Thomas HM. Calcaneal fracture in childhood. Br J Surg 1969;56:664–6.

[51] DeLee JC. Fractures and dislocations of the foot. In: Mann RA, Coughlin MJ, editors. Surgery of the foot and ankle. St. Louis (MO): Mosby; 1993.

[52] Christensen SB, Lorentzen JE, Krogsoe O, et al. Subtalar dislocation. Acta Orthop Scand 1977;48:707–11.

ELSEVIER
SAUNDERS

Clin Podiatr Med Surg
23 (2006) 257–282

CLINICS IN
PODIATRIC
MEDICINE AND
SURGERY

The Management of Lower Extremity Soft Tissue and Tendon Trauma

Theodoros B. Grivas, MD[a],*, Georgios E. Koufopoulos, MD[a],
Elias Vasiliadis, MD[a], Vasilios D. Polyzois, MD, PhD[b]

[a]Orthopaedic Department, Thriasio General Hospital, Genimata Avenue, 19600, Attica, Greece
[b]KAT Hospital, 2 Nikis str, 14561, Kifisia, Athens, Greece

Achilles, the warrior and hero of Homer's *Iliad*, lends his name to the Achilles tendon, the thickest and strongest tendon in the human body [1]. (Thetis, Achilles's mother, after learning of a prophecy that Achilles would die in battle, hoped to make him invulnerable to physical harm by holding him by the heel and immersing him in the river Styx. His heel, which was not immersed, remained vulnerable to injury, however.)

Hippocrates, in the first recorded description of an injury to the Achilles tendon, stated that "this tendon, if bruised or cut, causes the most acute fevers, induces choking, deranges the mind and at length brings death" [2].

Achilles tendon rupture

Background

Ruptures of the Achilles tendon most commonly occur spontaneously in healthy, young, active individuals who are aged 30 to 50 years and have no antecedent history of calf or heel pain. Unlike tears or ruptures at the musculo-tendinous junction of the Achilles tendon, Achilles tendon ruptures are located within the tendon substance itself, approximately 1 to 2 inches proximal to its

* Corresponding author. D. Bernardou 31st Street, Brilissia 152 35, Attica, Greece.
E-mail address: grivastb@panafonet.gr (T.B. Grivas).

0891-8422/06/$ – see front matter © 2006 Elsevier Inc. All rights reserved.
doi:10.1016/j.cpm.2006.01.002
podiatric.theclinics.com

insertion into the calcaneus. Poor conditioning, advanced age, and overexertion are risk factors for this injury. The common precipitating event, however, is a sudden eccentric force applied to a dorsiflexed foot. Ruptures of the Achilles tendon also may occur as the result of direct trauma or as the end result following Achilles peritenonitis with or without tendinosis [3].

Functional anatomy

The Achilles tendon is formed from the tendinous contributions of the gastrocnemius and soleus muscles coalescing approximately 15 cm proximal to its insertion. Along its course in the posterior aspect of the leg, the tendon spirals 30° to 150° until it inserts into the calcaneal tuberosity. The gliding ability of the Achilles tendon is aided by a thin sheath of paratenon rather than a true synovial sheath. The sheath of paratenon is composed of a visceral layer and a parietal layer. Tendons can receive their blood supply from vessels originating from three sources: the musculotendinous junction, the surrounding connective tissue, and the bone–tendon junction. The blood flow of the Achilles tendon depends on age, with a higher blood flow in younger individuals. The Achilles tendon is poorly vascularized, especially in its midportion, with blood vessels running from the paratenon into its substance [4].

There is a dispute concerning the distribution of blood vessels in the tendon. Some investigations have shown that the density of blood vessels in the middle part of the Achilles tendon is low compared with that in the proximal part. Others, using Doppler flowmetry, have shown that blood flow is evenly distributed throughout the Achilles tendon and may vary according to age, gender, and loading conditions [5].

History

Rupture most commonly occurs in the middle-aged male athlete (eg, the so-called "weekend warrior" engaging in a pickup game of basketball). Injury often occurs during recreational sports that require bursts of jumping, pivoting, and running, such as tennis, racquetball, basketball, and badminton. The patient often presents with a sensation of a sudden snap in the back of the calf or heel that is associated with acute, severe pain. This pain may be the result of an indirect injury (eccentric ankle contraction in a dorsiflexed foot) or a direct injury from blunt trauma to the tendon. Older recreational athletes usually have a relatively weakened tendon substance with muscles that are deconditioned. The patient should be questions about any changes in training and activity or intensity level.

A history of intratendinous steroid injections or the use of fluoroquinolone (eg, ciprofloxacin, levofloxacin) may lead to tendon weakness. The patient may have a history of prior Achilles tendon rupture on the affected side. The incidence of tendon rerupture after initial conservative management is relatively high.

Clinical tests

Calf-squeeze test

The description of the calf-squeeze test is often credited to Thompson, who described the test in 1962, 5 years after it was described by Simmonds [6]. With the patient prone on the examining table and the ankles clear of the table, the examiner squeezes the fleshy part of the calf. Squeezing the calf deforms the soleus muscle, causing the overlying Achilles tendon to bow away from the tibia, resulting in plantar flexion of the ankle if the tendon is intact. The affected leg should always be compared with the contralateral leg. A false-positive finding may occur in the presence of an intact plantaris tendon, although this possibility has not been proved scientifically.

Knee-flexion test

The patient is asked to flex the knees actively to 90° while lying prone on the examining table. During this movement, if the foot on the affected side falls into neutral or dorsiflexion, a rupture of the Achilles tendon can be diagnosed.

Needle test

A hypodermic needle is inserted through the skin of the calf, just medial to the midline and 10 cm proximal to the insertion of the tendon. The needle is inserted until its tip is just within the substance of the tendon. The ankle is then alternately placed in plantar flexion and dorsiflexion. If, on dorsiflexion, the needle points distally, the portion of the tendon distal to the needle is presumed to be intact. If the needle points proximally, there is presumed to be a loss of continuity between the needle and the site of the insertion of the tendon [7].

Sphygmomanometer test

For the sphygmomanometer test, a sphygmomanometer cuff is wrapped around the midpart of the calf while the patient is lying prone. The cuff is inflated to 100 mm Hg (13.33 kilopascals) with the foot in plantar flexion. The foot is then dorsiflexed. If the pressure rises to approximately 140 mm Hg (18.66 kilopascals), the musculotendinous unit is assumed to be intact. If, however, the pressure remains at around 100 mm Hg, a rupture of the Achilles tendon may be diagnosed [8].

Causes

The common precipitating event that causes an Achilles tendon rupture is a sudden eccentric force applied to a dorsiflexed foot. Ruptures of the Achilles tendon also may occur as the result of direct trauma or as the end result of Achilles peritendonitis with or without tendinosis. Risk factors associated with Achilles tendon rupture include participation in recreational athletics, relatively older age (30–50 years), prior Achilles tendon injury or rupture, prior tendon injections or fluoroquinolone use, and abrupt changes in training, intensity, or activity level [3].

Imaging studies

Radiographs of the ankle may show soft tissue swelling, increased ankle dorsiflexion, calcifications, calcaneal avulsion fractures, a Haglund deformity, or bony metaplasia; however, radiographs are more useful in ruling out concomitant bony injuries, anomalies, or fractures. Ultrasound is a relatively inexpensive, fast, repeatable, dynamic examination that helps determine tendon thickness and gap size. Ultrasound is operator dependent and requires an experienced ultrasound technician and radiologist for reliable imaging. In MRI the normal Achilles tendon is seen as an area of low signal intensity on all pulse sequences. The tendon is well delineated by the high signal intensity of the fat pad of Kager's triangle. Any increase in intratendinous signal intensity should be regarded as abnormal. T1- and T2-weighted images in the axial and sagittal planes should be used to evaluate suspected ruptures of the Achilles tendon. On T1-weighted images, a complete rupture of the Achilles tendon is identified as a disruption of the signal within the tendon. On T2-weighted images, the rupture is demonstrated as a generalized increase in signal intensity; the edema and hemorrhage at the site of the rupture are seen as an area of high signal intensity [9].

Treatment

The many techniques and procedures described for the treatment of an acutely ruptured Achilles tendon can be grouped under three headings: open operative, percutaneous operative, and nonoperative. Because there is no agreed-on protocol, the choice of treatment regimen is still based largely on the preference of the surgeon and the patient [10]. The exact type of operative procedure (open or percutaneous) remains controversial [11].

Nonoperative treatment has its supporters, but operative treatment has been the method of choice in the last 2 decades for athletes and young people and for patients who have a rupture for which treatment has been delayed. Acute ruptures in nonathletes may be treated nonoperatively.

Surgical intervention

The goal of the orthopedic surgeon is to restore tendon continuity and length to allow the patient to regain his or her functional and desired activity level. In general, operative intervention is recommended for younger, healthier, more active individuals who desire a reliable treatment method. Individuals participating in high school, college, semi-professional, or professional sports are strongly encouraged to have surgery to decrease the chance of rerupture. Acute ruptures, large partial ruptures, and reruptures are indications for surgical repair. On the other hand, patients who are older or more inactive and those who have systemic illnesses or poor skin integrity are not optimal candidates for operative treatment and are better served with nonoperative treatment [3]. Postoperatively, a posterior splint or short-leg cast is placed in gravity equinus for 10 to 14 days to reduce tension on the incision. With each cast change, the ankle is gradually dorsiflexed, with a neutral position being reached at approximately 4 weeks after surgery. At that time, the patient is allowed to begin weight bearing on the leg. At 6 weeks after surgery, use of the cast is discontinued, and the patient is referred to physical therapy.

The advantages of operative treatment include a lower rerupture rate (0–5%), a higher percentage of patients who return to participation in sports, and a greater return of strength, endurance, and power. Disadvantages of operative treatment include hospitalization, high operative costs, wound complications (eg, infection, skin slough, sinus formation), adhesions, and possible sural nerve injury (especially through a lateral longitudinal approach).

Nonoperative treatment

The most commonly used form of nonoperative treatment is immobilization in a plaster cast, usually for a period of 6 to 8 weeks. Immobilization has been advocated by those who think that it produces results similar to those achieved with operative treatment [12]. When the Achilles tendon ruptures, the paratenon generally remains intact. Stripping of the paratenon during an operation reduces the amount of reactive tissue that is produced later at the site of the injury because the paratenon provides a valuable blood supply to the damaged tendon. A short-leg cast is applied to the affected leg while the ankle is placed in slight plantar flexion (gravity equinus). In theory, keeping the foot in this position results in better apposition of the tendon ends. Cast immobilization is continued for about 6 to 10 weeks. Forced dorsiflexion is contraindicated. The ankle gradually may be dorsiflexed to a more neutral position after a period of immobilization (approximately 4–6 weeks). This position is sustained with serial casting or adjustable ankle orthotics. Walking in the cast is allowed at this time. After cast removal, a 2-cm heel lift in the shoe is worn for an additional 2 to 4 months. During this time, a rehabilitation program is initiated.

Achilles tendonitis

Background

"Achilles tendonitis' was the term originally used to describe the spectrum of tendon injuries ranging from inflammation to tendon rupture. Recently, a histopathologically determined nomenclature has evolved to classify this range of tendon inflammation and degeneration into the following three stages [13]:

Peritenonitis
Peritenonitis with tendinosis
Tendinosis

The occurrence of Achilles tendinopathy is highest among individuals who participate in middle- and long-distance running, track and field, tennis, badminton, volleyball, and soccer [14]. Johansson [15] reported an annual incidence of Achilles disorders that was between 7% and 9% in top-level runners.

History

The patient's history should provide most of the information needed to make the diagnosis of Achilles tendinopathy. The interval between the onset of symptoms and the first visit to a physician, as well as the onset of the symptoms, the injury mechanism in patients who have an acute case, and possible previous Achilles tendon problems and their treatment, must be recorded [16]. The course of events since the onset of symptoms, with special emphasis on the activities that seem to make the pain worse and the interventions that seem to relieve the pain, provides valuable additional information.

Histopathology

On the basis of a histopathologic examination, the findings in Achilles tendinopathy can be divided into peritendinous changes and intratendinous degeneration; frequently, these entities coexist [17].

Peritenonitis

In peritenonitis, the paratenon itself is inflamed, thickened, and typically adherent to the underlying unaffected tendon. Under the microscope, there is capillary proliferation and infiltration of inflammatory cells within the paratenon.

Tendinosis

With tendinosis, there are thickened and yellowish areas of mucoid degeneration within the tendon itself. The tendon loses its normal coloration and striation patterns. Hypocellularity, collagen disorganization, lack of inflammatory reaction, scattered vascular ingrowth, and intermittent areas of calcification or necrosis are hallmarks of this disease process. Pathology is usually found within the watershed area of the tendon.

Peritenonitis with tendinosis

Histologically and macroscopically, peritenonitis with tendinosis combines findings that occur in both tendinosis and peritenonitis.

Physical examination

Palpate the entire gastrocnemius-soleus complex for tenderness, nodules, swelling, warmth, atrophy, and tendon defects with the patient in a prone position with feet off the table. Localization of the tenderness should be differentiated between musculotendinous (tennis leg), intrasubstance (Achilles tendon injury), and insertional (eg, Haglund deformity, pump bump). Nodules should be palpated for tenderness, boundaries, mobility, and size. Calf atrophy, determined by calf circumference as compared with the contralateral side, may provide information as to the chronicity of the disease process (acute versus chronic). Gaps or areas of tendon discontinuity are often signs of partial or complete tendon rupture.

Patients who have peritenonitis typically present with warmth, swelling, and diffuse tenderness localized 2 to 6 cm proximal to the tendon's insertion. Crepitations also may be felt if peritenonitis presents acutely. As the condition becomes more chronic, symptoms may be provoked by decreased amounts of physical activity [18]. Tendinosis is often pain free. Typically, the only sign may be a palpable intratendinous nodule that accompanies the tendon as the ankle is placed through the range of motion (ROM). Occasionally, a thickening along the entire tendon may develop in chronic conditions. Peritenonitis with tendinosis is diagnosed in patients who have activity-related pain and swelling of the tendon sheath with tendon nodularity.

Perform a Thompson test to check for Achilles tendon rupture: with the patient prone and the knee flexed, squeeze the calf proximal to the affected area. If passive plantar flexion of the foot is achieved with this maneuver, the test is negative, and the Achilles tendon is at least partially intact. If no motion at the ankle is generated, the Thompson test is positive, and a complete rupture of the tendon has occurred. It is important to perform this test, because incomplete or complete ruptures may occur in patients who have a history of peritonitis with or without tendinosis. With acute partial or complete tendon ruptures, patients often report focal pain and swelling at the sight of injury.

Ascertain active and passive ROM of the knee, ankle, and subtalar joints. Patients who have overuse Achilles tendon injuries typically have decreased motion in the ankle or subtalar joints. Note resting alignment and motion of the forefoot and ankle. Forefoot and heel varus, pronated feet, cavus feet, and tibia vara are known predisposing risk factors for this disease process.

Determining if evidence of neurovascular compromise is present

Imaging methods

Radiographs usually are nondiagnostic but may show soft tissue swelling, calcifications, calcaneal avulsion fractures, increased dorsiflexion, Haglund deformity, and bony metaplasia.

Ultrasonography has been used increasingly to examine Achilles tendon injuries and other tendon disorders, because it provides a readily available, quick, safe, and inexpensive method to verify the existence and location of intratendinous lesions [19]. The primary disadvantages are that ultrasound is operator dependent, provides somewhat limited soft tissue contrast, and is not as sensitive as MRI. The results of ultrasonography have been found to be reliable when they demonstrate adhesions around an Achilles tendon. Ultrasound has been shown to be unreliable when it fails to detect adhesions, however, and patients who have few adhesions may have a false-negative result on ultrasonography. On the other hand, abnormalities detected by ultrasonography in an asymptomatic Achilles tendon can predict the development of Achilles tendinopathy very accurately [20].

In the acute phase of Achilles tendinopathy, ultrasonography reveals fluid surrounding the tendon. In its more chronic form, peritendinous adhesions can be seen as thickening of the hypoechoic paratenon with poorly defined borders [21]. Discontinuity of tendon fibers, focal hypoechoic intratendinous areas, and localized tendon swelling and thickening are the most characteristic ultrasonographic findings in patients who have a surgically verified intratendinous lesion (tendinosis) of the Achilles tendon.

MRI has been used extensively to visualize pathologic conditions of the tendon, because it satisfies two fundamental principles of imaging. First, it provides high intrinsic tissue contrast, which allows normal tendons to be distinguished from abnormal tendons. Second, it provides high spatial resolution that allows detailed anatomic structures to be identified [22]. The ability of MRI to acquire images in multiple planes (longitudinal, transverse, and oblique) is also a clear advantage. The disadvantages of MRI are its relatively high cost, limited availability in some countries, time-consuming scanning, and the slow and often incomplete resolution of signal changes after operative intervention.

In patients who have chronic Achilles tendinopathy, MRI frequently reveals tendon thickening on sagittal images and altered signal appearance within the tendon tissue. Movin and colleagues [23] suggested that the gadolinium-enhanced intratendinous signal abnormality in patients who had chronic Achilles tendinopathy was related to an increased amount of interfibrillar noncollagenous extracellular matrix and altered fiber structure.

Treatment

Conservative treatment

Initial conservative treatment should be directed toward relieving symptoms and should consist of a combination of strategies aimed at controlling inflammation and correcting training errors, limb malalignment, decreased flexibility, muscle weakness, and the use of poor equipment during sports [24]. In addition, injection of heparin to prevent edema or fibrin exudate in the paratenon (ie, prevention of the formation of adhesions between tendon and paratenon) and various modalities of physical therapy (heat, ultrasound, and electrical stimulation) are used in the treatment of some patients who have Achilles tendinopathy.

The control of inflammation is recommended in the early phase of Achilles tendon overuse injury. Inflammation is controlled by decreasing activity, the use of cold packs, and the administration of anti-inflammatory medication [25]. Decreasing the intensity, frequency, and duration of the activity that caused the injury, or modification of that activity may be the only action needed to control the inflammation and symptoms in the acute phase. Modified rest, which allows activity in the uninjured parts of the body, such as the upper extremities, has been recommended. Cryotherapy has been regarded as the single most useful intervention for tendon inflammation in the acute phase of this disorder. Cold therapy can control pain and edema as well as reduce regional blood flow and the metabolic demands of the tissue and thereby help prevent further tissue damage at the site of the injury. Cryotherapy also delays inflammation by decreasing the effects of histamine on vascular membranes, neutrophil activation, and leukocytes.

Nonsteroidal anti-inflammatory drugs, in the form of pills or topical gels, are frequently used in the treatment of acute as well as chronic forms of Achilles tendinopathy. The benefit of these drugs is controversial, however [26]. Healing of acute soft tissue injury is slightly more rapid, and inflammation is controlled slightly better with the use of nonsteroidal anti-inflammatory drugs than without them.

Steroid injections into and around the tendon are not advised because they have been shown to weaken the tendon.

Physical therapy. Instruct the patient in stretching, training modification/ re-evaluation, and muscle strengthening. Stretching exercises are believed to be the key modality in treatment because they provide better flexibility to the ankle. Stretching of the posterior gastroc-soleus complex should always be slow and deliberate. Each stretch should last for 20 to 30 seconds, with multiple repetitions in a set [27]. Three possible methods of stretching the gastroc-soleus complex include (1) use of an inclined board, (2) wall leans, and (3) foot-on-chair stretching. An inclined board is a fabricated ramp of 15° to 18° that allows the patient to stretch the heel cord complex gradually. A much simpler method is to have the patient stand and face a wall while leaning with knees extended and heels planted on the ground. The foot-on-chair method requires the athlete to place the foot flat on a chair and gradually bring the knee forward as far as possible without losing heel contact with the chair. Use orthotics to treat overpronation or heel cups to provide extra support and cushion to the tendon. Return to activities is gradual.

Surgical intervention

Operative treatment is indicated after a comprehensive conservative treatment program has failed in athletes who have peritonitis or tendinosis and who are unwilling to modify or stop their activity. Although there are no absolute indications, relative contraindications include noncompliant patients, patients who have an active infection site, and patients who have potential wound-healing problems (eg, patients who have diabetes mellitus or peripheral vascular disease and smokers). Lysis of adhesions through release of the Achilles tendon from the inflamed paratenon is the mainstay procedure for unrelieved peritonitis. Release is performed on the dorsal, medial, and lateral aspects of the tendon. Circumferential dissection to include the anterior sheath may jeopardize the vascular supply to the tendon and cause excessive scarring. This surgery is followed immediately with passive ROM and progressive weight bearing and strengthening for 2 to 3 weeks. When able to ambulate without pain, the patient may begin closed-chain activities, such as biking or stair climbing. Running may begin at 6 to 10 weeks after surgery. Participation in competitive sports can start after 3 to 6 months.

The relationship between operative treatment and healing of the tendon is still not well understood [26]. Although the results of uncontrolled studies have generally been good, the results may not have been caused by the operative treatment alone, because operative treatment usually was combined with a postoperative period of immobilization and rest and a prolonged period of controlled rehabilitation.

In most studies, operative treatment of Achilles tendinopathy has given satisfactory results in 75% to 100% of the patients [28]. Most of these reports were retrospective, however, and only a few had results that were based on objective evaluations, such as ROM of the ankle.

Maintenance phase

Physical therapy

Achilles tendonitis is best prevented, treated, and maintained by preserving good ROM in the heel cord complex. Such motion can be gained with the use of an inclined board, wall leans, or the foot-on-chair stretching exercises, as described. Moist heat or compresses before workouts and at night are beneficial. Cold modalities should be used after strenuous activities to provide pain relief and anti-inflammatory effects.

Complications

Patients who have long-standing tendonitis or tendinosis may progress to complete rupture of the tendon.

Prevention

A key to the prevention of Achilles tendonitis is maintaining good flexibility and strength of the heel cord complex and ankle. Proper warm-up is necessary before activity. In individuals who have faulty foot biomechanics (eg, overpronation), use of custom orthotics, heel cups, or arch supports may be recommended to prevent development of tendonitis.

Prognosis

In general, the prognosis is quite good for individuals who have Achilles tendonitis who comply with a period of relative rest and conservative treatment.

Education

Patients need to have a good understanding of the importance of proper warm-up techniques before participating is activities that may cause repetitive stress to the Achilles tendon. Wearing proper footwear in important, as is periodic changing of training surfaces. If athletes do demonstrate faulty foot biomechanics that may place them at risk, recommend that they consult with an orthotist or physical therapist for an evaluation and recommendation of proper orthotics [3].

Peroneal tendon syndromes

Injuries to the peroneal tendons are common but not always clinically significant. They are misdiagnosed as a lateral ankle sprain most of the time, because isolated injury to the peroneal tendons is rare. Injury can occur in one or both peroneus longus and brevis tendons and is typically classified as acute or chronic.

History

The histories for each type of peroneal injury have subtle differences. The key is to have a clinical suspicion and to listen carefully to the patient.

Peroneal tendonitis

In peroneal tendonitis, symptoms of pain behind and distal to the lateral malleolus usually occur when the patient returns to activity after a period of time off. Swelling and tenderness are also present.

Peroneal tendon subluxation

In peroneal tendon subluxation, snapping along the lateral ankle is present, with a sense of weakness or pain. A painful snapping sensation over the lateral ankle is the classic indication of peroneal tendon subluxation. Pain during toe walking or when cutting laterally while playing on a field is also observed. With acute injury, pain and swelling are noted over the posterolateral aspect of the ankle. Chronic injuries include recurrent inversion injury with lateral ankle instability and painful snapping across the ankle.

Peroneal tendon tears

With acute peroneal tendon tears, pain and swelling are inferior and posterior to lateral malleolus. The patient may have had pain before injury, but now the pain is debilitating, and strength is decreased. Chronic injury results in the subtle, insidious onset of pain posterior to the lateral malleolus that progressively worsens in terms of both function and the level of pain [30].

Anomalous peroneus brevis muscle injury

Anomalous peroneus brevis muscle injury can be acute or chronic. The patient may have debilitating pain in the push-off portion of the stance, without a history of ankle injury.

Clinical presentation

The patient who has peroneal tendon pathology typically complains of laterally based ankle or hindfoot pain. The pain usually worsens with activity. Presentation and diagnosis often is delayed, however. Patients may or may not recall a specific episode of trauma. Peroneal tendon subluxation or dislocation may present acutely after a traumatic injury to the ankle but may also present later with an uncertain history of trauma. Patients also may complain of snapping or popping in the ankle.

On physical examination, there usually is tenderness to palpation along the course of the peroneal tendons. Edema also may be present. These disorders require a high level of suspicion. Even frank dislocations may be missed if not specifically evaluated. A provocative test for peroneal pathology has been described. The patient's relaxed foot is examined hanging in a relaxed position with the knee flexed 90°. Slight pressure is applied to the peroneal tendons posterior to the fibula. The patient then is asked to dorsiflex and evert the foot forcibly. Pain may be elicited, or subluxation of the tendons may be felt [31].

Imaging studies

Radiography is useful to rule out fractures, arthritis, or loose bodies. Radiography is also useful to observe a migration of the os peroneum in a rupture of the peroneus longus. Most importantly, radiographs are used to identify a rim fracture, which is an avulsion of the superior peroneal retinaculum from the lateral malleolus. A talar stress view is helpful; if there is more than 15° of tilt, talar instability that can lead to peroneal instability may be present.

Ultrasonography is useful for detecting all types of peroneal lesions. In particular, real-time ultrasonography can be performed to assess dynamic stability. This approach is institution dependent, because not all facilities are proficient in musculoskeletal ultrasonography.

CT is useful, especially in the evaluation of a suspected calcaneal fracture. MRI is the criterion standard for identifying peroneal tendon injury. This injury is identified by the high signal intensity within tendon on T2-weighted axial views [32]. Tenography is useful for assessing large lesions of the tendons.

Other tests

Electromyelography may be useful in difficult cases with profound weakness and no significant damage to the peroneal tendons. Electromyelography should be used in instances of drop foot.

Medical therapy

Nonsteroidal anti-inflammatory medication to reduce pain and inflammation is often used. Any underlying medical problem (eg, diabetes, rheumatoid arthritis) should be medically controlled.

After medical therapy is initiated, nonoperative treatment usually is attempted. In general, conservative therapy may include activity modification, footwear changes, temporary immobilization, and corticosteroid injection. Lateral heel wedges can take stress off the peroneal tendons to allow healing. Nonoperative treatment of tenosynovitis alone is often successful, whereas a complete or partial tendon rupture often leads to surgery. Likewise, an acute injury is more likely to respond to conservative care than is a chronic process [29]. As with other disorders of the foot and ankle, the use of corticosteroid injection must be undertaken with extreme caution to avoid iatrogenic rupture.

Surgical intervention

For persistent symptoms with peroneal tendonitis, a tenosynovectomy is the procedure of choice. Chronic tears of the peroneal tendons with persistent pain and instability require surgical repair [33,34]. Tendinosis may cause nodules or scar tissue that may need débridement. Longitudinal tears that fail immobilization may be present.

Complications

Symptoms may recur after surgical treatment. Patients may complain of stiffness or tightness of the ankle after surgical repair. Surgical treatment also may be complicated by injury to the sural nerve or to the superficial peroneal nerve [30]. The sural nerve may be more at risk because of its variable position. Infections may complicate any surgical procedure. The potential for blood clots or pulmonary embolus, although uncommon with foot and ankle surgery, must not be underestimated.

Conclusion

The decision to use a specific procedure depends upon the specific pathology present and good surgical judgment. Also, the effectiveness of nonoperative versus operative treatment may be debated. The need for MRI evaluation and the timing of such, although becoming clearer, has yet to be convincingly defined. The need to proceed to surgery is always controversial.

Ankle sprain

Background

A large percentage of musculoskeletal injuries observed in the outpatient setting involve the ankle. Sprains constitute 85% of all ankle injuries. Of these, 85% are inversion sprains. Up to one sixth of participation time lost from sports results from ankle sprains. Proper rehabilitation begins with accurate diagnosis, because up to 40% of patients with untreated or misdiagnosed ankle injuries develop chronic symptoms. Most injuries respond to treatment. Pain reduction is essential, but improvement of any loss of motion, strength, or proprioception is equally important.

History

Determining the mechanism of injury is essential. Sudden intense pain and rapid onset of swelling and bruising suggest a ruptured ligament. Suspect neurovascular compromise if the patient complains of a cold foot or describes paresthesias. Determine presence of complicating conditions (eg, arthritis, connective tissue disease, diabetes, neuropathy, previous ankle sprain, trauma).

Frequency

Most ankle sprains probably are self-treated and are never reported to a health care provider. Therefore, many ankle sprains are not documented. Sprained ankles have been estimated to comprise approximately 15% of all sports-related injuries. More than 23,000 people per day, including athletes and nonathletes, require medical care for ankle sprains in the United States. Stated another way, incident cases have been estimated at 1 per 10,000 persons per day [35].

Pathophysiology

Most ankle sprains are caused by inversion during extension of the ankle. Thus, approximately 85% of injuries involve the three distinct lateral ligaments: the anterior talofibular ligament, the calcaneofibular ligament, and the posterior talofibular ligament. Of sprains caused by inversion, 65% are isolated to the anterior talofibular ligament. In some patients, the subtalar complex may also be injured. The calcaneofibular ligament is rarely injured in isolation. Isolated injury to the medial (deltoid) ligament is rare and usually involves malleolar fractures. Distal tibiofibular syndesmotic rupture is rare and is associated with dorsiflexion and external rotation. Recovery from this injury is significantly prolonged, unlike isolated lateral ligament sprains. Rupture of the superior peroneal retinaculum results in subluxation or dislocation of the peroneal tendons. The mechanism of injury is usually forced dorsiflexion with reflex contraction of the peroneal muscles. Patients complain of pain and a snapping sensation over the postero-lateral ankle with weakness of eversion.

Classification

Ankle sprains are classified into three grades. Grade 1 injuries involve stretching of the ligament with microscopic but not macroscopic tearing. Generally, little swelling is present, with little or no functional loss and no joint instability. Grade 2 injuries stretch the ligament with partial tearing, moderate-to-severe swelling, ecchymosis, moderate functional loss, and mild-to-moderate joint instability. Grade 3 injuries involve the complete rupture of the ligament with immediate and severe swelling, ecchymosis, an inability to bear weight, and moderate-to-severe instability of the joint [36].

Physical examination

Observe for edema, ecchymosis, or deformity. Palpate for tenderness, crepitation, or deformity. Assess active and passive ROM as well as weight-bearing ability.

Perform the talar-tilt test: place the foot in 20 to 30° of plantar flexion and apply slight adduction and gentle inversion stress to the calcaneal midfoot. If both the anterior talofibular and the calcaneofibular ligaments are ruptured, the examiner will detect talar tilt (ie, movement of the talus in the mortise).

Perform the anterior drawer test: place the foot in 10° to 15° of plantar flexion and apply gentle forward traction to the heel. With anterior talofibular ligament rupture, the deltoid ligament becomes the center of rotation, and a dimple may appear just anterior to the lateral malleolus. The examiner will detect forward motion of the talus. For this test, 3 mm of movement may be significant; 1 cm of movement is certainly significant. Perform and document a neuro-vascular examination, including checks of the dorsalis pedis and posterior tibial pulses [37].

Imaging studies

If the patient is aged 2 to 65 years, consider the Ottawa ankle rules when deciding whether to obtain a plain radiograph. These guidelines state that an examiner is unlikely to miss a clinically significant fracture if the patient has no bony tenderness and can bear weight for at least four steps. Obtain a radiograph if the history or physical is clinically suspicious for an injury other than an ankle sprain Injuries have been diagnosed as ankle sprains but are not improving as expected.

In chronic ankle instability that is not responding to treatment, a stress radiograph may be considered. Stress views include the talar-tilt test and the anterior drawer test. Because of the high variability of normal ankle laxity, comparison views of the uninjured side are usually needed. Although the figures used by clinicians vary, 3° to 5° more than the uninjured side or an absolute value of 10° is generally considered a positive finding.

Bone scanning is useful in evaluating stress fracture, infection, and tumors. CT scanning is useful in evaluating osteochondritis dissecans and stress fractures. MRI is useful in evaluating osteochondritis dissecans, fractures, ankle impingement, and soft tissue injury.

Medical issues/complications

Treatment goals during the acute phase of injury are to minimize swelling and allow the patient to begin walking. The acute phase of treatment should last 1 to 3 days after the injury. A combination of protection, relative rest, ice, compression, elevation, and support is used. Remember this approach with the mnemonic "PRICES" [38]:

Protection

Protective devices include air splints or plastic and braces using Velcro closure. Most sprains can be treated without casting. Depending on the severity of the sprain, protective devices are used for 4 to 21 days. Criteria to discontinue use of the device include minimal swelling and pain at the site of injury. The ROM should be smooth, particularly with dorsiflexion and plantarflexion.

Relative rest

Relative rest is advocated, because it promotes tissue healing. Advise the patient to avoid activities that cause increased pain or swelling. Advocate early pain-free movements during this time. Patient may perform alphabet exercises or towel stretches, if tolerated, to maintain ROM.

Ice

Use ice to control swelling, pain, and muscle spasm. As a rule, do not apply ice or a cold pack directly to the skin; wrap the pack in a towel before use. Recommend that the patient apply ice for 15 to 20 minutes, three times daily. Contrast baths can be used 24 to 48 hours after injury.

Compression

Recommend use of compression with an ACE wrap, elastic ankle sleeve, or lace-up ankle support. Advise the patient that wearing high-top, lace-up shoes can further support the ankle. These measures can help minimize edema.

Elevation

Encourage elevation of the injured ankle to facilitate reduction of swelling. Advise the patient to keep the ankle above the level of the heart.

Support

Support can include taping or the use of lace-up ankle supports with combination Velcro straps.

Surgical therapy

The two generally agreed-upon indications for surgical treatment of acute ankle sprains are (1) deltoid sprain with the deltoid ligament caught intra-articularly widening the medial ankle mortise, and (2) inferior tibiofibular syndesmosis sprain causing real or potential widening of the ankle mortise. Acute grade 3 tears of the interior tibiofibular ligament can occur with a normal radiographic appearance on images in which the patient is not bearing weight (the usual condition in acute ankle sprains because of the discomfort associated with bearing weight). Thus, normal radiographic findings may be compatible with the need for surgery. Pain and swelling localized over the inferior tibiofibular syndesmosis should alert the clinician to tears in the syndesmosis complex that may be best treated with surgical fixation. Controversy remains concerning the surgical treatment of complete anterior talofibular and fibulo-calcaneal tears (double ligament tears) or the rare cases in which all three lateral ankle ligaments are torn. In young patients with athletic requirements, surgical repairs of severe lateral ankle sprains are sometimes indicated [39]. Treatment of distal tibiofibular syndesmosis sprains consists of placement of a screw across the syndesmosis that remains in place for 6 weeks and is removed before weight bearing is allowed to avoid the difficult problem of screw breakage.

Further outpatient care

The recovery phase of rehabilitation begins after the third day of injury and may last up to 2 weeks. The goal during this period is to have the patient walk without a limp. Continue treatment with ice and elevation if swelling persists. Some pain is acceptable during this time; however, reevaluate the patient if pain persists. Initiate therapeutic exercises, including flexibility/ROM, strengthening, and proprioceptive/balance exercises. Encourage active ankle motion in inversion and eversion. Add standing lower leg stretches (gastroc-soleus complex and Achilles tendon) or non–weight-bearing towel stretches to the regimen. Begin strengthening exercises with isometrics. Then, recommend progressing to closed-chain loading (eg, toe raises). Add elastic bands or rubber tubing for open-chain loading. Recommend beginning proprioceptive or balance training on the injured leg. As an added challenge, have the patient stand on a pillow two to three times per day. A wobble board may be helpful during this time, depending on the patient's progress.

Rehabilitation-phase return-to-play criteria include

Full pain-free active and passive ROM
No pain or tenderness
Ankle muscles' strength 70% to 80% that of the uninvolved side
Ability to balance on one leg for 30 seconds with eyes closed

The functional phase of rehabilitation lasts 2 to 6 weeks. The goal is to return the patient to previous level of activity. Once this goal has been achieved, rehabilitation is complete. The three components addressed in the recovery phase reflect an advanced stage of rehabilitation. The ankle should move in full ROM. Strengthening continues with advanced open-chain and closed-chain exercises. Add exercises that promote agility and power, including line jumping, 5-point drill, jump rope, and plyometrics.

Supportive devices still can be used if the patient is participating in strenuous or competitive play. Functional-phase return-to-play criteria include [40]

Normal ROM of the ankle joint
No pain or tenderness
Satisfactory clinical examination
Ankle muscles' strength 90% of the uninvolved side
Ability to complete functional examination

Complications include functional or mechanical instability and chronic pain, stiffness, or edema.

Prognosis

With appropriate initial treatment, referral, and physical therapy, most patients have a favorable outcome.

Soft tissue defects and reconstruction

Foot diseases may affect normal life significantly, often requiring long care and expensive rehabilitation programs and representing a burden for society. Reconstruction of complex wounds of the foot and ankle, especially with exposure of bone, joint, or tendon, continues to pose a challenge in reconstructive surgery. The characteristics of the weight-bearing requirement of the foot, the lack of intervening muscle between the skeletal elements and the skin, and the limited mobility of the overlying skin make the reconstruction even more difficult [41].

Etiology

Foot defects can be classified according to cause into six main categories by cause: trauma, vascular disease, metabolic disease, tumor, infection, and malformation.

Trauma

Traumatic causes of foot defects are often related to motor vehicle accidents or work accidents. Traumas or injuries may be acute or continued, mild or severe. Hidalgo and Shaw [42] divided foot traumas into three classes according to dimension and extension of the lesion, as follows:

Type I–small soft tissue loss less than 3 cm^2
Type II–large tissue loss greater than 3 cm^2 without bone involvement
Type III–large tissue loss with bone involvement

Vascular disease

Vascular etiology may be caused mostly by the artery or the vein circulation. An ischemia or a venous stasis can cause a necrosis that often leads to an ulcer.

Metabolic diseases

Metabolic pathologies often induce neurovascular alteration to the whole body. Microangiopathy and neuropathy cause a nonpainful, craterlike ulceration localized on the plantar side of the foot, especially in the weight-bearing areas. Bacterial infection by anaerobes is fairly common. The most frequent causes are diabetes, alcoholism, phakomatosis, and gout (podagra).

Tumor

Melanomas, epitheliomas, and sarcomas of the bone or of the soft tissues are the most common neoplasms that can afflict this region, even though foot tumors are considered rare.

Infection

Infective ulcers often are secondary to traumas, vascular deficiencies, or diabetes. All these pathologies can result in low peripheral oxygenation and promote infection by anaerobes, gram-negative organisms, and saprophytes.

Malformation

Congenital diseases, such as the clubfoot or the bifid spine, are rare. They are associated with deformity of the skeletal and neurologic alterations and easily may cause ulcers on weight-bearing areas of the sole [42].

Clinical presentation

Presentation differs according to the causative agent. Traumatic ulcers are localized, with irregular shape and margins and with possible necrosis from vascular impairment caused by trauma. The surrounding tissue is normal and painful. Vascular ulcers caused by artery impairment are regular in shape (round) and margin. Vascular ulcers caused by venous impairment are irregular in shape with hypertrophic margins. Vascular ulcers of both causes have damaged surrounding tissue, are seen at different localizations (eg, dorsum of the foot or fingers), and are usually painful. Diabetic ulcers are irregular in shape, area numerous, have callous margins, are deep with damage to the surrounding tissue, are not painful, and are more frequent in weight-bearing areas.

Imaging studies

Obtain leg or foot radiographs for patients who have trauma-induced ulcers or for osteocutaneous free transfers. Obtain a chest radiograph if indicated by examination findings or the patient's history. Obtain leukocyte lymphoscintigraphy in patients who have osteomyelitis. Obtain baropodometric evaluation or gait analysis to identify eventual bone functional loss and to plan a repair of the arches. Nuclear magnetic resonance is indicated, especially to study ligaments and joints but also to evaluate the soft tissue damage.

Other tests

Perform Doppler, echo Doppler, or angiography to assess the vascular pattern of the foot and leg [43]. Perform an Allen test in patients who have radial free flaps. Obtain an EKG in elderly individuals or as indicated by operating room guidelines.

Surgical therapy

For dimensions smaller than 3 cm^2 in weight-bearing areas, a local flap is used. For dimensions smaller than 3 cm^2 in non–weight-bearing areas, a skin graft is used. For dimensions larger than 3 cm^2 in weight-bearing areas, a free flap (free fasciocutaneous, musculocutaneous flap or muscle free flap plus skin graft) is used. For dimensions greater than 3 cm^2 with soft tissue and bone loss, in weight-bearing areas, a free osteocutaneous flap is used [44].

Local flaps

Local flaps are dissected on the branches of the three major vessels of the leg and foot that provide blood supply to muscles and skin: the dorsalis pedis artery, the posterior tibial artery, and the peroneal artery.

Dorsalis pedis artery.   The dorsalis pedis flap consists of the skin, subcutaneous tissue, and the most superficial layer of fascia of the dorsum of the foot supplied by subcutaneous branches arising from the dorsalis pedis artery. The flap may include the skin of the entire dorsum of the foot extending from the webspace to the retinaculum. Sensory innervation can be maintained through the superficial and deep peroneal nerves. The flap is based proximally and turned laterally or medially to cover defects at both malleoli and lateral regions of the foot. The dissection is relatively quick, but its indications are limited by donor site morbidity. Grafting of donor defect of the foot is always required, and there is a potential for healing problems in the donor area if a complete paratenon cover of the extensor tendon is not maintained. Moreover, a sensory deficit of the entire dorsum of the foot always occurs. The flap can also be dissected as a reverse flap based on the reverse arterial flow coming from the lateral plantar artery anastomosing with the dorsalis pedis artery.

The extensor digitorum brevis muscle lies on the dorsum of the foot, arising mainly from the lateral surface of the calcaneus and running forward and medially to end in four tendons at the level of the tarsometatarsal joints. The vascular supply is a branch of the lateral tarsal artery that arises from the dorsalis pedis. This muscular flap is not of great use because of its limited mobility; nevertheless it is useful for Achilles tendon and heel defects. The dissection is easy, and it offers a reliable and effective reconstruction in infected wound and exposed fractures of the heel, because it consists of muscular tissue. Functional deficits are minimal, because the extensor hallucis and digitorum longus are more effective extensors, so a main artery such as dorsalis pedis can sometimes be sacrificed for small defects of the foot [45].

Posterior tibial artery.   The instep island flap consists of skin and subcutaneous tissue of the non–weight-bearing surface of the sole elevated on either the medial or lateral plantar vessels or both, ultimately based on the posterior tibial vessels. Although the dissection is quite difficult, it is especially indicated for defects of the plantar surface where the skin is uniquely adapted for weight bearing. It has a special vascularization, and its fibrous septation prevents displacement of subcutaneous fat and confers good sheer resistance. For reconstruction of defects of the sole it therefore is desirable to use similar tissue, such as the non–weight-bearing instep region of the sole between the heel and the metatarsal heads. After flap elevation, the donor area is resurfaced with a split-thickness skin graft. The flexor digitorum brevis muscle must not be included within the flap for three reasons: (1) the secondary defect is not as devastating aesthetically and functionally, (2) muscle function is preserved;(3) the deep surface of the flap, namely, the plantar fascia, gains attachment directly to the bone and prevents swivel, which might be expected to occur if muscle has been included.

This abductor hallucis brevis muscle arises from the medial process of the calcaneus and inserts with its tendon to the proximal phalanx of the big toe. Although a difficult dissection, this muscle can be used for small defects of the heel, especially for revascularization of the calcaneus after crush injuries [46].

Peroneal artery. The lateral calcaneal artery skin flap is an axial-pattern flap that can provide skin flap coverage over the exposed Achilles tendon or posterior heel defects. The pedicle consists of lateral calcaneal artery (the terminal branch of the peroneal artery), lesser saphenous vein, and sural nerve. There is a short version of this flap (vertical axis, approximately 8 cm long) and a long version (curved forward and up to 14 cm long). The shape is extremely reliable in providing viable skin flap coverage. In both cases, the flap is mobilized in a retrograde fashion, dissection is easy, and at the end a split-thickness skin graft is placed over the donor defect.

The superficial sural artery that accompanies the sural nerve supplies the sural fasciocutaneous flap flap. Because the artery anastomoses with septocutaneous branches from the peroneal artery in the lower part of the tibiofibular space, the flap can be distally based and vascularized by the peroneal artery. Dissection is easy and quick, and major arteries are not sacrificed. The flap can be raised anywhere in the lower two thirds of the leg, provided the center of the flap lies along the midline of the posterior aspect of the leg. The pivot point of the pedicle must be al least 5 cm above the lateral malleolus to allow anastomosis with the peroneal artery. The sural fasciocutaneous flap is a reliable and versatile solution for coverage of posterior defects of the heel, ankle, and dorsum of the foot. This flap is sometimes troublesome, however, because of the very small artery that provides its vascularization [46].

Microvascular flaps

A microvascular flap is a free transfer with microvascular anastomoses of the pedicle at the donor site. An artery and a vein must be anastomosed end-to-end or end-to-side. The advent of this technique has made the treatment of difficult situations more manageable, because wide defects in any area of the foot can be resurfaced [46].

Latissimus dorsi muscle or musculocutaneous flap. The latissimus dorsi muscle or musculocutaneous flap is a muscle flap, dissected in the back and based on the thoracodorsal vessels. The flap can also include a skin paddle (musculocutaneous unit).

Superficial temporal fascia flap. The superficial temporal fascia flap is a thin fascial flap, dissected in the temporal region and based on the superficial temporal vessels. After harvesting of the flap, donor-site morbidity is low, and the scar can be easily hidden by the hair.

Scapular fasciocutaneous flap. The scapular fasciocutaneous flap is a fasciocutaneous flap in the scapular region pedicled on the circumflex scapular vessels.

Decision making

Intrinsic muscle flaps are relative easy to dissect out, and their transfer leaves a minimal functional and aesthetic donor defect. The muscle brings an immediate increase of blood flow to the area, provides bulk to fill a soft tissue defect, and protects the underlying tendon, joint, and bone. Intrinsic muscle flaps, however, have high morbidity in the donor area and are not sufficient for large defects. Depending on the size of the defect, a pedicled or free flap is an ideal solution because the flap brings vascularized tissue over the bone defect. Wide defects including the weight- bearing areas are mostly repaired using free flaps. Free flaps, however, have characteristics of the transfer area (skin) [47]. The main goal is to give the patient a foot that is as normal as possible after the traumatic loss of tissue. The reconstruction must be aesthetically, psychologically, and functionally satisfactory, allowing use of normal footwear and the possibility of walking without pain and risk of skin ulceration.

Summary

Ruptures of the Achilles tendon most commonly occur spontaneously in healthy, young, active individuals who are aged 30 to 50 years. The calf-squeeze test (Thompson test) determines a rupture. Ultrasound and MRI are used to evaluate suspected ruptures of the Achilles tendon. Operative treatment has been the method of choice for athletes and young people.

The term "Achilles tendonitis" is used to describe the spectrum of tendon injuries, ranging from inflammation to tendon rupture. Palpate the entire gastroc-soleus complex for tenderness, nodules, swelling, warmth, atrophy, and tendon defects with the patient in a prone position. MRI has been used extensively to visualize pathologic conditions of the tendon. Initial conservative treatment should be directed toward relieving symptoms. Instruct the patient in stretching, training modification/re-evaluation, and muscle strengthening.

Operative treatment is indicated in athletes who still have peritonitis or tendinosis after undergoing a comprehensive conservative treatment program and who are unwilling to modify or stop their activity. Injuries to the peroneal tendons are common but are not always clinically significant. The patient who has peroneal tendon pathology typically complains of laterally based ankle or hindfoot pain. The pain usually worsens with activity. Ultrasonography is useful for detecting all types of peroneal lesions. Nonsteroidal anti-inflammatory medication to reduce pain and inflammation often is used. For persistent symptoms with peroneal tendonitis, a tenosynovectomy is the procedure of choice. Chronic tears of the peroneal tendons with persistent pain and instability require surgical repair.

Sprains constitute 85% of all ankle injuries. Most injuries respond to treatment. Pain reduction is essential, but improvement of any loss of motion, strength, or proprioception is equally important. A combination of protection, relative rest, ice, compression, elevation, and support is used. Remember this approach with the mnemonic "PRICES." The two indications that are generally agreed upon for surgical treatment of acute ankle sprains are (1) deltoid sprain

280

with the deltoid ligament caught intra-articularly, widening the medial ankle mortise and (2) inferior tibiofibular syndesmosis sprain causing real or potential widening of the ankle mortise.

Reconstruction of complex wounds of the foot and ankle, especially with exposure of bone, joint, or tendon, continues to pose a challenge in reconstructive surgery. Intrinsic muscle flaps are relative easy to dissect out, and their transfer leaves a minimal functional and aesthetic donor defect. The muscle brings an immediate increase of blood flow to the area, provides bulk to fill a soft tissue defect, and protects the underlying tendon, joint, and bone. These flaps have high morbidity in the donor area, however, and are not sufficient for large defects.

Depending on the size of the defect, a pedicled or free flap is an ideal solution, because the flap brings vascularized tissue over the bone defect. Wide defects, including the weight-bearing areas, are usually repaired using free flaps. Free flaps, however, have different characteristics of the transfer area (skin).

The main goal is to give the patient a foot that is as normal as possible after traumatic loss of tissue. The reconstruction must be aesthetically, psychologically, and functionally satisfactory, allowing use of normal footwear and the possibility of walking without pain and risk of skin ulceration.

References

[1] O'Brien M. Functional anatomy and physiology of tendons. Clin Sports Med 1992;11: 505–20.
[2] Carden DG, Noble J, Chalmers J, et al. Rupture of the calcaneal tendon. The early and late management. J Bone and Joint Surg [Br] 1987;69(3):416–20.
[3] Lin DY. Achilles tendon rapture. Emedicine 2005. Available at http://www.emedicine.com. Accessed January 21, 2005.
[4] Hattrup SJ, Johnson KA. A review of ruptures of the Achilles tendon. Foot Ankle 1985;6:34–8.
[5] Åström M, Westlin N. Blood flow in the human Achilles tendon assessed by laser Doppler flowmetry. J Orthop Res 1994;12:246–52.
[6] Thompson TC. A test for rupture of the tendo Achilles. Acta Orthop Scand 1962;32:461–5.
[7] O'Brien T. The needle test for complete rupture of the Achilles tendon. J Bone and Joint Surg [Am] 1984;66:1099–101.
[8] Copeland SA. Rupture of the Achilles tendon: a new clinical test. Ann R Coll Surg Engl 1990;72:270–1.
[9] Kabbani YM, Mayer DP. Magnetic resonance imaging of tendon pathology about the foot and ankle. Part I. Achilles tendon. J Am Podiatr Med Assn 1993;83:418–20.
[10] Leppilahti J, Orava S. Total Achilles tendon rupture. A review. Sports Med 1998;25:79–100.
[11] Assal M, Jung M, Stern R, et al. Limited open repair of Achilles tendon ruptures. J Bone Joint Surg 2002;84:161–70.
[12] Stein SR, Luekens Jr CA. Closed treatment of Achilles tendon ruptures. Orthop Clin North Am 1976;7:241–6.
[13] Saltzman C, Bonar S. Tendon problems of the foot and ankle. In: Lutter L, Mizel M, Pfeffer G, editors. Orthopaedic knowledge update: foot and ankle. American Orthopaedic Foot and Ankle Society 1994;1:236–73.
[14] Kvist M. Achilles tendon overuse injuries: a clinical and pathophysiological study in athletes [thesis]. Turku (Finland): University of Turku; 1991.
[15] Johansson C. Injuries in elite orienteers. Am J Sports Med 1986;14:410–5.

[16] Schepsis AA, Jones H, Haas AL. Achilles tendon disorders in athletes. Am J Sports Med 2002;30:287–305.

[17] Järvinen TA, Kannus P, Jᴏzsa L, et al. Achilles tendon injuries. Curr Opin Rheumatol 2001; 13:150–5.

[18] Saltzman CL, Tearse DS. Achilles tendon injuries. J Am Acad Orthop Surg 1998;6(5):316–25.

[19] Fornage BD. Achilles tendon: US examination. Radiology 1986;159:759–64.

[20] Fredberg U, Bolvig L. Significance of ultrasonographically detected asymptomatic tendinosis in the patellar and Achilles tendons of elite soccer players: a longitudinal study. Am J Sports Med 2002;30:488–91.

[21] Kainberger FM, Engel A, Barton P, et al. Injury of the Achilles tendon: diagnosis with sonography. AJR Am J Roentgenol 1990;155:1031–6.

[22] Pope CF. Radiologic evaluation of tendon injuries. Clin Sports Med 1992;11:579–99.

[23] Movin T, Gad A, Reinholt FP, et al. Tendon pathology in long standing achillodynia. Biopsy findings in 40 patients. Acta Orthop Scand 1997;68:170–5.

[24] Alfredson H, Lorentzon R. Chronic Achilles tendinosis: recommendations for treatment and prevention. Sports Med 2000;29:135–46.

[25] Hess GP, Cappiello WL, Poole RM, et al. Prevention and treatment of overuse tendon injuries. Sports Med 1989;8:371–84.

[26] Sandmeier R, Renström PA. Diagnosis and treatment of chronic tendon disorders in sports. Scand J Med Sci Sports 1997;7:96–106.

[27] Khan KM, Cook JL, Taunton JE. Overuse tendinosis, not tendinitis. Phys Sportsmed 2000; 28(5):38–48.

[28] Paavola M, Kannus P, Orava S, et al. Surgical treatment for chronic Achilles tendinopathy: a prospective 7-month follow-up study. Br J Sports Med 2002;36:178–82.

[29] Scanlan RL, Gehl RS. Peroneal tendon injuries. Clin Podiatr Med Surg 2002;19(3):419–31.

[30] Krause JO, Brodsky JW. Peroneus brevis tendon tears: pathophysiology, surgical reconstruction, and clinical results. Foot Ankle Int 1998;19(5):271–9.

[31] Hort K. Peroneal tendon pathology. Emedicine 2005. Available at http://www.emedicine.com. Accessed March 18, 2005.

[32] Rosenberg ZS, Beltran J, Cheung YY, et al. MR features of longitudinal tears of the peroneus brevis tendon. AJR Am J Roentgenol 1997;168(1):141–7.

[33] Redfern D, Myerson M. The management of concomitant tears of the peroneus longus and brevis tendons. Foot Ankle Int 2004;25(10):695–707.

[34] Jones E. Operative treatment of chronic dislocations of the peroneal tendons. J Bone Joint Surg 1932;14A:574–6.

[35] Trevino SG, Davis P, Hecht PJ. Management of acute and chronic lateral ligament injuries of the ankle. Orthop Clin North Am 1994;25(1):1–16.

[36] Richards CF. Ankle injury, soft tissue. Emedicine 2004. Available at http://www.emedicine.com. Accessed July 20, 2004.

[37] Ankel F. The ankle. In: Hart RG, Rittenberry TJ, Uehara DT, editors. Handbook of orthopaedic emergencies. Philadelphia: Lippincott Williams & Wilkins; 1999.

[38] Renstrom PAFH, Kannus P. Injuries to the foot and ankle. Orthop Sports Med 1994:1705–67.

[39] Foster R. Acute ankle sprains. Emedicine 2004. Available at http://www.emedicine.com. Accessed July 20, 2004.

[40] Kibler WB. Rehabilitation of the ankle and foot. Functional rehabilitation of sports and musculoskeletal injuries. Aspen Publishers; 1998.

[41] Chang SM, Zhang F, Yu GR, et al. Modified distally based peroneal artery perforator flap for reconstruction of foot and ankle. Microsurgery 2004;24:430–6.

[42] Hidalgo DA, Shaw WW. Reconstruction of foot injuries. Clin Plast Surg 1986;13(4):663–80.

[43] Ogun TC, Arazi M, Kutlu A. An easy and versatile method of coverage for distal tibial soft tissue defects. J Trauma 2001;50:53–9.

[44] Santanelli F. Lower extremity reconstruction, foot. Emedicine 2003. Available at http://www. emedicine.com. Accessed February 26, 2003.

[45] Young HL. Distally based lateral supramalleolar adipofascial flap for reconstruction of the dorsum of the foot and ankle. Plast Reconstr Surg 2004;114:1478.

[46] Grazia SU. Plastic and reconstructive surgery of the foot. Foot Ankle Surg 2005;11:69–73.

[47] Attinger CE. The role of intrinsic muscle flaps of the foot for bone coverage in foot and ankle defects in diabetic and non diabetic patients. Plast Reconstr Surg 2002;110:1047–54.

ELSEVIER
SAUNDERS

Clin Podiatr Med Surg
23 (2006) 283–301

CLINICS IN
PODIATRIC
MEDICINE AND
SURGERY

Fractures of the Forefoot

Vincent J. Mandracchia, DPM, MS*, Denise M. Mandi, DPM,
Patris A. Toney, DPM, MPH, Jennifer B. Halligan, DPM,
W. Ashton Nickles, DPM

*Division of Podiatric Surgery, Department of Surgery, Broadlawns Medical Center,
1801 Hickman Road, Des Moines, IA 50314, USA*

Metatarsal fractures are common injuries of the forefoot, second only to digital fractures, and are the most common injuries sustained in motorcycle accidents [1,2]. An extensive research study by Iwamoto and Takeda [3] contrastingly found metatarsals to be the third most commonly fractured site in the body and the most common fracture site of the foot. The mechanism of injury resulting in metatarsal fractures includes both direct and indirect traumatic forces, such as crush injuries, high-impact motor vehicle accidents, inversion injuries, eversion injuries, and jamming, with direct injuries being the most common cause of injury, particularly in the industrial setting [2,4–9]. Fracture pattern and location are generally associated with the position of the foot and the nature of the energy imparted at the time of injury [5]. High-energy impacts typically result in crush injuries with a comminuted presentation of the fracture, whereas low-energy injuries usually present with a single fracture line [10].

Transverse fractures are seen when the causative forces are transmitted perpendicular to the long axis of the bone; oblique fractures stem from torsional forces [10]. Avulsion fractures typically result from inversion or torque injury, with the peroneus brevis and the peroneus longus being deforming forces [5,6,10,11]. The pull of the peroneus longus results in a fracture of the lateral base of the first metatarsal, whereas the pull of the peroneus brevis along with the long plantar ligament and the plantar aponeurosis results in a fracture of the styloid

* Corresponding author.
E-mail address: vmandracchia@broadlawns.org (V.J. Mandracchia).

doi:10.1016/j.cpm.2006.01.009
podiatric.theclinics.com

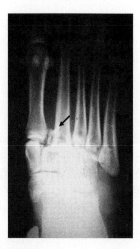

Fig. 1. Fleck fracture (*arrow*) off the medical base of the second metatarsal in a Lisfranc fracture injury.

process of the fifth metatarsal [7,12]. Fractures of the medial base of the second metatarsal ("fleck" fracture) result from the pull of Lisfranc's ligament (Fig. 1) [10]. Fractures of the base of the lateral border of the first metatarsal are attributed to the pull of the tarsometatarsal ligament connecting the first metatarsal and the medial cuneiform [13]. Stress fractures are more commonly seen in the second metatarsal, followed by the third metatarsal, and are attributable to repeated microtrauma, poor physical condition or training conditions (eg, in military recruits and ballet dancers), hallux valgus, hallux rigidus, following implants or resectional arthroplasty of the hallux, or secondary to structural malalignment or iatrogenic factors such as poor metatarsal osteotomies (Fig. 2) [3,5,8,10,14–17].

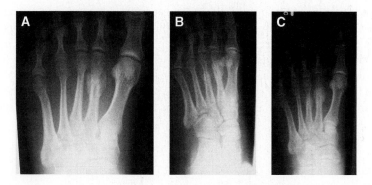

Fig. 2. (*A*) Stress fracture of the second metatarsal that went undiagnosed. (*B, C*) Subsequent development of a second stress fracture to the third metatarsal caused by transferred weight bearing and noncompliance.

Compartment syndrome

In cases involving high-energy trauma, especially crush injuries, compartment syndrome needs to be considered. A high index of suspicion for compartment syndrome is raised by the classic clinical picture of progressive pain, numbness in the toes, and decreased motor function. Tense, bulging tissue (gross edema) may be the most reliable sign. Pallor, delayed capillary filling time, and an inability to palpate pedal pulses are indications that progressive compartment syndrome is present. Compartment pressure measurements may be performed in the face of an index of suspicion, but decompression should not be delayed if there is strong clinical evidence that compartment syndrome exists. Compartment pressures in the foot above 30 mm Hg or 10 to 30 mm Hg below the diastolic pressure are considered diagnostic. Fascial decompression is the treatment of choice, and all compartments should be adequately opened (Fig. 3). Although

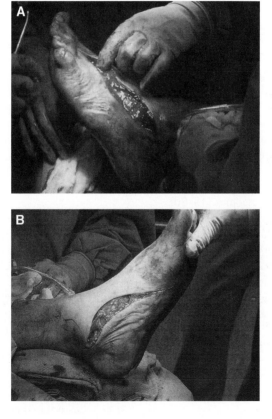

Fig. 3. (*A*) A dorsal incisional approach used to facilitate decompression in compartment syndrome affecting the foot. (*B*) A medial incisional approach.

Box 1. Compartments of the foot

1. Intrinsic
   Four intrinsic muscles between the first and
   fifth metatarsals
2. Medial
   Abductor hallucis
   Flexor hallucis brevis
3. Central
   Flexor digitorum brevis
   Quatratus plantae
   Adductor hallucis
4. Lateral
   Flexordigiti minimi brevis
   Abductor digiti minimi

---

there is some discussion as to the number of compartments in the foot, it is generally agreed that there are four major compartments with as many as nine subsections (Box 1).

The approaches for compartment decompression generally include two dorsal incisions to access the forefoot compartments and one medial incision to access the calcaneal, superficial, and lateral compartments. Long-term sequelae of foot compartment syndromes include contractures, deformity, weakness, paralysis, and sensory neuropathy. These complications are poorly tolerated and often necessitate multiple surgical procedures. Consequently, the threshold for considering compartment syndrome and performing fasciotomy must be low to minimize such outcomes [18–20].

Patients suffering from metatarsal fractures may complain of difficulty ambulating or painful ambulation, present with swelling, ecchymosis, blisters, and motor or sensory deficits, and exhibit tenderness and pain upon range of motion [2,4,5]. A palpable fracture fragment may be noted on physical examination if dislocation is present [5]. Standard radiographs aid in diagnosing overt fractures, but the diagnosis of stress fractures is based on suspicion. Because of to the 10- to 14-day lag time of osteoblastic activity following the osteoclastic resorptive response to the microtrauma, CT, MRI, and bone scan may be helpful in diagnosis of stress fractures [4,5,7,10,21,22].

Classification

Salter [23] classified fractures of metatarsals two, three, and four based on (1) site, (2) extent, (3) configuration, (4) relationship of fragments to each other, and (5) relationship of fragments to outside environment. Each category is classified as follows:

1. Site: epiphyseal, metaphyseal, diaphyseal, or intra-articular
2. Extent: complete or incomplete
3. Configuration: transverse, spiral, oblique, or comminuted
4. Fragment relationship: displaced, malaligned, impacted, or angulated
5. Environmental relationship: open or closed

A sixth category was added by Gudas [24], the neutralization of the intrinsic musculature.

Treatment

Typically, nondisplaced fractures are held in good alignment by surrounding ligamentous structures, do well with conservative treatment, and are allowed to heal by secondary bone healing [5,7,25,26]. Armagan and Shereff [22] believe that 3 to 4 mm of medial or lateral transverse plane deformity and 10° or less of angulation are well tolerated and need not undergo corrective measures. In addition to rest, ice, compression, and elevation, other conservative measures include immobilization in a cast, stiff-soled shoe, or cam walker device with partial or complete absence of weight bearing [24,5,14,25]. In displaced or dislocated fractures, closed reduction may be attempted, but it is usually unsuccessful; thus, surgical reduction and maintenance of the reduction may be warranted [4,5,10].

Surgical correction may be performed through use of crossed Kirschner wires, percutaneous pinning, circlage wire, interfragmentary screw, plate and screw fixation, external fixation, or intramedullary fixation using a Steinmann pin or double-threaded compression screw [1,4,5,7,10,26]. When used for fixation of metatarsal fractures, interfragmentary screw fixation lends static compression using the lag technique. On the other hand, intramedullary nail fixation works by allowing limited fragmentary motion secondary to a tight fit of the nail within the metatarsal's internal canal (Figs. 4,5) [27]. Steinmann pins are used for intramedullary fixation, with pin size based on the medullary canal size. A 1/8-inch pin can be used in the second metatarsal. For the third, fourth and fifth metatarsals, 3/32-inch and 7/74-inch pins can be used [10].

Open reduction and internal fixation is indicated in metatarsal fractures that are irreducible, involve a joint, or are significantly displaced [10]. This fixation method can be challenging because of the small size of the bone but is necessary to provide insurance against rotational forces that may continue to deform the fracture site [21]. Plate fixation is almost always an inadequate choice when addressing metatarsal neck fractures, because it is nearly impossible to follow the Arbeitsgemeinshaft fur Osteosynthesefragen/Association for the Study of Internal Fixation (AO/ASIF) rule of cortices (ie, three or four cortical threads in each fragment distally and five or six proximally). The limited amount of bone available may allow the use of only one or two screws for stabilization. Plates can also

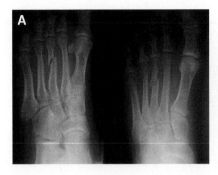 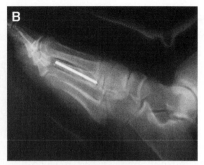

Fig. 4. (*A*) Displaced and angulated metatarsal shaft fracture of the third metatarsal. (*B*) Metatarsal fracture after fixation by intramedullary rod placement.

become irritating to the patient in shoe gear because of the limited amount of soft tissue coverage in the dorsal forefoot [10].

Kirschner wire fixation can also be difficult to perform. The proper placement of the wire depends on the attitude of the fracture [10], and the distal fragments are often displaced plantarly because of the strong pull of the flexor tendons [24]. Single Kirschner wires retrograded distally from the fracture site through the metatarsal head and toe are not stable, and crossed Kirschner wires are recommended [10]. In multiple metatarsal fractures percutaneous pinning can be used successfully by driving a 0.062-inch Kirschner wire transversely through the metatarsals. Donahue and colleagues [28] reported that placing the wire through the lateral side of the foot makes use of the uninjured fifth metatarsal as an added stabilizing force during healing. This approach has the added advantage of minimal soft tissue and vascular injury, because only one incision is needed. The risk of pin-tract infection is an ever-present disadvantage whenever wire fixation is used.

Fractures at the base of the metatarsals are inherently more stable than their distal counterparts. This stability can be attributed to the large number of soft

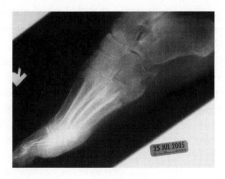

Fig. 5. Fracture of the proximal fifth metatarsal depicting a Jones fracture at the location of the metaphyseal–diaphyseal junction.

tissue attachments to this area of the bone. Caution should be taken when selecting treatment for fractures of the proximal fourth metatarsal because delayed healing time has been observed, as in a Jones fracture of the neighboring fifth metatarsal [29]. The authors also encourage the reader not to overlook the possibility of a fracture of a metatarsal base as a cause for unresolved midfoot pain. Fortin and colleagues [16] described the base of the second metatarsal as particularly venerable to fracture because of the stresses it may receive when biomechanical abnormalities are present in the hallux (eg, hallux abducto valgus, hypermobility). These fractures are usually nondisplaced and may be difficult to diagnose on plain radiographs. Immobilization remains the criterion standard of treatment [30].

Interfragmentary screws offer another choice for fixation of metatarsal fractures. When used in a lag fashion, they provide static compression, but several factors beyond the surgeon's control often make their placement difficult. Unfortunately, the anatomic location and orientation of the fracture, along with inadequate exposure of the metatarsals (especially the central three), may complicate screw fixation [10].

Intramedullary nailing

Intramedullary nail fixation of metatarsal fractures has become increasingly popular in the last 5 years. Intramedullary fixation maintains fracture reduction through the tight fit of the nail against the internal surface of the medullary canal. Translation, rotation, and angulation of the fracture fragments are prevented by this close contact. Once inserted, the rigid nail acts more like a splint, limiting the motion of the bone rather than providing rigid fixation. The metatarsal is a long bone and anatomically lends itself well to the intramedullary nailing of both head and shaft fractures. Using intramedullary nailing to fixate fractures at the distal neck of the metatarsal can be difficult. Other internal fixation is often required to secure the head of the metatarsal. In 2003, Aguado and colleagues [31] proposed the Metaizeau technique of anterograde placement of an elastic endomedullar. This technique demonstrated good reduction of the metatarsal head without the need for secondary fixation.

Another advantage of intramedullary nail fixation is that the reaming process pushes cancellous and cortical bone to the inner cortex, providing an autograft deposition directly to the fracture site. This mixture of bone and marrow elements has been shown to have excellent osteoinductive and osteoconductive properties [10]. Kouzelis and colleagues [32] demonstrated that reaming 1 mm less than the minimal canal diameter provides the highest viable bone mass percentage. The patient's vascular supply must always be carefully evaluated when considering this method of fracture reduction. Reaming of the metatarsal shaft partially obliterates the medullary afferent and efferent blood supply.

A 1982 study by Rhinelander and colleagues [33] showed that revascularization in the medullary canal takes place in 2 to 3 weeks. The intact periosteum can provide adequate blood supply during the initial stages of healing [10]. A study by Crowl and colleagues [34] in 2000, however, reported that patients who have less than optimal vascular perfusion at the time of intramedullary fixation demonstrated a twofold increase in postoperative complications. Several other concerns about using intramedullary nailing for fracture stabilization have been voiced in recent literature. Thermal injury to the bone and soft tissues during nail placement may be a valid consideration. A study by Frolke and colleagues [35] in 2001 demonstrated that much higher temperatures are conducted through reaming of the medullary canal than were previously assumed. They suggest that the surgeon pay close attention and use only moderate power and speed when placing the nail. Furthermore, there has been some concern about fat embolism syndrome, a rare but possible complication of intramedullary nailing. This phenomenon is well documented in orthopedic literature with intramedullary fixation of the tibia and femur [36]. There may be increased risk during nailing of multiple metatarsals. Most literature regarding intramedullary fixation complications deals with long bones that are significantly larger than the metatarsals. Although much can be learned from these studies, research that addresses these issues on a more applicable scale is needed.

Complications encountered from improperly treated or misdiagnosed fractures may result in metatarsalgia secondary to displaced fracture fragments or transferred weight bearing, malunion, claw toe secondary to interosseous muscle bleeding after traumatic injury, arthritis, pin-tract infection, joint stiffness, non-union, intractable plantar keratosis, neuroma or nerve impingement, or soft tissue irritation from bony prominences [2,4,7,10,17].

Jones fractures

Fractures of the proximal fifth metatarsal are given special attention within the literature. Like the other metatarsals, the fifth metatarsal is susceptible to fracture injury and is considered the most commonly fractured metatarsal when avulsion fractures are included [2]. Altogether there are considered to be three prevailing types of fractures commonly affecting the base of the fifth metatarsal [2,37,38]. Sir Robert Jones is credited with the first description of a fifth metatarsal fracture in 1902, which he described as being at the diaphyseal portion of the fifth metatarsal distal to the proximal tuberosity [39]. Today, there is still great debate as to the true location of a Jones fracture, with two subsets of fractures identified. Torg [40] describes two proximal fifth metatarsal fractures including the tuberosity and the more proximal portion of the diaphysis 1.5 cm distal to the tuberosity.

Torg's [40] classification of fifth metatarsal fractures is based on both clinical and radiographic presentations. Radiographically, the fractures are classified as acute, delayed, and non-united. Type I acute fractures display no previous history of trauma, no sclerosis within the medullar canal, no widening of the fracture site or radiolucency, and only minimal signs of periosteal reaction or cortical hypertrophy. Type II delayed fractures are associated with a history of previous trauma or fracture with periosteal changes, widening of the fracture line, medullar sclerosis, and radiolucency at the fracture site. Type III non-united

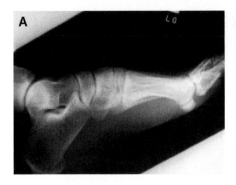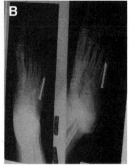

Fig. 6. (*A*, *B*) A Jones fracture that underwent surgical fixation with (*B*) interfragmentary screw placement.

fractures manifest in the presence of repetitive trauma with recurring symptoms along with periosteal new bone formation and radiolucency in addition to widening of the fracture site and replacement of the medullar canal by sclerotic bone (Fig. 6). A second classification system for Jones fractures developed by Stewart [41] classifies Jones fractures based upon the relationship of the fracture line to the articular surface, the fracture type, and the fracture site. The Stewart classification consists of five types, which are summarized as follows:

   Type I: supra-articular fracture (true Jones fracture)
   Type II: intra-articular avulsion fracture
   Type III: extra-articular avulsion fracture
   Type IV: intra-articular, comminuted avulsion fracture
   Type V: extra-articular avulsion epiphyseal fracture

Direct and indirect mechanisms of injury result in fifth metatarsal fractures and include avulsion injuries, forefoot adduction on a plantar-flexed ankle, stress fractures, and inversion injuries [39,41]. Avulsion fractures are considered the most common fracture type and are typically extra-articular, involving the styloid process, and are attributed to the pull of the peroneus brevis, long plantar ligament, and the plantar aponeurosis [12,15]. Jones fractures are considered to be acute in nature as compared with the less frequent stress fracture of the fifth metatarsal [15]. Stress fractures of the fifth metatarsal are thought to occur at the more distal diaphyseal portion and to be extra-articular and transverse in orientation, whereas the acute Jones fracture is most often described as occurring at the metaphyseal–diaphyseal junction and involving the intermetatarsal articular space (Fig. 7) [12,14,15,39,42,43]. The location of the Jones fracture at the more proximal metaphyseal–diaphyseal junction between the tendinous insertion of the peroneus brevis and peroneus tertius is thought to be at the watershed area; disruption to the blood supply causes concern regarding the best effective treatment to assure good healing, because the area is prone to delayed union and to non-union [15,40,42,43].

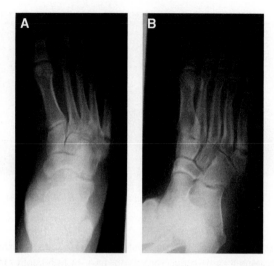

Fig. 7. (*A*) A non-united Jones fracture. (*B*) Note the medullary sclerosis and widening of the fracture site.

Treatment for fifth metatarsal fractures, particularly Jones fractures, is much debated. Conservative treatment measures include icing, elevation, immobilization, non–weight bearing, and orthosis [40,44,45]. Surgical treatment has been advocated as the treatment of choice to expedite the healing process in athletes and highly active individuals who have acute Jones fractures [15]. Surgical treatment is also considered for delayed unions and non-unions as well as for displaced and intra-articular fractures [2,40]. Reports indicate that acute Torg type I and Jones fractures heal successfully with immobilization and non–weight bearing [39–41]. Torg [40] further believed that delayed unions treated conservatively eventually heal, although healing time averaged roughly 14 weeks.

Surgical treatment includes circlage wires, external fixation, intramedullary screw, plate with screw fixation, and crossed Kirschner wires [14,35,39,40, 44–50]. For avulsion fractures, Husain and colleagues [51] found that screw fixation was better for treatment than tension band wiring. Intramedullary screw fixation is thought to be advantageous because it provides stability and compression across the fracture site without disrupting the periosteum or fractures site and allows primary bone healing (Fig. 8) [44,46,52]. For interfragmentary screw fixation, both cannulated and malleolar screws have been used, with screw sizes varying from 4.5 mm to 5.0 mm and 6.5 mm [10,42,44,48]. Comparable outcomes were noted for use of 4.5-mm cannulated screws and 4.5-mm malleolar screws [44]. Kelly and colleagues [42] demonstrated a significant difference in the pull-out strength of 5.0-mm and 6.5-mm screws in fixation of Jones fractures. No significant difference in the load needed to cause screw failure was found between the 4.5-mm and the 5.5-mm cannulated screws [48]. Horst and colleagues [53] found no significant difference in resistance to torsional forces

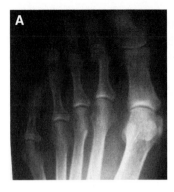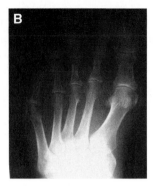

Fig. 8. Displaced proximal phalanx fracture of the second digit (*A*) before and (*B*) after closed reduction. Note the realignment.

between the use of a 5.0-mm screw and a 6.5-mm screw. In delayed unions and non-unions, curettage of the medullar canal and application of bone graft are done in addition to screw fixation [14,40,44,45,54,55]. Bone stimulation has also been used in cases of delayed union or non-union [54,56]. Nolte and colleagues [56] noted an 86% success rate in the treatment of non-unions using low-intensity pulsed ultrasound. When avulsion injury is present, surgical excision of the fracture fragment with advancement of the peroneus brevis is performed in cases recalcitrant to conservative treatment and of insufficient size for fixation [2,22].

Complications associated with Jones fracture include soft tissue irritation from the prominent screw head, deformation of the screw, penetration of distal cortices, refracture, delayed union, and non-union [39,40,42,45,50,54,57]. Refracture is thought to occur in the face of weaker sclerotic bone across the fracture site [40]. Delayed union and non-union are noted to occur at the plantar lateral border of the fracture site [39,44].

Digital and sesamoidal fractures

Digital fractures are the most common forefoot injuries; fractures of the sesamoid are the least common fractures of the forefoot. Digital fractures may also manifest as fracture dislocations [58,59]. Digital fractures typically result from stubbing injuries, running/push-off injuries, or a direct crush injury [2,8, 22,59]. On the other hand, sesamoidal fractures are seen in avulsion or hyperextension injuries of the forefoot and axial loading of the foot and may also manifest as stress fractures secondary to prolonged standing [8,15,58,59]. Sesamoidal injuries are common, particularly in football players and especially in those playing on turf fields [9]. Patients who have digital or sesamoidal fractures may complain of tenderness and pain with ambulation and present with swelling, local pain upon palpation, ecchymosis, and subungal hematoma, particularly with distal phalangeal fractures [2,58,59]. Patients who have a sesamoid fracture or fracture dislocation may complain of great toe pain as well as demonstrate pain localized to the sub-first metatarsal head, with notable pain upon first meta-tarsophalangeal joint range of motion [58].

Standard radiographs suffice for diagnosing digital fractures, but sesamoidal fractures may require a more diagnostic evaluation. When a sesamoidal fracture is suspected, axial sesamoidal radiographs are useful for looking at the sesamoids. The medial oblique view of standard radiographs is useful for assessing the tibial sesamoid, and the lateral oblique is useful for looking at the fibular sesamoid [59]. Nevertheless, contralateral radiographs should be considered to rule out a bipartite sesamoid [25]. Bipartite sesamoids typically have rounded edges with

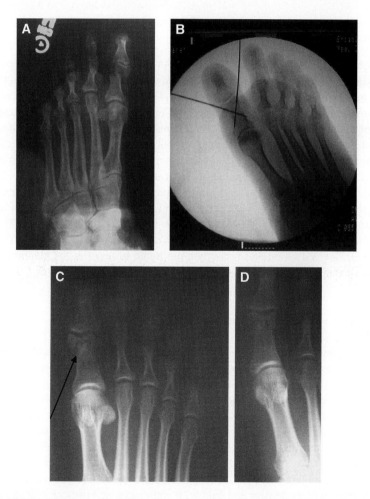

Fig. 9. (*A*) Digital fractures of the hallux and second digit, which are displaced dorsally and medially. (*B*) Second digit was amenable to closed reduction, whereas closed reduction of the hallux did not hold. Therefore crossed Kirshner wires were used. (*C*, *D*) Intra-articular split fracture involving the proximal phalanx of the hallux.

equal spacing between the two pieces, whereas sesamoidal fractures character-
istically have sharp, jagged edges with uneven spacing between the fracture
fragments [15,58,59]. Because of the surrounding soft tissue and important
attachments about the sesamoidal complex, soft tissue damage must be
considered when patients complain of pain in the sub-first metatarsal head. CT,
bone scans, and MRI are helpful in further evaluating and diagnosing sesamoid
fractures and the integrity of the soft tissue [58,59].

Nondisplaced digital fractures are treated with buddy taping and placed in a
stiff-soled shoe for 4 to 6 weeks [2,22,58]. If the fracture is displaced, closed
reduction should be attempted with concomitant immobilization (Fig. 9) [2,59]. If
closed reduction fails, or the fracture line violates the joint, surgical fixation
should be employed (Fig. 10). Means of surgical correction include percutaneous
pinning, mini-screw fixation, a plate with screw fixation, and circlage wires
[2,7,11,22,59]. Subungal hematomas are often seen with distal phalanx fractures.
If a digital fracture is identified in the presence of nail bed bleeding or laceration,
the fracture should be treated as an open fracture, and the nail bed should be
decompressed, depending on the extent of the damage [22,59]. For chip fractures,
fragments that fail to heal or cause irritation or pain may be excised [22,60].

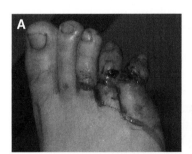
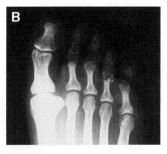
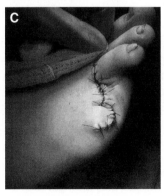

Fig. 10. (A) Open fracture of the fourth and fifth digits with extensive soft tissue injury resulting from
an electric saw injury. Third toe was affected by simple laceration with tendons intact. (B) Radiograph
depicting osseous damage from the electric saw. (C) Treatment of the open fracture in which the third
digit was amenable to soft tissue repair. The fourth and fifth digits were surgically amputated.

The base of the first metatarsal should not be overlooked when evaluating a patient who has an inversion-type injury. Just as other avulsion fractures (eg, anterior process of the calcaneus, tuberosity of the fifth metatarsal) have been well documented, avulsion fractures of the base of the hallux have been reported several times in the literature [6]. Avulsion fractures are possible because of the pull of the peroneus longus as it inserts on the lateral aspect of the base of the first metatarsal. Surgical fixation is often indicated for successful reduction, and a variety of methods can be used (multiple Kirshner wires, screw fixation, and other means) [6,11]. Chip fractures off the peripheral rim of the first metatarsal are not as common. When they do occur, traditional cast immobilization may not be optimal in the active patient. Surgical removal can offer a much quicker return to pervious levels of activity [45].

Treatment of sesamoidal fractures may vary slightly, particularly in the face of a fracture dislocation. Icing, offloading, immobilization, closed reduction, reduced activity, and orthosis are some conservative methods for treatment [58,59]. Surgical treatments include excision of the affected sesamoid in addition to surgical reconstruction of the sesamoidal complex for sesamoidal fracture dislocations [58,59]. The long-term, negative sequelae of untreated or poorly treated fractures are more detrimental in sesamoidal fractures than in digital fractures; complications include arthritis, hallux varus, hallux rigidus, cocked-up hallux, and irritation of the adjacent nerve [58,59].

Open fractures about the forefoot

Gustilo [61] describes an open fracture as "one in which the bone ends have penetrated to the outside skin and there is injury to the underlying soft tissue of varying severity." Gustilo [61–64] and colleagues have developed a classification system for open fractures based on three types of wound presentation. The three types of open fractures are categorized as follows:

- Type I: open fracture with clean wound more than 1 cm long
- Type II: open fracture with laceration more than 1 cm long without extensive soft tissue involvement; moderate crushing injury, moderate comminution, and moderate contamination
- Type III: open fracture with extensive soft tissue damage including muscle, skin, and neurovascular structures, traumatic amputation, or open segmental fracture; highly contaminated

Type III is further divided into subtypes A, B, and C. Type III-A has adequate bony soft tissue coverage and includes gunshot wounds. Type III-B open fractures include farm injuries and entail periosteal stripping with exposed bone. Type III-C open fractures are associated with arterial injuries necessitating repair and include traumatic amputations (see Fig. 10). Open fractures more than 8 hours old are typically considered type III-C open fractures.

Treatment of open fractures has come a long way since the descriptions by Hippocrates, Theodoric of Salerno, Joseph Desault, and Lister. Nevertheless, many of the core principles of treatment have been maintained and improved upon. Hippocrates, in the fourth century BC, is credited with detailing five principles of healing for open fractures [65]. These principles included antisepsis, bandaging, reduction, splinting, and traction. Centuries later, Joseph Desault described débridement of open fractures, and the concept was popularized by Dominique-Jean Larrey, Surgeon-in-Chief of Napoleon's Grand Army. In the mid 1800s, Lister employed the idea of the prevention of sepsis [65]. Today, treatment of open fractures centers around three main goals: prevention of wound sepsis, healing of fracture, and return to normal function [64]. Present treatment evolved from core principles of treatment as described by Gustilo [61], Anderson and Gustilo [66], and Gustilo and colleagues [63,64]. The principles of treatment include

1. Treating all open fractures as emergencies
2. Thorough full-body assessment
3. Appropriate antibiotic coverage
4. Débridement and irrigation
5. Stabilization of open fracture
6. Appropriate coverage of wound
7. Early cancellous bone grafting
8. Rehabilitation of the affected extremity
9. Rehabilitation of the patient

Débridement and irrigation is considered the most important step and is the first step in treating open fractures [61–66]. Additionally, type III and some type II open-fracture wounds must be closely monitored for 24 to 48 hours after injury and initial wound débridement, because further tissue necrosis may occur secondary to unfolding damage from circulatory embarrassment [61].

For antibiotic coverage, cephalosporins are generally given to patients who have open fractures to ensure coverage of gram-positive organisms [62,64,66–69]. Typically 2.0 g of cefazolin sodium is given intravenously every 6 hours for type I fractures and is continued for 2 to 3 days. Type II and type III open

Table 1
Tetanus wound classification

Clinical features	Tetanus prone	Non-tetanus prone
Age of wound	>6 h	<6 hours
Configuration	Stellate, avulsion	Linear
Depth	>1 cm	<1 cm
Mechanism of Injury	Missile, crush, burn, frostbite	Sharp knife
Devitalized tissue	Present	Absent
Contaminants	Present	Absent

Table 2
Tetanus prophylaxis

	Immunization schedule			
History of tetanus immunization	Dirty tetanus -prone wound		Clean non–tetanus-prone wound	
	TD	TIG	TG	TIG
Unknown or < three doses	Yes	Yes	Yes	Yes
Three or more doses	No (yes if >5 y since last booster)	No	No (yes if >10 y since last booster	No

fractures are treated with cefazolin sodium plus an aminoglycoside such as tobramycin or gentamycin to ensure adequate coverage of gram-negative organisms. Aminoglycosides are administered intravenously: 1.5 mg/kg is administered initially, and 3.0 to 5.0 mg/kg/d is administered for 3 days total [62,67–69]. Tetanus status must also be assessed and treated in cases of open fractures, because disruption of the integument increases susceptibility to *Clostridium tetani* infection (Tables 1 and 2) [67]. Sandusky [70] developed a guideline for tetanus prophylaxis:

- If the patient has previously been immunized with a booster within 1 year, no treatment
- If immunization occurred less than 10 years ago with no booster, or immunization occurred more than 10 years ago with a booster within 10 years, or there has been no immunization or booster within 10 years, but the would is minor and clean and treatment is prompt, give 0.5 mL of tetanus and diphtheria toxoid (Td)
- If immunization occurred more than 10 years ago, with no booster within 5 years, and the wound is unclean wound or treatment is delayed, give 0.5 mL Td and 250 to 500 units of tetanus immune globulin (human) [TIG(H)]
- If there is no history of immunization, but the wound is clean and relatively minor and treatment is prompt, give 0.5 mL Td and schedule future immunizations
- If there is no history of immunization, and the wound is unclean or treatment is delayed, give 250 to 500 units of TIG(H) and begin immunization with 0.5 mL of Td

Wound and fracture care in open fractures varies depending on the fracture type. Gustilo and colleagues [63,64] state that the goal of soft tissue coverage for open fractures is 7 to 10 days to optimize wound healing and minimize infection. Primary or delayed primary closure may be used, based on physician preference and the presenting situation [61,62,64]. Early amputation is deemed acceptable and is indicated in the presence of injury to muscle and skin, in the presence of an intact neurovascular system but with such severe muscular damage and bone loss that function is unlikely, or in the presence of an intact vascular system or a disrupted vessel amenable to repair but with loss of movement or sensation with nerve damage not amenable to primary or secondary repair [61,62,64].

Summary

Fractures of the forefoot are common injuries of various causes. Although not crippling, forefoot fractures can be debilitating if they go undiagnosed or are mistreated. Whenever patients complain of foot pain with ambulation or difficulty ambulating, radiographs should be taken as part of a standard routine to assess for bony pathology. This measure may also serve as precaution to avoid the unfortunate mistake of potentially (and unnecessarily) misdiagnosing a patient, along with the negative sequelae of untreated or poorly treated fractures. For open fracture, tetanus status needs to be assessed and treated accordingly, antibiotics must be administered, and the wound must be debrided and irrigated.

References

[1] Jeffers RF, Tan HB, Nicolopoulos C, et al. Prevalence and patterns of foot injuries following motorcycle trauma. J Orthop Trauma 2004;18:87–91.
[2] Shereff MJ. Fractures of the forefoot. Instr Course Lect 1990;29:133–40.
[3] Iwamoto J, Takeda T. Stress fractures in athletes: review of 196 cases. J Orthop Sci 2003;8: 273–8.
[4] Campbell JT. Foot and ankle fractures in the industrial setting. Foot Ankle Clin 2002;7:323–50.
[5] Sammarco GJ, Carrasquillo HA. Intramedullary fixation of metatarsal fracture and nonunion. Orthop Clin North Am 1995;26:265–72.
[6] Yoho RM, Hatchett H, Olson K, et al. Avulsion fracture of the plantar lateral base of the first metatarsal. J Am Podiatr Med Assoc 2000;90:101–3.
[7] Rammelt S, Heineck J, Zwipp H. Metatarsal fractures. Injury 2004;35:S-B77–S-B86.
[8] Schenk RC, Heckman JD. Fractures and dislocations of the forefoot: operative and nonoperative treatment. J Am Acad Orthop Surg 1995;3:70–8.
[9] Abidi NA. Sprains about the foot and ankle encountered in the Workman's Compensation patient. Foot Ankle Clin 2002;7:305–22.
[10] Pendarvis JA, Mandracchia VJ, Haverstock BD, et al. A new fixation technique for metatarsal fractures. Clin Podiatr Med Surg 1999;16:643–57.
[11] Kwak HY, Bae SW. Isolated avulsion fracture at the plantar lateral base of the first metatarsal. Foot Ankle Int 2000;21:864–7.
[12] Theodorou DJ, Theodorou SJ, Kakitsubata Y, et al. Fractures of proximal portion of fifth metatarsal bone: anatomic and imaging evidence of a pathogenesis of avulsion of the plantar aponeurosis and the short peroneal muscle tendon. Radiology 2003;226:857–65.
[13] Gumman G, Engle AJ, Snowdy HA. Comminuted intra-articular fracture of the first metatarsal base. J Am Podiatr Assoc 1982;72:521–4.
[14] Tuan K, Wu S, Sennett B. Stress fractures in athletes: risk factors, diagnosis, and management. Orthopedics 2004;27:583–91.
[15] Harmath C, Demos TC, Lomasney L, et al. Radiologic case study. Orthopedics 2001;24:204–8.
[16] Fortin PT, Myerson MS. Second metatarsophalangeal joint instability. Foot Ankle Int 1995; 16:306–12.
[17] Peris P. Stress fractures in rheumatologic practice: clinical significance and localizations. Rheumatol Int 2002;22:77–9.

[18] Myerson MS. Experimental basis for fasciotomy of the foot and decompression in acute compartment syndromes. Foot Ankle 1988;8:308–14.

[19] Myerson M. Compartment syndromes of the foot. Bull Hosp Jt Dis Orthop Inst 1987;47: 251–61.

[20] Fulkerson E, Razi A, Tejwani N. Review: acute compartment syndrome of the foot. Foot Ankle Int 2003;24:180–7.

[21] Schenk R, Willenegger H. Morphological findings in primary fracture healing. Symp Biol Hung 1967;7:75–86.

[22] Armagan OE, Shereff MJ. Injuries to the toes and metatarsal. Foot Ankle Trauma 2001;32:1–10.

[23] Salter R. Disorders and injuries of the musculoskeletal system. Philadelphia: WB Saunders; 1970.

[24] Gudas CJ. Traumatic fractures and dislocations of the foot and ankle. In: Proceedings of the Seventh Annual Northlake Surgical Seminar. Chicago: 1977.

[25] Goldman FD, Morris G, Nix K. Fracture of the second metatarsal base. J Am Podiatr Med Assoc 2003;93:6–10.

[26] DeHeer PA. Forefoot applications of external fixation. Clin Podiatr Med Surg 2003;20:27–44.

[27] Trafton PG. Tibial shaft fractures. In: Browner BD, Jupiter JB, Levine AM, et al, editors. Skeletal trauma: fractures, dislocations, ligamentous injuries, vol. 2. Philadelphia: WB Saunders; 1992. p. 1809–12.

[28] Donahue MP, Manoli A. Technical tip: transverse percutaneous pinning of metatarsal neck fractures. Foot Ankle Int 2004;25:438–9.

[29] Erickson S, Krisdakumtorn T, Saxena A. Proximal fourth metatarsal injuries in athletes: similarity to proximal fifth metatarsal injury. Foot Ankle Int 2001;22:603–8.

[30] Fakhouri AJ, Manoli A. Acute foot compartment syndromes. J Orthop Trauma 1992;6:223–8.

[31] Aguado HJ, Herranz PG, Rapariz JM. Metaizeau's technique for displaced metatarsal neck fractures. J Pediatr Orthop B 2003;12:350–3.

[32] Kouzelis AT. Does reaming affect the composition of reaming products in intramedullary nailing of long bones? Orthopedics 2004;27:852–6.

[33] Rhinelander FW, Stewart CL, Wilson JW, et al. Growth of tissue into a porous, low modulus coating in intramedullary nails: an experimental study. Clin Orthop Relat Res 1982;164: 293–305.

[34] Crowl AC, Young JS, Kahler DM, et al. Occult hypoperfusion is associated with increased morbidity in patients undergoing early femur fracture fixation. J Trauma 2000;48:260–7.

[35] Frolke JP, Peters R, Boshuizen K, et al. The assessment of cortical heat during intramedullary reaming of long bones. Injury 2001;32:683–8.

[36] Madan S, Blakeway C. Radiation exposure to surgeon and patient in intramedullary nailing of the lower limb. Injury 2002;33:723–7.

[37] Vertullo CJ, Glisson RR, Nunley JA. Torsional strains in the proximal fifth metatarsal: implications for Jones and stress fracture management. Foot Ankle Int 2004;25:650–6.

[38] Johnson JT, Labib SA, Fowler R. intramedullary screw fixation of the fifth metatarsal: an anatomic study and improved technique. Foot Ankle Int 2004;25:274–7.

[39] Portland G, Kelikian A, Kodros S. Acute surgical management of Jones' fractures. Foot Ankle Int 2003;24:829–33.

[40] Torg JS, Balduini FC, Zelko RR, et al. Fractures of the base of the fifth metatarsal distal to the tuberosity. J Bone Joint Surg [Am] 1984;66:209–14.

[41] Stewart IM. Jones fracture: fracture of base of fifth metatarsal. Clin Orthop 1960;16:190–8.

[42] Kelly IP, Glisson RR, Fink C, et al. Intramedullary screw fixation of Jones fractures. Foot Ankle Int 2001;22:585–9.

[43] Arangio GA, Xiao D, Salathe EP. Biomechanical study of stress in the fifth metatarsal. Clin Biomech (Bristol, Avon) 1997;12:160–4.

[44] Porter DA, Duncan M, Meyer SJ. Fifth metatarsal Jones fracture fixation with a 4.5 mm cannulated stainless steel screw in the competitive and recreational athlete. Am J Sports Med 2005;33:1–8.

[45] Rehman S, Kashyap S. Proximal fifth metatarsal stress fracture treated by early open reduction and internal fixation. Orthopedics 2004;27:1196–8.

[46] Reese K, Litsky A, Kaeding C, et al. Cannulated screw fixation of Jones fractures. Am J Sports Med 2004;32:1736–42.

[47] Larson CM, Almekinders LC, Taft TN, et al. Intramedullary screw fixation of Jones fractures. Am J Sports Med 2002;30:55–60.

[48] Shah SN, Knoblich GO, Lindsey DP, et al. Intramedullary screw fixation of proximal fifth metatarsal fractures: a biomechanical study. Foot Ankle Int 2001;22:581–4.

[49] Carpenter B, Garrett A. Using a hook plate as alternative fixation for fifth metatarsal base fracture. J Foot Ankle Surg 2003;42:315–6.

[50] Lombardi CM, Connolly FG, Silhanek AD. The use of external fixation for treatment of the acute Jones fracture: a retrospective review of 10 cases. J Foot Ankle Surg 2004;43:173–8.

[51] Husain ZS, DeFronzo DJ. Relative stability of tension band versus tow-cortex screw fixation for treating fifth metatarsal base avulsion fractures. J Foot Ankle Surg 2000;39:89–95.

[52] Bonutti PM, Bell GR. Compartment syndrome of the foot. J Bone Joint Surg [Am] 1986;68:1449–51.

[53] Horst F, Gilbert BJ, Glisson RR, et al. Torque resistance after fixation of Jones fractures with intramedullary screws. Foot Ankle Int 2004;25:914–9.

[54] Low K, Noblin JD, Brown JE, et al. Jones fractures in the elite football player. J Surg Orthop Adv 2004;13:156–60.

[55] Rosenburg GA, Sferra JJ. Treatment strategies for acute fractures and nonunions of the proximal fifth metatarsal. J Am Acad Orthop Surg 2000;8:332–8.

[56] Nolte PA, van der Krans A, Patka P, et al. Low-intensity pulsed ultrasound in the treatment of nonunions. J Trauma 2001;51:693–703.

[57] Wright RW, Fischer DA, Shively RA, et al. Refracture of proximal fifth metatarsal (Jones) fracture after intramedullary screw fixation in athletes. Am J Sports Med 2000;28:732–6.

[58] Cortes ZE, Baumhauer JF. Traumatic lateral dislocation of the great toe fibular sesamoid. Case report. Foot Ankle Int 2004;25:164–7.

[59] Mittlemeier T, Haar P. Sesamoid and toe factures. Injury 2004;35:S-B87–S-B97.

[60] Kohles SS, McKinney PF. Chip fractures of the first metatarsal head. Primary fragment excision versus immobilization: a report of 4 cases. J Foot Ankle Surg 2001;40:50–3.

[61] Gustilo RB. Principles of the management of open fractures. In: Sledge CB, editor. Saunders monographs in clinical orthopaedics, vol. 4. Philadelphia: WB Saunders; 1982. p. 15–54.

[62] Gustilo RB. Current concepts in the management of open fractures. Instr Course Lect 1987;36:359–66.

[63] Gustilo RB, Gruninger RP, Davis T. Classification of type III (severe) open fractures relative to treatment and results. Orthopedics 1987;10:1781–8.

[64] Gustilo RB, Merkow RL, Templeman D. Current concepts review: the management of open fractures. J Bone Joint Surg [Am] 1990;72:299–304.

[65] Anderson JT. History of the treatment of open fractures. In: Sledge CB, editor. Saunders monographs in clinical orthopaedics, vol. 4. Philadelphia: WB Saunders; 1982. p. 1–14.

[66] Anderson JT, Gustilo RB. Immediate internal fixation in open fractures. Orthop Clin North Am 1980;11:569–78.

[67] Kind AC, Williams DN. Antibiotics in open fractures. In: Sledge CB, editor. Saunders monographs in clinical orthopaedics, vol. 4. Philadelphia: WB Saunders; 1982. p. 55–69.

[68] Dellinger EP, Caplan ES, Weaver LD, et al. Duration of preventive antibiotic administration for open extremity fractures. Arch Surg 1988;123:333–9.

[69] Dellinger EP, Miller SD, Wertz MJ, et al. Risk of infection after open fracture of the arm or leg. Arch Surg 1988;123:1320–7.

[70] Sandusky WR. Prophylaxis of infection in trauma. In: Mandell GI, Douglas RG, Bennett JE, editors. Principles and practice of infectious disease. New York: Churchill Livingstone; 1979. p. 837.

ELSEVIER
SAUNDERS

Clin Podiatr Med Surg
23 (2006) 303–322

CLINICS IN
PODIATRIC
MEDICINE AND
SURGERY

Lisfranc Fracture-Dislocations: Current Treatment and New Surgical Approaches

Thomas Zgonis, DPM*, Thomas S. Roukis, DPM,
Vasilios D. Polyzois, MD, PhD

*Podiatry Division, Department of Orthopaedics,
University of Texas Health Science Center at San Antonio, 7773 Floyd Curl Drive,
San Antonio, TX 78229, USA*

Non-neuropathic fracture-dislocations about the tarso-metatarsal joints are referred to as Lisfranc injuries after the French field surgeon in the Napoleonic Wars [1]. Lisfranc fracture-dislocations are difficult to treat and are frequently overlooked in the emergency room and clinical setting because they occur at an area of complex, poorly visualized, and highly articulated osseous anatomy [2–6].

Clinical signs that should raise the level of suspicion for an occult Lisfranc injury include ecchymosis about the plantar aspect of the midfoot, which is indicative of severe soft tissue disruption about the tarsometatarsal region [7]; asymmetrical gapping between the first and second toes with weight bearing, which is suggestive of intercuneiform disruption [8]; pain with abduction or pronation of the forefoot on the midfoot, which stresses the plantar ligamentous complex supporting the medial three articulations of the Lisfranc complex [9]; and an inability to rise onto the toes with severe pain localized to midfoot region, which produces peak compression across the Lisfranc complex [10]. The use of multiplane (ie, anterior-posterior, oblique, and lateral) weight-bearing radiographs of the injured side compared with the contralateral uninvolved side is a useful technique to evaluate subtle injuries and represents a stress view when image intensification is not readily available [11]. Several constant anatomic relationships between the osseous components of the Lisfranc complex have been shown to exist. On the anterior-posterior view, the distance between the first and second metatarsal bases should be 3 mm or less; the medial border of the

---

* Corresponding author.
E-mail address: zgonis@uthscsa.edu (T. Zgonis).

second metatarsal should be in line with the medial border of the intermediate cuneiform; the first metatarsal should be in line with medial and lateral borders of the medial cuneiform; and the first and second intermetatarsal space should be continuous with the intertarsal space of the medial and intermediate cuneiforms [12]. On a 30° oblique view, the medial border of the fourth metatarsal should be in line with the medial border of the cuboid; the lateral border of the third metatarsal should be in line with the lateral border of the lateral cuneiform; and the third and fourth intermetatarsal space should be contiguous with the intertarsal space of the lateral cuneiform and cuboid [12]. On the lateral view, failure of the metatarsal bases to align directly with their respective tarsal bones (ie, dorsal subluxation) and asymmetrical collapse of the medial longitudinal arch with plantar widening between the tarsometatarsal articulations are strongly suggestive of disruption of the Lisfranc complex [12,13]. Finally, the presence of the so-called "fleck-sign" or avulsion of the Lisfranc's ligament at the base of the second metatarsal is usually diagnostic of a Lisfranc fracture-dislocation but can be confused with an os intermetatarsium (one or two accessory ossicles), which usually presents bilaterally [14]. The advent of readily available and low-cost CT scanning and MRI affords complete evaluation of the entire Lisfranc osseous and ligamentous complex. These evaluations should be obtained for each patient suspected of having an occult Lisfranc fracture-dislocation, because diastasis of 2 mm or less between the first and second metatarsal bases is readily identified with these modalities but not with radiographs. CT and MRI studies should also be obtained for patients who have obvious pathology to evaluate the adjacent osseous and soft tissue structures and to aid in preparation for intervention [3,5,15].

Myriad conservative and surgical methods of treating this complicated injury have been described [16–22]. Although no formal consensus regarding the optimal treatment of displaced Lisfranc fracture-dislocations exists, it has been proven that prompt and early intervention with complete restoration of the normal anatomic alignment of the entire Lisfranc's complex in all three cardinal planes is paramount to limit the development of painful posttraumatic osteoarthritis [23–34]. In severe Lisfranc fracture-dislocations, especially open fractures and those with extensive soft tissue injuries, strong consideration should be given to primary arthrodesis [35]. This approach is technically demanding and should be performed only by experienced foot and ankle surgeons who have specialized training in trauma [36], because there is little tolerance for malalignment at this level in the foot [37–39]. Unlike other traumatic injuries in the foot, posttraumatic arthrosis or arthrodesis procedures about the Lisfranc complex are difficult to accommodate with pedorthic-type shoe and insole therapy [40].

Internal fixation: literature review

The surgical treatment of Lisfranc fracture-dislocations has undergone a series of evolutionary changes. Closed reduction with cast immobilization was initially attempted, but this approach is no longer used because of the high incidence of loss of reduction, extended immobilization, and frequent need for late arthrodesis [1,9,14,18,20,23,24,26,29,32].

Limited open reduction with Kirschner-wire fixation followed by cast immobilization has been shown to be effective if anatomic reduction can be achieved and maintained throughout the immobilization period [1,14,19,24,26,27]. A review of the literature regarding this technique, however, reveals that most fracture-dislocations treated in this fashion were those that could be treated with closed reduction and were of minimal severity [1,14,19,24,26,27]. Therefore, this approach should be reserved for injuries that are primarily ligamentous in nature, can be close reduced, and seem to be stable following insertion of the Kirschner wires and application of a well-padded short-leg cast.

Limited open reduction with internal transarticular screw fixation followed by cast immobilization has become one of the most widely applied techniques for managing Lisfranc fracture-dislocations [1,14,21,26–28,30]. This technique affords rigid fixation about the intercuneiform and medial three metatarsal-cuneiform articulations; the lateral tarsometatarsal articulations usually are either left alone (ie, reduced using the Vassal principle) or stabilized with percutaneous Kirschner wires followed by cast immobilization. A recent cadaveric biomechanical study comparing the stiffness and amount of displacement following reduction of simulated Lisfranc fracture-dislocations with longitudinal Kirschner-wire fixation of the entire tarsometatarsal complex, rigid cortical screw fixation of the medial three tarsometatarsal articulations with Kirschne-wire fixation of the lateral tarsometatarsal articulations, and cortical screw fixation of the entire tarsometatarsal complex revealed that the use of cortical screw fixation for the medial three tarsometatarsal articulations resulted in the greater stiffness and less displacement than seen with Kirschner-wire stabilization of these articulations [21]. The screw orientation for the medial three tarsometatarsal articulations was slightly different in the two groups in which screws were used. Each group had a screw from the first metatarsal base into the medial cuneiform and a screw from the medial cuneiform into the second metatarsal base. The variation occurred with the stabilization of the third metatarsal cuneiform articulation: in one group the screw was oriented from the third metatarsal base into the intermediate cuneiform; in the other group the screw was oriented from the third metatarsal into the lateral cuneiform. The latter construct was shown to produce greater stiffness about the medial three tarsometatarsal articulations. This group, however, had screw fixation across the entire Lisfranc complex, which may have caused the increased stiffness. Nonetheless, the use of screw fixation across the lateral tarsometatarsal articulations did not produce a statistically significant difference in stiffness when compared with Kirschner-wire stabilization [21]. Because the lateral column of the foot is usually quite immobile, screw fixation across the lateral tarsometatarsal articulations should probably be reserved for situations in which Kirschner-wire fixation fails to maintain sufficient stability to allow some mobility about the lateral column of the foot [1,14, 21,26–28,30].

Despite the stability achieved with internal transarticular screw fixation, there has been some recent concern regarding the additional damage to the already traumatized articular cartilage because of transarticular nature of the screws [21,28,41]. For this reason, most authors recommend removal of the internal transarticular screw fixation between 6 and 12 months after operation to allow full repair of the ligamentous structures while limiting the potential for screw breakage and articular cartilage damage.

In an effort to limit the need for a secondary surgery to remove the retained hardware, the use of absorbable internal transarticular screws has been advocated [17,18]. Although the sample sizes were small and the studies retrospective in nature, the use of one to four absorbable screws for stabilization of Lisfranc fracture-dislocations about the medial three tarsometatarsal joints did not result in any soft tissue reaction, osteolysis, or loss of reduction over the mean 20-month follow-up period (range, 3–45 months). Although these reports are of interest, the increased expense associated with the use of absorbable screws and the transarticular location of the screws, as well as the small sample size and lack of long-term follow-up of this technique, raise some questions concerning its ultimate role in the surgical management of Lisfranc fracture-dislocations.

Both plantar [41] and dorsal [21] plate-and-screw fixation have been shown to afford greater stiffness and less deformation than transarticular cortical screw fixation of the medial three tarsometatarsal joint articulations. The potential difficulties in closing the resultant incisions because of the thickness of the plates, the additional dissection required to properly seat them, and the increased expense of these devices, and the small sample size and lack of long-term follow-up of this technique [28] raise some questions as to its ultimate role in the surgical management of Lisfranc fracture-dislocations. Although there is interest in alternative fixation techniques, the use of internal transarticular screw fixation followed by cast immobilization seems to be the most widely used technique for the surgical stabilization of Lisfranc fracture-dislocations, especially about the medial three tarsometatarsal articulations.

Operative technique: percutaneous internal fixation

Percutaneous reduction and internal transarticular screw placement is primarily useful for ligamentous Lisfranc fracture-dislocations that can be passively reduced. The sequence of events described here can also be used in isolation when more extensive open procedures are necessary to reduce the deformity fully.

Under general or spinal anesthesia, the patient is positioned on the operating room table in the supine position with the entire affected lower extremity draped free to afford unlimited access to the entire foot, ankle, and lower extremity. A tourniquet is usually not used because of the percutaneous nature of the technique. Intraoperative image intensification is positioned opposite the surgeon to

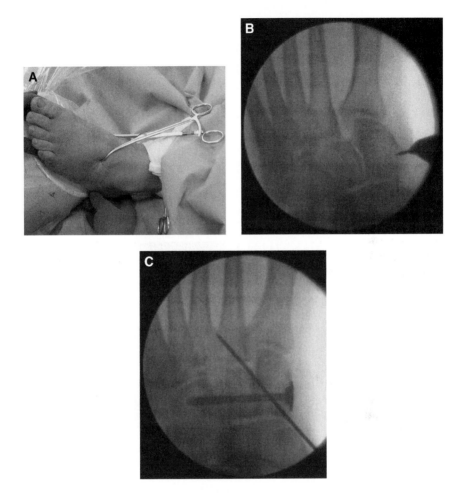

Fig. 1. Intraoperative photographs. (A) The location and application of a Weber large, pointed reduction clamp to maintain reduction of the Lisfranc fracture-dislocation. (B) Image-intensification view demonstrating the location of the insertion point for the guide wire used to stabilize the intercuneiform articulations. (C) Anterior-posterior image-intensification view demonstrating the position of the guide wire used to stabilize the second tarsometatarsal dislocation. Note the location and orientation of both the guide wire and the initial screw and washer used to stabilize the intercuneiform articulations. (D) The technique used to align and stabilize the first metatarsal medial cuneiform articulation during initial drill application and subsequent screw fixation. (E) Anterior-posterior image intensification view demonstrating the location and orientation of the path for the solid cortical screw fixation of the first metatarsal medial cuneiform articulation. (F) Image-intensification view demonstrating the location and orientation of the guide wire used to stabilize the third tarsometatarsal articulation. (G) The guide-wire cage created when the tandem technique is employed for repair of Lisfranc fracture-dislocations. (H) Anterior-posterior and (I) lateral image-intensification views demonstrating the final percutaneous internal transarticular screw fixation construct and (J) resultant soft tissue incisions needed to place the internal fixation properly.

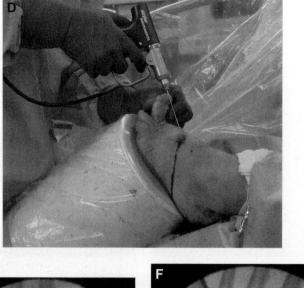

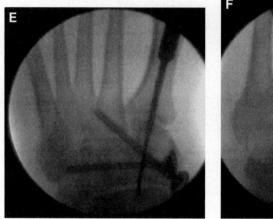

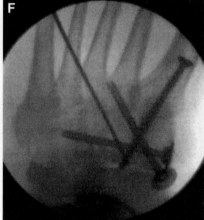

Fig. 1 (*continued*).

afford direct visualization without impeding access to the entire foot. Under direct image intensification the surgeon assesses the extent of the injury to the tarso-metatarsal joint complex by simultaneously abducting and everting the forefoot on the midfoot. The degree and location of the instability is compared with the preoperative radiographs to make certain that no occult injury pattern to the tarsometatarsal and midfoot articulations exists. The ability to reduce the deformity anatomically is assessed by simultaneously adducting the forefoot on the midfoot and dorsiflexing the toes at the metatarsophalangeal joints, a maneuver that engages the plantar fascia and long flexor tendons and creates stability about the tarsometatarsal and midfoot articulations.

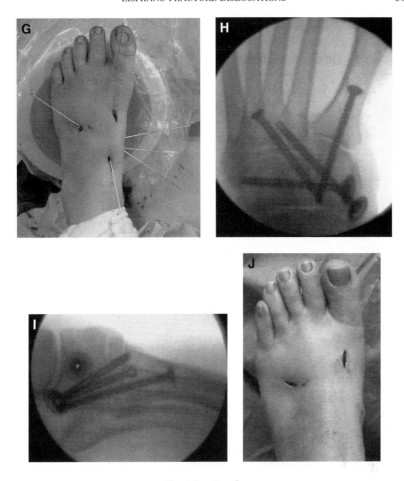

Fig. 1 (*continued*).

Once the fracture is fully reduced, a Weber large, pointed reduction clamp is applied between the plantar medial aspect of the medial cuneiform and the dorsal lateral aspect of the third metatarsal to stabilize the medial three tarso-metatarsal articulations (Fig. 1A). Through a percutaneous incision, the guide wire from a small-fragment screw-fixation system is driven from the medial aspect of the medial cuneiform about its central portion across the intercunei-form articulations into the lateral cuneiform with a slight dorsal-to-plantar orientation to create a solid block of fixation proximally and to reduce the intercuneiform instability usually present in tarsometatarsal joint fracture-dislocations (Fig. 1B). A washer is usually used with this screw to create additional stability and avoid sinking of the screw head into the relatively soft bone of the medial cuneiform.

Next, through a percutaneous incision, another guide wire is driven from the plantar medial aspect of the medial cuneiform into the dorsal lateral aspect of the second metatarsal base (Fig 1C). This orientation allows the threads of the subsequent screw to purchase the dense bone within the second metatarsal base rather than the relatively softer bone of the medial cuneiform and allows the second metatarsal base to be lagged against the base of the first metatarsal and

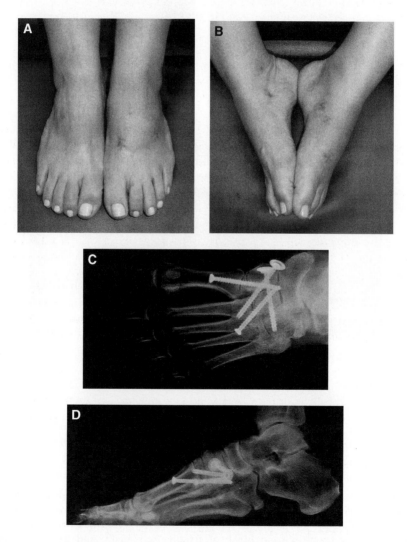

Fig. 2. Long-term clinical (*A*) dorsal and (*B*) medial photographs along with the (*C*) anterior-posterior and (*D*) lateral weight-bearing radiographs following percutaneous internal transarticular screw fixation of a Lisfranc fracture-dislocation as described in the text. Note the limited edema and lack of any failure of the internal fixation or development of degenerative changes about the tarsometatarsal joint complex.

medial cuneiform. The Weber clamp is removed at this time, and the stability of the reduction is assessed, because anatomically reducing and stabilizing the second metatarsal within its recess is considered the most essential component of the procedure.

Once stability has been verified through stress manipulation under image intensification, the remaining Lisfranc articulations are addressed. Through a 1-cm incision, with the great toe held in full dorsiflexion at the metatarsophalangeal joint for the reasons already discussed (Fig. 1D), the drill from a solid, small-fragment screw-fixation system is driven from the dorsal central aspect of the first metatarsal at the junction of the proximal and middle thirds into the plantar central aspect of the medial cuneiform (Fig. 1E). Through a percutaneous incision, another guide wire is driven from the dorsal lateral aspect of the third metatarsal base into either the intermediate or lateral cuneiform in a slight dorsal-to-plantar orientation (Fig. 1F).

As an alternative to this sequential reduction technique, each guide wire can be sequentially placed and followed by step-wise screw placement in the order already described (Fig. 1G). This technique allows a more rapid reduction because the same instruments are used in tandem rather than in a disrupted fashion as occurs with the previously described technique.

Regardless of which technique is employed, the final fixation should provide anatomic reduction of each articulation involved (Fig. 1H, I) with a minimum of soft tissue dissection (Fig. 1J). This percutaneous reduction technique is followed by cast immobilization for 2 to 3 weeks until soft tissue edema has subsided and the incision sites have healed fully. A gradual increase in weight bearing in a removable walking boot is then allowed for the next 3 to 4 weeks, during which time passive range of motion of the toes and ankle is permitted. A formal physical therapy program is then initiated, and the patient is usually fitted with soft, accommodative pedorthic-type insoles to afford shock absorption, along with a sturdy shoe to provide stability. Unless the screw fixation becomes painful, the authors elect to leave the internal transarticular fixation intact rather than remove it, avoiding the need for a secondary surgery and potential late loss of reduction. This technique affords anatomic reduction with minimal disruption of the soft tissue and seems to be well tolerated with minimal complications (Fig. 2).

Operative technique: primary arthrodesis with internal fixation

Primary arthrodesis is indicated in severe Lisfranc fracture-dislocations with extensive soft tissue and articular damage (Fig. 3A–C) in which use of the percutaneous repair technique described previously is impossible because of bone and cartilage loss or in which the interposition soft tissue limits reduction without an open technique (Fig. 3D).

Under general or spinal anesthesia, the patient is positioned on the operating room table in the supine position with the entire affected lower extremity draped free to afford unlimited access to the entire foot, ankle, and lower extremity. In

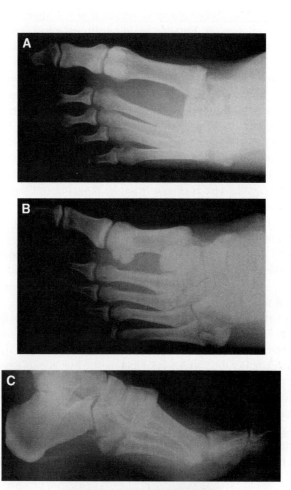

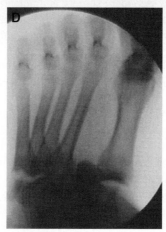

the presence of an open fracture, appropriate soft tissue technique and adherence to the principles of open fractures should be employed but are beyond the scope of this article.

A two- or three-incision technique is most commonly used to access the entire tarsometatarsal joint complex. A medial incision located just dorsal to the abductor hallucis muscle belly is used to access the first metatarsal medial cuneiform articulation, because this approach respects the regional vasculature [42,43], allows complete reduction of the deformity, facilitates removal of any interposed soft tissues from the articulation, allows complete decompression of any associated pedal compartment syndrome, and allows the abductor hallucis muscle belly to be used as a muscle flap with subsequent skin graft coverage should soft tissue coverage be necessary. The second incision is placed at the level of the second and third metatarsal cuneiform articulations and affords complete access to these articulations as well as further access to the first metatarsal medial cuneiform articulation, if necessary. A third incision placed at the level of the fourth and fifth metatarsal base cuboid articulations is used if access to these areas is necessary.

Once the tarsometatarsal articulations are accessed, any interposed soft tissues are either resected (ie, capsule, ligament, adipose tissue) or repositioned and repaired (ie, tendon, neurovascular structures) (Fig. 4A, B). The articular cartilage is then resected from the adjacent joint surfaces, and the subchondral bone plates of the resected surfaces are fenestrated multiple times using a small osteotome and mallet (ie, fish-scaling or shingling technique). Rather than autogenous bone graft harvest, the authors prefer to interpose a specialized cortico-cancellous allograft material with an inert biologic carrier impregnated with autogenous platelet-rich plasma concentrate to facilitate tarsometatarsal joint arthrodesis. Although the use of allogenic bone graft impregnated with autogenous platelet-rich plasma concentrate is not imperative, it has been shown to possess excellent osteoinductive and osteoconductive properties [44–47]. This technique also avoids the morbidity and mortality associated with harvest of autogenous iliac crest bone graft [48]. Limited quantities of autogenous bone graft can be harvested from regional sources when the platelet-rich plasma–impregnated allogenic bone graft mixture is either unavailable or deemed unnecessary [49,50].

The tarsometatarsal joint articulations and any associated osseous pathology are then repaired and stabilized using either solid cortical or cannulated screws following the guidelines presented previously (Fig. 4C). The patient is placed into a well-padded short-leg splint to accommodate edema and is seen according to the needs of any adjunctive soft tissue procedures until a short-leg non–weight-

Fig. 3. (A) Anterior-posterior, (B) oblique, and (C) lateral radiographs revealing a severe Lisfranc fracture-dislocation with extensive osseous disruption. During intraoperative image intensification the fracture-dislocation could not be closed, mandating open reduction that revealed (D) soft tissue interposition of the tibialis anterior tendon medially and of the neurovascular bundle centrally.

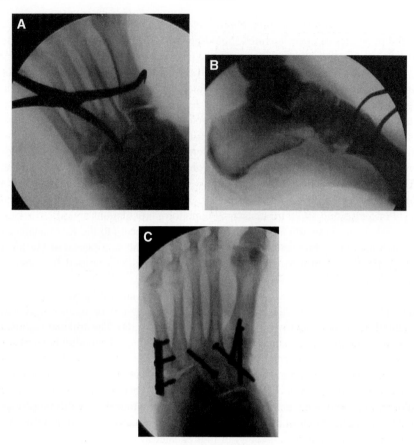

Fig. 4. (*A*) Anterior-posterior and (*B*) lateral intraoperative image-intensification views after open reduction and stabilization of the Lisfranc fracture-dislocation demonstrated in Fig. 3 revealing extensive comminution of the tarsometatarsal articulations and fracture of the fifth metatarsal base. (*C*) Intraoperative image-intensification view after primary arthrodesis of the medial three tarso-metatarsal articulations using internal transarticular screw fixation with platelet-rich plasma–impregnated allogenic bone grafting as described in the text. Note the open reduction and internal fixation of the fifth metatarsal base fracture with plate and screws, which was also packed with the bone graft mixture, and the variation on internal transarticular screw orientation necessary because of soft-tissue limitations.

bearing cast can be applied. The cast is changed at regular intervals and is converted to a short-leg weight-bearing cast until osseous consolidation is achieved as demonstrated by sequential radiographic evaluation of the arthrodesis sites.

An aggressive physical therapy program is initiated after this time, and the patient is usually fitted with soft, accommodative pedorthic-type insoles to afford shock absorption along with a sturdy shoe to provide stability.

Unless the screw fixation becomes painful, the authors elect to leave the internal fixation intact rather than remove it, avoiding the need for a secondary

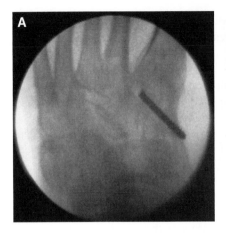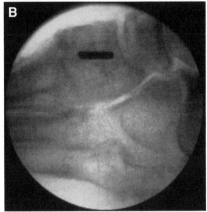

Fig. 5. Long-term (*A*) anterior-posterior and (*B*) lateral intraoperative image-intensification views after removal of the internal fixation shown in Fig. 4. Note the sound arthrodesis throughout the medial tarsometatarsal articulations and the presence of a fractured screw that was left unretrieved.

surgery and potential late loss of reduction. Primary arthrodesis, however, seems to require internal hardware removal at a higher rate than with the percutaneous technique (Fig. 5). Hardware removal allows the surgeon to revise any malalignment about the tarsometatarsal joint complex, if necessary.

Primary arthrodesis of Lisfranc fracture-dislocations affords anatomic reduction and permanent stability [35] but is associated with a higher rate of malunion and gait abnormality [25,31] than when a secondary arthrodesis is performed following failed initial open or percutaneous reduction with internal transarticular screw fixation [37–39]. For these reasons, this technique should be reserved for severe Lisfranc fracture-dislocations with extensive soft tissue and articular damage in which a limited open or percutaneous technique is either impossible or is associated with soft tissue interposition that would limit reduction without an open technique.

External fixation: literature review

Even though there is enough evidence in the literature for the use of internal fixation in the treatment of Lisfranc fracture-dislocations, there are few descriptions of the use of external fixation as a primary or a supplement tool in the surgical treatment of Lisfranc injuries. Mittlmeier and colleagues [25] described the use of external fixation to supplement internal fixation for Lisfranc fracture-dislocations associated with severe injuries and open fractures. To authors' knowledge there are no written reports on the use of external fixation in the treatment of the acute or chronic non-neuropathic Lisfranc fracture-dislocations.

Operative technique: limited open reduction and internal fixation and percutaneous ring-type fine-wire external fixation for the chronic instability of the Lisfranc's joint

Under general or spinal anesthesia, the patient is positioned on the operating room table in the supine position with the entire affected lower extremity draped free to afford unlimited access to the entire foot, ankle, and lower extremity. A tourniquet is usually not used because of the percutaneous nature of the technique. Intraoperative image intensification is positioned opposite the surgeon to afford direct visualization without impeding access to the entire foot. Under direct image intensification the surgeon assesses the extent of the injury to the tarsometatarsal joint complex by simultaneously abducting and everting the forefoot on the midfoot. The ability to reduce the deformity anatomically is assessed by simultaneously adducting the forefoot on the midfoot and dorsiflexing the toes at the metatarsophalangeal joints; this maneuver engages the plantar fascia and long flexor tendons and creates stability about the tarsometatarsal and midfoot articulations.

Once the fracture is fully reduced, a Weber large, pointed reduction clamp is applied between the plantar medial aspect of the medial cuneiform and the dorsal lateral aspect of the third metatarsal, stabilizing the medial three tarsometatarsal articulations (see Fig. 1A). Next, through a percutaneous incision, a guide wire is driven from the plantar medial aspect of the medial cuneiform into the dorsal lateral aspect of the second metatarsal base. This orientation allows the threads of the subsequent Lisfranc screw to purchase the dense bone within the second metatarsal base rather than the relatively softer bone of the medial cuneiform and allows the second metatarsal base to be lagged against the base of the first metatarsal and medial cuneiform. The Weber clamp is removed at this time, and the stability of the reduction assessed, because anatomically reducing and stabilizing the second metatarsal within its recess is considered the most essential component of the procedure.

Once stability has been verified through stress manipulation under image intensification, the prebuilt circular fixator is applied to compress the tarso-metatarsal complex. Two tibial rings and a footplate are applied for a maximum stability during the weight-bearing status. Between 110 and 130 kg of tension is applied to the tibial rings, between 90 and 110 kg is applied to the calcaneus, and between 70 and 90 kg is applied to the metatarsals. Medial and lateral olive wires are applied to the medial cuneiform and to the base of the fifth metatarsal, respectively. Tension is applied carefully to the medial and lateral olive wires under direct image intensification, making sure that the Lisfranc complex is adequately reduced. The circular frame is kept in place for 6 to 8 weeks. The patient is allowed to start minimal weight bearing with assistance at the first postoperative week. After frame removal, the patient is encouraged to start physical therapy and slowly advance into a surgical postoperative shoe or a normal shoe (Fig. 6).

In cases of severe comminution at the tarso-metatarsal complex, a primary arthrodesis at that joint is preferred. The authors' method includes the use of a circular multiplane external fixator and providing compression by bending-wire techniques across the Lisfranc joint. Modifications of the skin incisions are shown in Fig. 7A, B. The same techniques and principles are applied to the primary arthrodesis site by adding a tensioned wire to the Lisfranc joint. Temporary fixation can also be incorporated into the circular external fixator. The advantages of this procedure are minimal dissection, use of one incision, early weight bearing, avoidance of multiple screws that must be removed later, and faster return to work with minimal assistance (Fig. 8A, B). The circular frame is kept in place for 6 to 8 weeks, and the patient is allowed to start minimal weight bearing with assistance at the first postoperative week. After frame removal, the patient is encouraged to start physical therapy and slowly advance into a surgical postoperative shoe or a normal shoe.

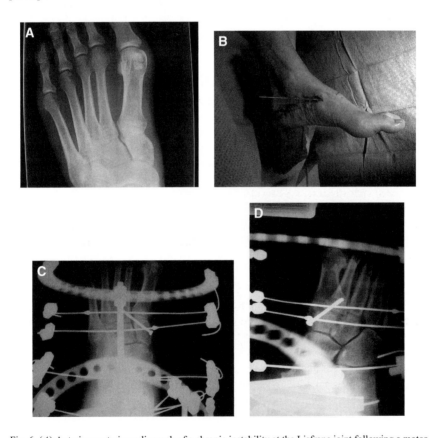

Fig. 6. (A) Anterior-posterior radiograph of a chronic instability at the Lisfranc joint following a motor vehicle accident. (B) Intraoperative picture of the percutaneous Lisfranc screw placement. Post-operative (C) anterior-posterior and (D) medial oblique views showing the technique described in the text for providing stability at the Lisfranc joint. Clinical pictures of the (E) circular external fixator and (F) early weight-bearing status. (G) Clinical and (H, I) radiographic pictures after frame removal. Notice (H) the minimal amount of edema and (I) the orientation of the second metatarsal base lagged against the base of the first metatarsal and medial cuneiform.

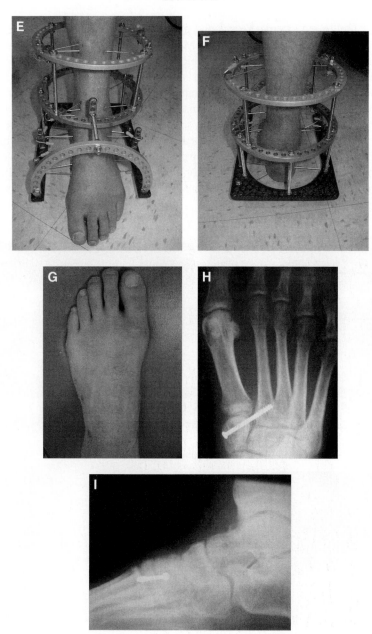

Fig. 6 (*continued*).

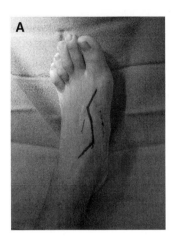
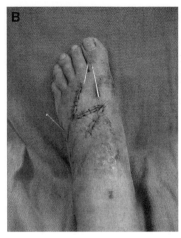

Fig. 7. (*A*, *B*) Proposed incisional approaches for primary arthrodesis at the Lisfranc joint using circular external fixation.

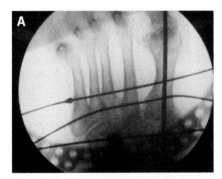

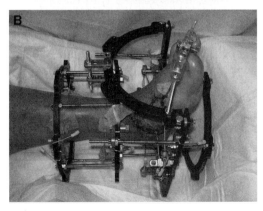

Fig. 8. (*A*) Intraoperative image-intensification showing placement of olive and tensioned wires across the primary Lisfranc arthrodesis site. (*B*) Postoperative picture of the circular external fixator used in Lisfranc arthrodesis.

Discussion

Lisfranc fracture-dislocation is a serious injury. Common complications include wound dehiscence and infection, chronic edema, complex regional pain syndrome, forefoot abduction, bony exostosis, and posttraumatic arthrosis. Anatomic reduction with the use of internal or external fixation is necessary to decrease the morbidity of these injuries. The new surgical approaches for the chronic instability and severe comminution at the Lisfranc joint, and the application of external fixation and multiplane Ilizarov frames in particular, should be used with caution by an experienced surgeon [51,52].

References

[1] Buzzard BM, Briggs PJ. Surgical management of acute tarsometatarsal fracture dislocation in the adult. Clin Orthop Rel Res 1998;353:125–33.

[2] Englanoff G, Anglin D, Hutson HR. Lisfranc fracture-dislocation: a frequently missed diagnosis in the emergency department. Ann Emerg Med 1995;26(2):229–33.

[3] Peicha G, Preidler KW, Lajtai G, et al. Diagnostic value of conventional roentgen image, computerized and magnetic resonance tomography in acute sprains of the foot: a prospective clinical study. Unfallchirurg 2001;104(12):1134–9.

[4] Peicha G, Labovitz J, Seibert FJ, et al. The anatomy of the joint as a risk factor for Lisfranc dislocation and fracture-dislocation. J Bone Joint Surg [Br] 2001;84(7):981–5.

[5] Haapamaki V, Kiuru M, Koskinen S. Lisfranc fracture-dislocation in patients with multiple trauma: diagnosis with multidetector computed tomography. Foot Ankle Int 2004;25(9):614–9.

[6] Mittlmeier T, Beck M. Tarsometatarsal injuries: an often neglected entity. Ther Umsch 2004; 61(7):459–65.

[7] Ross G, Cronin R, Hauzenblas J, et al. Plantar ecchymosis sign: a clinical aid to diagnosis of occult Lisfranc tarsometatarsal injuries. J Orthop Trauma 1996;10(2):119–22.

[8] Davies MS, Saxby TS. Intercuneiform instability and the "gap" sign. Foot Ankle Int 1999; 20(9):606–9.

[9] Curtis MJ, Myerson M, Szura B. Tarsometatarsal joint injuries in the athlete. Am J Sports Med 1993;21(4):497–502.

[10] Kadel N, Boenisch M, Teitz C, et al. Stability of Lisfranc joints in ballet pointe position. Foot Ankle Int 2005;26(5):394–400.

[11] Coss HS, Manos RE, Buoncristiani A, et al. Abduction stress and anterior-posterior weightbearing radiography of purely ligamentous injury in the tarsometatarsal joint. Foot Ankle Int 1998;19(8):537–41.

[12] Stein RE. Radiological aspects of the tarsometatarsal joints. Foot Ankle 1983;3(5):286–9.

[13] Faciszewski T, Burks RT, Manaster BJ. Subtle injuries of the Lisfranc joint. J Bone Joint Surg [Am] 1990;72(10):1519–22.

[14] Myerson MS, Fisher RT, Burgess AR, et al. Fracture dislocations of the tarsometatarsal joints: end results correlated with pathology and treatment. Foot Ankle 1986;6(5):225–42.

[15] Lu J, Ebraheim NA, Skie M, et al. Radiographic and computed tomographic evaluation of Lisfranc dislocation: a cadaver study. Foot Ankle Int 1997;18(6):351–5.

[16] Thordarson DB, Hurvitz G. PLA screw fixation of Lisfranc injuries. Foot Ankle Int 2002;23(11): 1003–7.

[17] Thordarson DB. Lisfranc ORIF with absorbable fixation. Techniques in Foot and Ankle Surgery 2003;2(1):21–6.

[18] Thompson MC, Mormino MA. Injury to the tarsometatarsal joint complex. J Am Acad Orthop Surg 2003;11(4):260–7.

[19] Owens BD, Wixted JJ, Cook J, et al. Intramedullary transmetatarsal Kirschner wire fixation of Lisfranc fracture-dislocations. Am J Orthop 2003;32(8):389–91.

[20] Sands AK, Grose A. Lisfranc injuries. Injury 2004;35:S-B71–6.

[21] Lee CA, Birkedal JP, Dickerson EA, et al. Stabilization of Lisfranc joint injuries: a biomechanical study. Foot Ankle Int 2004;25(5):365–70.

[22] Alberta FG, Aronow MS, Barrero M, et al. Ligamentous Lisfranc joint injuries: a biomechanical comparison of dorsal plate and transarticular screw fixation. Foot Ankle Int 2005;26(6):462–73.

[23] Babst R, Simmen BR, Regazzoni P. Clinical significance and treatment concept of Lisfranc dislocation and dislocation fracture. Helv Chir Acta 1989;56(4):603–7.

[24] Jarde O, Trinquier-Lautard JL, Filloux JF, et al. Lisfranc's fracture-dislocations. Rev Chir Orthop Reparatrice Appar Mot 1995;81(8):724–30.

[25] Mittlmeier T, Krowiorsch R, Brosinger S, et al. Gait function after fracture-dislocation of the midtarsal and/or tarsometatarsal joints. Clin Biomech (Bristol, Avon) 1997;12(3):S16–7.

[26] Mulier T, Reynders P, Sioen W, et al. The treatment of Lisfranc injuries. Acta Orthop Belg 1997;63(2):82–90.

[27] Randt T, Dahlen C, Schikore H, et al. Dislocation fractures in the area of the middle foot: injuries of the Chopart and Lisfranc joint. Zentralbl Chir 1998;123(11):1257–66.

[28] Kuo RS, Tejwani NC, Digiovanni CW, et al. Outcome after open reduction and internal fixation of Lisfranc joint injuries. J Bone Joint Surg [Am] 2000;82(11):1609–18.

[29] Brinsden MD, Smith SR, Loxdale PH. Lisfranc injury: surgical fixation facilities an early return to work. J R Nav Med Serv 2001;87(2):116–9.

[30] Yuen JS, Ying SW, Wong MK. Open reduction and temporary rigid internal fixation of Lisfranc fracture-dislocations. Singapore Med J 2001;42(6):255–8.

[31] Teng AL, Pinzur MS, Lomasney L, et al. Functional outcome following anatomic restoration of tarsal-metatarsal fracture dislocation. Foot Ankle Int 2002;23(1):922–6.

[32] Modrego FJ, Garcia-Alvarez F, Bueno AL, et al. Results of the surgical treatment of Lisfranc fracture-dislocations. Chir Organi Mov 2002;87(3):189–94.

[33] O'Connor PA, Yeap S, Noäl J, et al. Lisfranc injuries: patient and physician-based functional outcomes. Int Orthop 2003;27(2):98–102.

[34] Calder JD, Whitehouse SL, Saxby TS. Results of isolated Lisfranc injuries and the effect of compensation claims. J Bone Joint Surg [Br] 2004;86(4):527–30.

[35] Mulier T, Reynders P, Dereymaeker G, et al. Severe Lisfranc's injuries: primary arthrodesis or ORIF? Foot Ankle Int 2002;23(1):902–5.

[36] Cutler L, Boot DA. Complex fractures: do we operate on enough to gain and maintain experience? Injury 2003;34(12):888–91.

[37] Johnson JE, Johnson KA. Dowel arthrodesis for degenerative arthritis of the tarsometatarsal (Lisfranc) joints. Foot Ankle 1986;6(5):243–53.

[38] Sangeorzan BJ, Veith RG, Hansen ST. Salvage of Lisfranc's tarsometatarsal joint by arthrodesis. Foot Ankle 1990;10(4):193–200.

[39] Zwipp H, Rammelt S, Holch M, et al. Lisfranc arthrodesis after malunited fracture healing. Unfallchirurg 1999;102(12):918–23.

[40] Wachtl S, Elsig JP. Orthopedic technique following arthrodesis of the Lisfranc joint. Schweiz Rundsch Med Prax 1993;82(22):655–60.

[41] Marks R, Parks B, Schon LC. Midfoot fusion technique for neuroarthropathic feet: biomechanical analysis and rationale. Foot Ankle Int 1998;19(8):507–10.

[42] Attinger C, Cooper P, Blume P. Vascular anatomy of the foot and ankle. Operative Techniques in Plastic and Reconstructive Surgery 1997;4:183–98.

[43] Attinger C, Cooper P, Blume P, et al. The safest surgical incisions and amputations applying the angiosome principles and using the Doppler to assess the arterial-arterial connections of the foot and ankle. Foot Ankle Clin 2001;6(4):745–99.

[44] Slater M, Patava J, Kingham K, et al. Involvement of platelets in stimulating osteogenic activity. J Orthop Res 1995;13(5):655–63.

[45] Marx RE, Carlson ER, Eichstaedt RM, et al. Platelet-rich plasma: growth factor enhancement for bone grafts. Oral Surg Oral Med Oral Pathol Oral Radiol Endod 1998;85(6):638–46.

[46] Dugrillon A, Eichler H, Kern S, et al. Autologous concentrated platelet-rich plasma (cPRP) for local application in bone regeneration. Int J Oral Maxillofac Surg 2002;31(6):615–9.

[47] Bibbo C, Bono CM, Lin SS. Union rates using autologous platelet concentrate alone and with bone graft in high-risk foot and ankle surgery patients. J Surg Orthop Adv 2005;14(1):17–22.

[48] DeOrio JK, Farber DC. Morbidity associated with anterior iliac crest bone grafting in foot and ankle surgery. Foot Ankle Int 2005;26(2):147–51.

[49] Geideman W, Early JS, Brodsky J. Clinical results of harvesting autogenous cancellous graft from the ipsilateral proximal tibia for use of foot and ankle surgery. Foot Ankle Int 2004;25(7): 451–5.

[50] Raikin SM, Brislin K. Local bone graft harvest from the distal tibia or calcaneus for surgery of the foot and ankle. Foot Ankle Int 2005;26(6):449–53.

[51] Zgonis T, Burns P, Gehl R. Lisfranc arthrodesis. Clin Podiatr Med Surg 2004;21(1):113–28.

[52] Zgonis T, Jolly GP, Blume P. External fixation use in arthrodesis of the foot and ankle. Clin Podiatr Med Surg 2004;21(1):1–15.

ELSEVIER
SAUNDERS

Clin Podiatr Med Surg
23 (2006) 323–341

CLINICS IN
PODIATRIC
MEDICINE AND
SURGERY

Midfoot Fractures

Theodoros B. Grivas, MD[a],*, Elias D. Vasiliadis, MD[a],
Georgios Koufopoulos, MD[b], Vasilios D. Polyzois, MD, PhD[b],
Demetrios G. Polyzois, MD[c]

[a]Orthopaedic Department, Thriasio General Hospital, Genimata Avenue, 19600, Attica, Greece
[b]KAT Hospital, 2 Nikis str, 14561, Kifisia, Athens, Greece
[c]Metropolitan Hospital, E. Makariou and E. Venizelou 1, 18547, N. Faliro, Attica, Greece

The midfoot consists of five small bones (tarsal scaphoid, cuboid, and three cuneiforms) with multiple articular surfaces that comprise seven or fewer joints.

The tarsal scaphoid is located in the medial aspect of the midfoot anterior to the talus and articulates proximally with the talar head by a concave articular surface and distally with the three cuneiforms by a convex articular surface that has three impressions which correspond to the three cuneiform bones and share a common synovial joint. The blood supply of the tarsal scaphoid is relatively poor. The surface area available for nutrient blood vessels is limited, because it is largely covered with articular cartilage; thus it is more vulnerable to avascular necrosis than are the other bones of the midfoot.

The cuboid is located in the lateral midfoot and is an important stabilizer of the lateral column. It has a small medial articulation with the lateral cuneiform. It articulates proximally with the calcaneus and distally with the base of fourth and fifth metatarsals and occasionally with the tarsal scaphoid. It is involved in almost all motions of the midfoot. The three cuneiforms articulate distally with the base of the first three metatarsals.

The naviculocuneiform, intercuneiform, and cuneocuboid articulations are relatively rigid, with little motion occurring between them. Significant motion is provided by the talonavicular and cuboid-metatarsal articulations.

* Corresponding author. D. Bernardou 31st Street, Brilissia 152 35, Attica, Greece.
E-mail address: grivastb@panafonet.gr (T.B. Grivas).

The Chopart and Lisfranc joint complexes outline the boundaries of the midfoot. The Chopart or midtarsal joint includes the talonavicular and calcaneocuboid articulations. This joint lies in a plane transverse to the medial and lateral longitudinal arches of the foot. The Lisfranc joint consists of the tarsometatarsal joint complex. The cuboid, which articulates to the fourth and fifth metatarsal bases, acts as a linkage across the three naviculocuneiform joints. With the first, second, and third metatarsal bases the three cuneiforms form a rigid and stable articulation at the junction of the mid- and forefoot. The middle cuneiform is smaller than the medial and lateral ones, creating a recession that locks the second metatarsal base into a stable position. Transverse intermetatarsal, dorsal, and plantar ligaments traversing the tarsometatarsal joint contribute to stability. The tibialis anterior, peroneus longus, the intrinsic muscles, and the plantar fascia serve as accessory stabilizers.

The unique three-dimensional anatomy of the midfoot creates the longitudinal and transverse arches. Alignment of the cuboid and the three cuneiforms creates the transverse arch of the foot. The tarsal scaphoid is the keystone for the medial longitudinal arch, and the cuboid is the central bone of the lateral longitudinal arch of the foot. Plantar and interosseous ligaments, capsular structures, and fascia directly support the bony morphology of the arches. The plantar intertarsal and capsular structures, located on the tension side of the arch, are significantly stronger than their dorsal counterparts [1]. The medial and central bands of the plantar fascia span the longitudinal arch, providing additional indirect support, whereas the lateral band stabilizes the calcaneocuboid and cubometatarsal regions [2]. The lateral side of the midfoot is more stable than the medial side, which is more dynamic and mobile.

The transverse tarsal joint complex is supported by the bifurcate ligament, which lies between the distal lateral aspect of the calcaneus to both the tarsal scaphoid and cuboid, and the stout spring ligament that supports the medial longitudinal arch and the talonavicular joint. The short and long plantar cubometatarsal ligaments support the cubometatarsal joint complex. Adjunct dynamic support is provided by tendons of the anterior tibialis, posterior tibialis, and peroneus longus muscles.

Midfoot biomechanics

The midfoot cannot be isolated from overall foot biomechanics. Mid- and forefoot function are theoretically related to a three-column basis of function [3]. The first metatarsal and the medial cuneiform comprise the medial column. The second and third metatarsals and corresponding cuneiforms make up the middle column. The lateral column is comprised of the cuboid and fourth and fifth metatarsals. The central column is rigid; lateral and medial columns have variable flexibility [3]. The lateral column serves as the shock absorber for the foot, because this portion of the Lisfranc region demonstrates considerable sagittal motion [4]. Therefore, the lateral Lisfranc joint complex is an essential midfoot structure whose functional integrity should be preserved if possible [5].

The Chopart joint is mobile when the heel is pronated and is relatively fixed when the heel is supinated. Such alternating flexibility and rigidity are essential for normal bipedal gait. The talonavicular joint is a ball-and-socket joint that contributes to three-dimensional motion. Its function is critical to normal foot biomechanics; therefore, talonavicular joint function should also be preserved if possible [1].

For efficient ambulation all components of the midfoot must function properly. Alterations in gait caused by the impairment of one function put excessive stress on the entire foot structure to compensate for this deficiency, and with time this excessive stress may lead to deterioration of the uninjured parts.

Injury patterns of the midfoot

The configuration of multiple constrained joints in the midfoot minimizes susceptibility to injury, as reflected in the small number of injuries reported to occur in this region. When injury does occur, more than one structure is frequently involved, and many fracture–dislocation patterns have been reported in the literature [6]. Although isolated fractures, dislocations, and sprains can occur, the clinician must search carefully for associated injuries in the region whenever an apparently isolated injury is identified.

For simplicity, traumatic midfoot injuries are categorized here as injuries to the Chopart joint, tarsal scaphoid fractures, cuboid fractures, cuneiform fractures, and injuries to the Lisfranc joint.

Chopart joint injuries

Injuries of the Chopart joint are relatively uncommon and are often under-diagnosed even after a thorough radiographic evaluation. Commonly they occur in conjunction with associated fractures of the foot. The entire foot must be carefully examined to estimate the full extent of the injury. Neurovascular assessment of the foot should be performed, and a possible compartment syndrome should be detected.

Main and Jowett [7] in a review of 71 midtarsal joint injuries, identified five patterns of injury based on the direction of the applied force, the presumed mechanism of injury, the extent of injury, and the consequent direction of displacement of the forefoot (medial, longitudinal, lateral, plantar, and crush) (Table 1). Although this classification is not universally accepted, it can be useful, because it classifies injuries on a continuum of displacement from sprain to complete dislocation.

Table 1
The five injury patterns of the midtarsal joint*

Stress Injury Patterns	Subtypes	Mechanism of Injury
Medial	Fracture sprains	Foot inversion
	Fracture subluxations	Forefoot adduction
	and dislocations	Medial rotation of the foot
	Swivel dislocations	without inversion or eversion
Longitudinal	Vertical fractures	Force transmitted proximally
	Fracture sprains	along the rays with the foot in
		varying degrees of plantarflexion
		Foot eversion
Lateral	Fracture subluxations	Forefoot abduction
	and dislocations	Lateral rotation of the foot
	Swivel dislocations	
Plantar	Fracture sprains	Plantarly directed forces with
	Fracture subluxations	foot inversion or eversion
	and dislocations	Plantarly directed forces with
		foot abduction or adduction
Crush	Inconstant fracture	Crushing
	patterns	

* Based on the direction of the applied force, the presumed mechanism of injury, the extent of injury, and the consequent direction of displacement of the forefoot.
Data from: Main BJ, Jowett RL. Injuries of the midtarsal joint. J Bone Joint Surg [Br] 1975;57:89–97.

Medial stress injury

Medial stress injuries had a prevalence of 30% in the series of Main and Jowett [7]. Medial stress injuries are divided into three subgroups: fracture sprains, fracture subluxations, and dislocations and swivel dislocations.

Most injuries are fracture sprains of the midtarsal joint caused by inversion of the foot, with no dislocation. Radiographs show avulsion fractures of the dorsal margins of the talus or tarsal scaphoid and of the lateral margins of the calcaneus or cuboid. In addition, fracture subluxation or fracture dislocation of the joint may be found.

In fracture subluxations and dislocations, the forefoot is displaced medially as a result of injuries to both the talonavicular joint and the calcaneocuboid joint. The hindfoot remains in normal alignment with the tibia.

In swivel dislocations, a medial force applied to the forefoot disrupts the talonavicular joint but leaves the calcaneocuboid joint and the subtalar joint intact. The foot rotates medially but does not invert or evert.

Longitudinal stress injury

Longitudinal injuries were the most common (41%) injuries in the series of Main and Jowett [7]. These injuries occur with the foot in varying degrees of plantarflexion, with the force being applied to the metatarsal heads and transmitted proximally along the rays to disrupt the midtarsal joint and fracture the cuboid or the tarsal scaphoid. With this mechanism, fractures tend to occur vertically through the tarsal scaphoid in line with the intercuneiform joints. Injuries of this type are usually severe, with a high incidence of associated fracture and significant residual displacement of the fracture fragments.

Lateral stress injury

Lateral stress injuries occur less frequently (17%). The characteristic feature of these injuries is crushing of the cuboid or anterior calcaneus as the forefoot is driven laterally. Avulsion fractures of the tarsal scaphoid tuberosity are seen frequently, and the tarsal scaphoid may subluxate laterally on the talar head. This injury is frequently misdiagnosed as an ankle sprain.

Lateral stress injuries are subdivided into the same three subgroups as medial stress injuries: fracture sprains, fracture subluxations and dislocations, and swivel dislocations. When an eversion force is applied to the foot, a fracture sprain pattern occurs, which causes a small avulsion fracture of the tarsal scaphoid tuberosity or creates a flake of bone from the dorsum of the tarsal scaphoid or medial talus. An impaction fracture of the cuboid or calcaneus may be present.

An abduction force applied to the forefoot produces lateral subluxation of the talonavicular joint, avulsion fracture of the tarsal scaphoid tuberosity, and collapse of the lateral column of the foot, with possible comminution of the calcaneocuboid joint.

In swivel dislocations there is a lateral dislocation of the talonavicular joint, but the calcaneocuboid and talocalcaneal joints remain intact.

Dewar and Evans [8] suggested that the mechanism is crushing of the cuboid between the calcaneus and the bases of the fourth and fifth metatarsals by a forced abduction of the forefoot. Subluxation of the midtarsal joint was frequent, and four of the five patients sustained avulsion fractures of the tarsal scaphoid tuberosity. Hermel and Gershon-Cohen [9] presented five similar cases of cuboid fracture and appropriately applied the term "nutcracker fracture" to this injury. Similarly, in separate reports, Howie and colleagues [10] and Tountas [11] proposed a mechanism of abduction and dorsiflexion at the midtarsal joint. All were characterized by avulsion fracture of the tarsal scaphoid tuberosity and damage to the calcaneocuboid joint, with fracture of one of these two bones.

Plantar stress injury

Plantarly directed forces are applied to the forefoot on rare occasions (7%). They area divided into two subgroups: fracture sprains and fracture subluxations and dislocations.

Fracture sprains are responsible for disruption of the midtarsal joint with avulsion fractures at the dorsum of the tarsal scaphoid or talus and from the anterior process of the calcaneus.

Crush injury

Crushing is the final mechanism of injury described by Main and Jowett [7]. Open wounds are frequent with this type of injury, and inconstant fracture patterns, which are difficult to classify, occur.

Injuries to the midtarsal joint are frequently misdiagnosed as ankle sprains. An isolated avulsion fracture of one of the bones (particularly the tarsal scaphoid tuberosity) is clearly visible on routine radiographic assessment; often, careful attention is not given to the entire joint complex. These errors lead to incomplete diagnoses, inadequate treatment, and persistent problems.

The main principles for treatment of midfoot fractures include maintaining medial and lateral column length, maintaining the appropriate anatomic relationship between the hindfoot and the forefoot, preserving motion of the talonavicular and the cuboid-metatarsal articulation, and ensuring a plantigrade foot. Usually open reduction and internal fixation (ORIF) is required to maintain the anatomic reduction, and a proper period of time is required for bone or soft tissue healing.

Initial treatment should be initiated only after accurate diagnosis is made. A high index of suspicion is required, especially if the patient is suffering from other major injuries or is unconscious. Treatment should aim at prompt restoration of the anatomy of the midtarsal joint by reduction of dislocations or subluxations and anatomic restoration of the bony architecture whenever possible.

Restoration of the medial and lateral column length might be extremely difficult when a comminution exists. A shortened medial column results in cavus deformity, whereas a shortened lateral column results in planus deformity. In a severely traumatized foot an external ring fixator provides a safe indirect reduction without interfering with the soft tissues. It can be applied to distract the medial column through the talus and first metatarsal or to distract the lateral column through the calcaneus and fourth or fifth metatarsals. Eastaugh-Waring and Saleh [12] describe an effective method of supplementing Kirschner wire fixation with a circular external fixation frame in severely comminuted fracture dislocation of the midtarsal region.

The role of primary arthrodesis is controversial. Early local or triple arthrodesis can relieve pain caused by late degenerative changes but may significantly alter normal foot function. Arthrodesis of the cuboid-metatarsal articulation is not well tolerated by the patient, whereas fusion of the talonavicular joint compromises the function of the foot. Primary arthrodesis of calcaneocuboid, naviculocuneiform, intercuneiform, and cuneiform-metatarsal articulations can be performed if necessary, with minimal loss of function [13]. In most cases adequate initial reduction and fixation may lead to an acceptable result preserving the function of the midtarsal joint. Arthrodesis can be reserved for the treatment of patients who have residual disability [14] or in cases where comminution is so extensive and the cancellous bone so severely crushed that reduction cannot be achieved. A corticocancellous iliac bone graft should be undertaken early to restore the longitudinal arch of the foot. Primary midtarsal arthrodesis is also recommended for acute fractures or dislocations in feet that have inadequate circulation (eg, in diabetics) to prevent later collapse [15].

The fracture sprain subgroups of Main and Jowett's [7] classification are stable injuries but have the potential for late displacement with unprotected weight bearing. They should be treated by use of a short-leg walking cast for 4 weeks followed by use of a hard-soled shoe with a longitudinal arch support until the patient is free of pain in the foot.

In fracture subluxations and dislocations and swivel dislocations, a closed or open reduction under anesthesia is required as well as adjacent stabilization with Kirschner wires. A short-leg non–weight-bearing cast is worn for 6 weeks, after which protected partial weight bearing begins in a walking cast. Kirschner wires should be removed at 6 weeks. After this initial period, the patient is allowed to ambulate in a good shoe with a longitudinal arch support for an additional 9 to 12 months.

In longitudinal stress injuries nondisplaced fractures are treated in a short-leg walking cast for 6 weeks or until healing occurs. Displaced fractures are treated with ORIF, followed by use of a short-leg non–weight-bearing cast for 6 to 8 weeks. In Main and Jowett's [7] series of 24 displaced fractures, 18 patients had fair or poor results at long-term follow-up.

In lateral stress injuries any subluxation or dislocation should be reduced and held with Kirschner wires. ORIF with bone grafting of the cuboid may be necessary to restore the lateral column. Application of an external fixation to restore the length of the lateral column is another treatment option. If the avulsed tarsal scaphoid tuberosity is significantly displaced, it should be reattached to the tarsal scaphoid to prevent late planovalgus deformity of the foot as a result of tibialis posterior dysfunction [16]. Postoperatively, the foot should be immobilized as in medial stress injury.

Plantar stress injuries are managed similarly to fracture sprains and fracture dislocations the other injury patterns.

In crush injuries, closed reduction can be attempted, and the fragments can then be stabilized with Kirschner wires. For particularly severe crush injuries, external fixation may also be used to maintain the length of the medial and lateral columns.

A short-leg non–weight-bearing cast is applied postoperatively. Kirschner wires should be removed at 6 weeks. A non–weight-bearing cast or cast-boot should then be applied for an additional 4 to 6 weeks. The patient should then be instructed to wear a good shoe with a longitudinal arch support for 9 to 12 months.

Tarsal scaphoid fractures

Tarsal scaphoid fractures are subdivided into four types [17]: avulsion fractures of the dorsal lip, fractures of the tuberosity, displaced and nondisplaced fractures of the body, and stress fractures (Table 2).

Table 2
Classification of tarsal scaphoid fractures

Types	Mechanism of Injury
Avulsion fractures of the dorsal lip	Talonavicular ligament stress in inversion and plantarflexion Deltoid ligament stress in eversion
Fractures of the tuberosity	Posterior tibial tendon stress after a forced eversion of the foot
Displaced and nondisplaced fractures of the body	Direct or indirect forces applied to the tarsal scaphoid
Stress fractures	Repetitive forceful loading of the midfoot

Avulsion fractures of the dorsal lip

Capsular avulsion fractures from the dorsal talonavicular ligament and the anterior division of the deltoid ligament are common (47% of tarsal scaphoid fractures) [18]. The talonavicular ligament is stressed in inversion and plantarflexion, whereas the deltoid ligament is stressed in eversion of the foot and excessive tension; either may avulse a variably sized fragment of bone. Two accessory ossicles, the os supranaviculare and the os supratalare, can occur in this region. Patients present with pain, swelling, and pinpoint tenderness over the fracture site.

An associated midtarsal injury should be excluded first. Treatment is immobilization with a short-leg walking cast for 4 to 6 weeks or until symptoms resolve. Excision should be considered for small, displaced symptomatic fragments especially those that affect shoe wear. If the articular fragment is larger than one quarter of the articular surface, ORIF with a Kirschner wire is recommended to restore the articular surface of the talonavicular joint [13].

Fractures of the tuberosity

Approximately one fourth of tarsal scaphoid fractures are fractures of the tarsal scaphoid tuberosity. The tarsal scaphoid tuberosity is avulsed by the anterior slipping of the posterior tibial tendon after a forced eversion of the foot. The anterior fibers of the deltoid ligament may contribute to injury [18].

A thorough evaluation of the midtarsal joint is necessary. Often such an avulsion fracture is seen in conjunction with compression fractures of the cuboid or anterior calcaneus [7], and it is important to determine whether the Chopart joint is subluxated. During radiographic control an accessory tarsal scaphoid (os tibiale externum) should be distinguished from a fracture. Accessory tarsal scaphoids, found in up to 12% of the population, are smooth and often are bilateral (64%). Occasionally bone scanning and MRI may be helpful.

Nondisplaced or minimally displaced tuberosity fractures are considered stable and can be managed by a short-leg walking cast, well molded under the longitudinal arch with the foot in a neutral position, for 4 to 6 weeks. Displaced fractures are less common, are considered unstable, and require prompt open reduction to prevent displacement and to avoid dysfunction of the posterior tibial tendon.

Should an asymptomatic non-union occur, no additional treatment is required. If the non-union causes discomfort, the tuberosity can be excised, and the tendon can be reattached to the fracture bed under the same tension that existed before excision of the tarsal scaphoid tubercle. The lower leg is then placed in a short-leg cast for 4 to 6 weeks.

Non-union is the most frequent complication. Asymptomatic non-unions should be left untreated. If a non-union is painful, excision of the fragment is recommended through a dorsal incision just above the tuberosity of the tarsal scaphoid. The posterior tibial tendon is reattached to the remaining freshen to bleeding bone by strong sutures or by bone anchors [15], followed by use of a short -leg cast for 4 to 6 weeks.

Displaced and nondisplaced fractures of the body

Fractures of the tarsal scaphoid body are the most infrequent tarsal scaphoid fractures and are commonly associated with other midtarsal injuries. Indirect forces applied to the tarsal scaphoid as the result of a fall from a height or a motor vehicle accident produce a high-energy displaced fracture of the body. Isolated fractures of the tarsal scaphoid body are usually secondary to direct forces that produce a comminuted but usually not displaced fracture [17].

Any tenderness on the medial side of the midfoot or pain produced during passive motion of the foot should be radiographically assessed. Anteroposterior, oblique, and lateral radiographs should be obtained, because the fracture line might be obvious on only one of the views. A preoperative CT scan to determine fracture planes and the degree of comminution is also recommended [19]. A high index of suspicion is required for early detection of associated injuries of the entire midtarsal joint. The possibility of compartment syndrome should be considered, especially for high-energy fractures. Sangeorzan and colleagues [19] classified tarsal scaphoid body fractures into three types based on fracture orientation, pattern of adjacent joint disruption, and direction of forefoot displacement (Table 3). In type I, the fracture is in the coronal plane producing dorsal and plantar fracture fragments, with no angulation of the forefoot. In type II, the major fracture line is dorsolateral to plantarmedial, and the forefoot is displaced medially. In type III, the fracture is comminuted, the medial border of the foot is disrupted at the cuneonavicular joint, and the forefoot is displaced laterally. This useful classification scheme provides guidance in fracture management and prognosis. Prognosis is good for type I, intermediate for type II, and poor for type III fractures.

Nondisplaced fractures of the tarsal scaphoid body, comminuted or not, are treated with a short-leg walking cast worn for 6 weeks or until there is a radiographic evidence of union, followed by use of a longitudinal arch support orthosis.

Table 3
Classification of tarsal scaphoid body fractures based on fracture orientation, pattern of adjacent joint disruption, and direction of forefoot displacement

Type	Mechanism of Injury
Type I	Fracture line in the coronal plane producing dorsal and plantar fracture fragments, with no angulation of the forefoot
Type II	Major fracture line is dorsolateral to plantarmedial with medial displacement of the forefoot
Type III	Comminuted fracture with disruption of the medial border of the foot at the cuneonavicular joint and lateral displacement of the forefoot

Adapted from: Sangeorzan BJ, Benirschke SK, Mosca V, et al. Displaced intra-articular fractures of the tarsal navicular. J Bone Joint Surg [Am] 1989;71:1504–10.

For displaced type I, fractures Sangeorzan and colleagues [5,19] recommend ORIF with lag-screw fixation through an anteromedial approach in the interval between the anterior and posterior tibial tendons beginning just distal to the medial malleolus. The periosteum over the tarsal scaphoid is not divided, so the remaining blood supply to the bone is preserved. The articular surfaces of the talonavicular and calcaneonavicular joints should be inspected and reduced with a combination of direct and indirect reduction techniques. Bone graft taken from the iliac crest or distal tibia can be used as necessary to fill in any central defects once the articular surfaces have been elevated.

In type II fractures, a comminution makes the plantar lateral fragment difficult to reduce. The large medial fragment of the tarsal scaphoid must be reduced through an anteromedial incision [5] so that the talonavicular joint can be inspected. Treatment options are screw fixation of the tarsal scaphoid fragments to other tarsal bones, especially to adjacent cuneiforms, or the use of a mini-external fixator. It is important to preserve talonavicular joint alignment.

Restoration of normal anatomy is a challenge for type III fractures. Bone grafting and use of multiple Kirschner wires for transfixion of the naviculo-cuneiform and talonavicular joints are required. A further incorporation of the Kirschner wires on a ring external fixator for maintenance of the overall alignment of the midfoot is a good solution. The transfixion wires should be removed at 6 to 8 weeks, and a custom-made shoe with medial arch support should be fitted. Alternatively, primary arthrodesis of the talonavicular or naviculocuneiform joints should be considered if there is an extensive damage to the articular surface.

Avascular necrosis, degenerative arthritis, and malunion are the most common complications of fractures of the tarsal scaphoid body. Avascular necrosis occurs in 25% of these fractures [19]. Excessive soft tissue detachments should be avoided to avoid devascularization of the tarsal scaphoid, which is poorly supplied with blood. If the tarsal scaphoid collapses because of avascular necrosis, or if degenerative arthrosis occurs, the length and orientation of the medial column should be restored by use of a tricortical bone and arthrodesis.

Stress fractures

Stress fractures of the tarsal scaphoid have been reported in athletes. An increased index of suspicion among orthopedic surgeons and greater participation in sports have resulted in more frequent diagnosis of this injury in recent years. A long second metatarsal or, on the contrary, a short first metatarsal seems to be a risk factor for developing a stress fracture [20,21]. Poorly localized tenderness at the midnavicular region and pain at the longitudinal arch worsened by activity and relieved by rest are the most common symptoms, especially in persons who engage in sports that result in repetitive forceful loading of the midfoot, such as basketball players, sprinters, and high jumpers.

The fracture line is usually sagitally oriented in the middle third of the bone and is not visible on plain radiographs. A bone scan should be performed when there is clinical suspicion; if the bone scan is positive, a CT scan should be performed to confirm the diagnosis. The possible role of MRI has recently been described [22].

Diagnosis is usually delayed, with a mean interval of 7 months between the onset of symptoms and diagnosis [20]. Stress fractures of the tarsal scaphoid must be differentiated from other overuse syndromes.

Early diagnosed tarsal scaphoid stress fractures are treated conservatively by use of a non–weight-bearing cast for 6 to 8 weeks. Absence of local tenderness is a clinical sign of union. Delay in diagnosis or persistent weight bearing seems to lead to non-union, delayed union, or fracture recurrence [20]. Delayed union or non-union of stress fractures may require débridement; bone grafting, and internal fixation followed by additional cast immobilization. Fitch and colleagues [21] recommend autologous bone grafting for all complete and comminuted fractures, for incomplete fractures that do not heal in in 8 to 10 weeks with the use of a non–weight-bearing cast, and for all non-unions characterized by marginal sclerosis or the presence of a medullary cyst.

Athletes should be instructed to return to full activity gradually. A CT documentation of union [23], although not routinely recommended [24], is a valuable tool as an adjunct to clinical evaluation of healing in highly competitive athletes.

Cuboid fractures

Cuboid fractures are uncommon. They occur only in 5% of all tarsal fractures. Cuboid fractures are further categorized as avulsion, body fracture dislocations [2], and stress fractures (Table 4) [25]. Sixty-six percent of cuboid fractures are chip or avulsion types from the plantar calcaneocuboid ligament. A direct force applied to the cuboid may result in a fracture of the body. Indirect forces, which most commonly are applied to the cuboid through strong ligaments and capsular attachments, may result after the cuboid is compressed between the calcaneus and the fourth and fifth metatarsals as a consequence of violent forefoot abduction. This compression fracture, which leads to lateral column shortening,

Table 4
Classification of cuboid fractures

Types	Mechanism of Injury
Avulsion	Plantar calcaneocuboid ligament stress
Body	Direct force
	Violent forefoot abduction results in compression of the cuboid between the calcaneus and the fourth and fifth metatarsals (nutcracker fracture)
Fracture dislocations	Indirect force
Stress fractures	Repetitive forceful loading of the midfoot

has been referred to as a "nutcracker fracture" [9] and is often associated with an avulsion fracture of the tarsal scaphoid tuberosity or a tear of the posterior tibial tendon [5].

Although the bony support of adjacent tarsal bones prevents displacement, there are rare reports of cuboid subluxation [26,27] and total dislocation [28,29].

A positive history of direct or indirect trauma to the foot accompanied by local tenderness, significant swelling of the midfoot, and a high index of suspicion should lead to the diagnosis. Associated injuries to the midfoot region should be recognized, because cuboid fractures are commonly part of a more complex injury of the midtarsal joint. Radiographic evaluation of the entire foot, especially a 30° medial oblique projection, is required to determine the fracture line and the anatomic relations between all the tarsal bones. A high index of suspicion for complex injuries is essential. CT scanning might be helpful if surgery is planned, and a bone scan using technetium-99m should be performed when the possibility of a stress fracture is considered. Cuboid fractures, if left untreated, may lead to severe disruption of foot biomechanics and degenerative arthritis.

Isolated nondisplaced fractures of the cuboid should be treated by use of a short-leg walking cast for 4 to 6 weeks, followed by a longitudinal arch support [17].

For displaced fractures that heal with residual articular incongruity, ORIF with a structural iliac-crest bone graft is recommended through a longitudinal incision over the cuboid, superior to the peroneal tendons and sural nerve [30]. The muscle belly of the extensor digitorum brevis is retracted superiorly, sparing the stabilizing ligaments of the calcaneocuboid joint and the two lateral tarsometatarsal ligaments. A small distractor can be placed in the calcaneus and in one of the lateral metatarsals to aid in indirect reduction of the articular surfaces. The cuboid is then held out to length using a buttress technique, with a small plate strutting the defect, which is packed with cancellous or cortical cancellous bone graft [5,1]. Longitudinal fractures can be fixed with a lag screw. Postoperatively, the foot is immobilized in a below-knee non–weight-bearing cast for 6 weeks.

A key to successful treatment is the maintenance of lateral column length and preservation of mobility at the fourth and fifth tarsometatarsal joints. Distraction can be provided using a lateral-based half-pin external fixator [12] or by transarticular fixation for stabilization of associate subluxations and attachment of the Kirschner wires to the rings of the circular external fixator that acts as a neutralization device.

Total dislocations have been successfully treated with closed reduction and percutaneous pinning [28].

Stress fractures of the cuboid heal well with 4 to 6 weeks of protected weight bearing and activity restriction [25].

Severe comminution and residual displacement may require arthrodesis of the involved joints to restore alignment of the foot and minimize late complications [8]. With healing of the cuboid fracture, scarring and irregularity of the peroneal groove can lead to impaired function of the peroneus longus tendon [32].

Fracture of the os peroneum

The os peroneum is present in 5% to 14% of the population and lies within the substance of the peroneus longus tendon plantar to the cuboid. Supination and plantarflexion forces on the foot can cause fracture of the os perineum [31]. Cast immobilization is sufficient, but often a painful fibrous union persists that requires late excision of the painful bone fragments [31].

Cuneiform fractures

Cuneiform fractures are approximately 4.2% of all tarsal bone fractures and can be further categorized as small, minimally displaced chip-type fractures caused by partial avulsion of the tibialis anterior tendon and as crush-type fractures caused by a direct blow (Table 5) [33].

Isolated fractures of the cuneiforms are uncommon and are considered high-energy injuries [34]. The medial cuneiform seems to be the most commonly injured [5]. Dislocations are extremely rare because of the stability of the strong ligaments, which are augmented by the tendons of anterior tibialis, posterior tibialis, and peroneus longus. Occasionally dislocations or subluxations occur in association with injuries of the Lisfranc or Chopart joint [35].

The entire foot should be clinically evaluated, and soft tissue trauma and neurovascular status should be determined. A gap sign (an abnormal space be-

Table 5
Classification of cuneiform fractures

Types	Mechanism of Injury
Chip type fractures	Partial avulsion of the tibialis anterior tendon
Crush type fractures from direct blow	Direct blow
Dislocations or subluxations	In association to Lisfranc or Chopart joint injuries

tween the first and second toe with weight bearing) may represent occult inter-cuneiform instability [36]. Standard anteroposterior, lateral, and oblique radiographs and a CT scan should be obtained.

Stable, nondisplaced chip-type fractures are treated with walking-cast immobilization until the patient is asymptomatic followed by use of a shoe with longitudinal arch support [37].

Nondisplaced crush fractures resulting from indirect mechanisms are treated with a short-leg, non–weight-bearing cast with frequent, intermittent radiographic evaluation to make sure that the foot alignment remains anatomic under weight-bearing stresses [37].

High-energy crush injuries require anatomic reduction that occasionally can be performed closed. A combined medial-dorsal approach has been described [30]. The medial approach is directly medial, overlying the anterior tibial tendon along the medial side of the foot and dorsal to the posterior tibial tendon. A second incision on the dorsal side of the foot, medial to the neurovascular bundle, is used to help visualize the reduction. After reduction, cuneiform fractures can be stabilized with screws or Kirschner wires. Dislocations should be reduced and held with at least two orthogonally placed Kirschner wires [5]. In fractures or dislocations of the intermediate cuneiform, its position should be restored, because it serves as a cornerstone of the transverse arch of the midfoot [5].

The leg should be protected in a non–weight-bearing short-leg cast for 6 weeks postoperatively if there is not an associated ligamentous injury and for 10 weeks if an indirect injury is involved. Kirschner wires must be removed at 6 weeks postoperatively [5].

Lisfranc injuries

Injuries to the Lisfranc joint compromise approximately 0.2% of all skeletal injuries. Twenty percent of Lisfranc fractures may be missed [38], because these injuries may be misdiagnosed or unrecognized.

Two main mechanisms of trauma, direct and indirect, have been described [39], although the exact mechanism of injury is often difficult to identify. Indirect force, the most common mechanism of injury, may result from a forceful abduction and twisting of the forefoot on the tarsus or an axial loading on a plantarflexed foot. Indirect stress to the Lisfranc ligament may cause a purely ligamentous injury when applied to a plantarflexed foot. A direct blow or a high-energy crush may also cause this injury.

A radiographic classification according to the presentation of the incongruity shown on radiographs [39] and based on Quenu and Kuss's system [40] is currently used. In this classification, type A injuries are injuries with total incongruity (lateral and dorsal or plantar subtypes), type B injuries are injuries with partial incongruity (medial or lateral subtypes), and type C injuries are the divergent types (partial or total displacement subtypes) caused by a lack of direct structural support between the first and second metatarsal bases (Table 6).

Table 6
Hardcastle et al Classification of Lisfranc joint injuries according to the presentation of incongruity shown on radiographs

Classification	Presentation
Type A	Total incongruity (lateral and dorsoplantar subtypes)
Type B	Partial incongruity (medial or lateral subtypes)
Type C	Divergent types (partial or total displacement subtypes)

Adapted from: Hardcastle PH, Reschauer R, Kutscha-Lissberg E, et al. Injuries to the tarsometatarsal joint. Incidence, classification and treatment. J Bone Joint Surg [Br] 1982;64:349–56.

Any injury to the midfoot should be evaluated with suspicion, especially if there is excessive swelling in the area. Adjacent serious soft tissue injuries often occur.

A thorough radiographic evaluation must include anteroposterior, lateral, and 30° oblique views. Congruity between the medial base of the second metatarsal and the middle cuneiform is the most reliable radiographic relationship. A widening between the base of the first and second metatarsals should also be viewed with suspicion. If an injury to the Lisfranc joint is suspected, an abduction stress view can provide definite diagnosis [41]. Even with these radiographs, however, these fractures can still be overlooked. In a recent study the initial radiographic diagnosis was missed in 39% of patients who had a Lisfranc injury [42]. CT scanning provides more detailed information because of the variety of views and reconstructions available [43], whereas MRI may demonstrate ligamentous disruption, especially of the Lisfranc ligament.

Stable, nondisplaced injuries may be treated with immobilization using a non–weight-bearing cast for a minimum of 6 weeks.

For unstable or displaced injuries, early diagnosis and appropriate treatment are necessary to obtain good functional results [44]. Criteria for satisfactory reduction are (1) a gap of no less than 3 mm between the first and second metatarsals, and (2) no evidence of lateral translation of the lesser metatarsals [33]. A controversy exists concerning the method of fixation after anatomic reduction [45]. Optimal results cannot be achieved with closed reduction and a plaster cast because the initial reduction often is lost when soft tissue swelling diminishes [46]. Closed reduction with percutaneous pin fixation under fluoroscopy has been used successfully, with pin removal in 6 to 8 weeks [33].

Although closed fixation is less traumatic for swollen, traumatized soft tissue than ORIF, it is often unlikely to be successful where there is soft tissue interposition, severe comminution, or diastasis between the medial and intermediate cuneiform bones, suggesting interposition of the tibialis anterior tendon [39]. Migration of Kirschner wires and infection of pin tracts are also common causes of unstable or unsuccessful reduction.

Currently, ORIF seems to be the most reliable method to secure and maintain an anatomic reduction [5,41,47]. Preservation of anatomic medial column alignment and fourth and fifth tarsometatarsal joint mobility and accurate assessment of ligamentous damage are associated with good outcomes. Trans-articular bony stabilization indirectly provokes ligamentous healing. Advantages of ORIF include visual assessment of articular damage, débridement, and lavage of intra-articular loose bodies and accurate interpretation of intraoperative stress tests.

Buzzard and Briggs [48] reported that surgery normally is performed through two longitudinal incisions, one in the first and second metatarsal interspace and the other in the third and fourth metatarsal interspace. All fractures and dislocations are reduced before fixation. Fixation of the first, second, and third metatarsals is with lagged transarticular cortical screws between the bases of the metatarsals and the cuneiforms. The Lisfranc joint is stabilized with a screw placed between the medial cuneiform and the base of the second metatarsal. The fourth and fifth metatarsals may be stabilized adequately with Kirschner wires. Injuries to the other tarsal bones or the metatarsal shafts also require treatment to restore and maintain metatarsal and foot length. Buzzard and Briggs [48] also reported that wound complications can be minimized with appropriate soft tissue care. Early fixation of open injuries, within the first 6 hours, aids stabilization of the soft tissues. In closed injuries, early surgery is preferred, but significant foot swelling makes ORIF more difficult and increases the risk of wound complications. A delay of 1 to 2 weeks before open surgery, allowing resolution of foot swelling, may be appropriate in many cases and does not seem to compromise the long-term result.

Primary tarsometatarsal arthrodesis is an excellent salvage procedure and should be reserved for significant traumatic chondral injury, comminuted fractures, or a failed primary treatment [49,50]. A non–weight-bearing cast is applied for 6 to 12 weeks postoperatively, depending on the complexity of the foot injury. A well-padded arch support is worn for approximately 3 months or until the patient is asymptomatic. Internal fixation should not be removed before 4 months.

Lisfranc injuries are commonly associated with many complications. Skin necrosis, infection, redislocation, compartment syndrome, iatrogenic nerve injury, vascular compromise, ligamentous instability, and iatrogenic or injury-related tendon or chondral lesions are early complications [51]. The most common late complications are degenerative arthritis, non-union, bony exostosis, abnormal gait patterns, and chronic pain caused by reflex sympathetic dystrophy [39,52].

Summary

Fractures of the midfoot are uncommon because of the constrained configuration of multiple articular surfaces, which is augmented by capsular attachments and strong ligaments and tendons. Injury patterns usually involve more than one structure, although isolated fractures, dislocations, and sprains can occur. The key to optimal treatment of midfoot fractures is a high index of clinical suspicion because of their rareness. The traumatic midfoot injuries described in this article are categorized as Chopart joint injuries, tarsal scaphoid fractures, cuboid fractures, cuneiform fractures, and Lisfranc joint injuries.

References

[1] Solan MC, Moorman III CT, Miyamato RG, et al. Ligamentous restraints of the second tarsometatarsal joint: a biomechanical evaluation. Foot Ankle Int 2001;22:637–41.

[2] Steven LJ. Midfoot trauma, bony and ligamentous: evaluation and treatment. Curr Opin Orthop 2002;13(2):99–106.

[3] Myerson MS. The diagnosis and treatment of injuries to the Lisfranc joint complex. Orthop Clin North Am 1989;20:655–64.

[4] Ouzounian TJ, Shereff MJ. In vitro determination of midfoot motion. Foot Ankle 1989;10: 140–6.

[5] Pinney SJ, Sangeorzan BJ. Fractures of the tarsal bones. In: Sangeorzan BJ, editor. The traumatized foot. American Academy of Orthopedic Surgeons monograph series. Rosemont, Illinois: American Academy of Orthopedic Surgeons; 2001. p. 41–53.

[6] Heckman JD. Fractures and dislocations of the foot. Injuries of the midtarsal region. In: Rockwood Jr CA, Green DP, editors. 2nd edition. Fractures in adults, vol. 2. Philadelphia: JB Lippincott; 1984. p. 1786–95.

[7] Main BJ, Jowett RL. Injuries of the midtarsal joint. J Bone Joint Surg [Br] 1975;57:89–97.

[8] Dewar FP, Evans DC. Occult fracture-subluxation of the midtarsal joint. J Bone Joint Surg [Br] 1968;50:386–8.

[9] Hermel MB, Gershon-Cohen J. The nutcracker fracture of the cuboid by indirect violence. Radiology 1953;60:850–4.

[10] Howie CR, Hooper G, Hughes SPF. Occult midtarsal subluxation. Clin Orthop 1986;209:206–9.

[11] Tountas AA. Occult fracture-subluxation of the midtarsal joint. Clin Orthop 1989;243:195–9.

[12] Eastaugh-Waring SJ, Saleh M. The management of a complex midfoot fracture with circular external fixation. Injury 1994;25:61–3.

[13] Peterson DA, Stinson W. Excision of the fractured os peroneum: a report on five patients and review of the literature. Foot Ankle 1992;13:277–81.

[14] Fogel FR, Katoh Y, Rand JA, et al. Talonavicular arthrodesis for isolated arthrosis—9.5-year results and gait analysis. Foot Ankle 1982;3:105–13.

[15] Lesko P, Maurer RC. Talonavicular dislocations and midfoot arthropathy in neuropathic diabetic feet: natural course and principles of treatment. Clin Orthop 1989;240:226–31.

[16] Davis CA, Lubowitz J, Thordarson DB. Midtarsal fracture-subluxation: case report and review of the literature. Clin Orthop 1993;292:264–8.

[17] DeLee JC. Fractures and dislocations of the foot. In: Mann RA, Coughlin MJ, editors. 6th edition. Surgery of the foot and ankle, vol. 2. St. Louis (MO): Mosby-Year Book; 1993. p. 1465–703.

[18] Eichenholtz SN, Levine DB. Fractures of the tarsal navicular bone. Clin Orthop 1964;34: 142–57.

[19] Sangeorzan BJ, Benirschke SK, Mosca V, et al. Displaced intra-articular fractures of the tarsal navicular. J Bone Joint Surg [Am] 1989;71:1504–10.

[20] Torg J, Pavlov H, Cooley L, et al. Stress fractures of the tarsal navicular: a retrospective review of 21 cases. J Bone Joint Surg [Am] 1982;64:700–12.

[21] Fitch KD, Blackwell JB, Gilmour WN. Operation for non-union of stress fracture of the tarsal navicular. J Bone Joint Surg [Br] 1989;71:105–10.

[22] Steinbach LS. Painful syndromes around the ankle and foot: magnetic resonance imaging evaluation. Top Magn Reson Imaging 1998;9:311–26.

[23] Kiss ZS, Khan KM, Fuller PJ. Stress fractures of the tarsal navicular bone: CT findings in 55 cases. J Radiol 1993;160:111–5.

[24] Khan KM, Fuller PJ, Brukner PD, et al. Outcome of conservative and surgical management of navicular stress fracture in athletes: eighty-six cases proven with computerized tomography. Am J Sports Med 1992;20:657–66.

[25] Beaman DN, Roeser WM, Holmes JR, et al. Cuboid stress fractures: a report of two cases. Foot Ankle 1993;14:525–8.

[26] Marshall P, Hamilton WG. Cuboid subluxation in ballet dancers. Am J Sports Med 1992; 20:169–75.

[27] Everson LI, Galloway HR, Suh JS, et al. Cuboid subluxation. Orthopedics 1991;14:1044–8.

[28] Drummond DS, Hastings DE. Total dislocation of the cuboid bone: report of a case. J Bone Joint Surg [Br] 1969;51:716–8.

[29] Jacobsen FS. Dislocation of the cuboid. Orthopedics 1990;13:1387–9.

[30] Sangeorzan BJ, Swiontkowski MF. Displaced fractures of the cuboid. J Bone Joint Surg [Br] 1990;72:376–8.

[31] Sangeorzan BJ, Mayo KA, Hansen ST. Intraarticular fractures of the foot: talus and lesser tarsals. Clin Orthop 1993;292:135–41.

[32] Phillips RD. Dysfunction of the peroneus longus after fracture of the cuboid. J Foot Surg 1985;24:99–102.

[33] Lee EW, Donatto KC. Fractures of the midfoot and forefoot. Curr Opin Orthop 1999;10(3): 224–30.

[34] Patterson RH, Petersen D, Cunningham R. Isolated fracture of the medical cuneiform. J Orthop Trauma 1993;7:94–5.

[35] Brown DC, McFarland Jr GB. Dislocation of the medial cuneiform bone in tarsometatarsal fracture–dislocation: a case report. J Bone Joint Surg [Am] 1975;57:858–9.

[36] Davies MS, Saxby TS. Intercuneiform instability and the "gap" sign. Foot Ankle Int 1999; 20:606–9.

[37] Miller CM, Winter WG, Bucknell AL, et al. Injuries to the midtarsal joint and lesser tarsal bones. J Am Acad Orthop Surg 1998;6:249–58.

[38] Gossens M, De Stoop N. Linsfranc fracture dislocations: etiology, radiology and results of treatment. A review of 20 cases. Clin Orthop 1983;176:154–62.

[39] Hardcastle PH, Reschauer R, Kutscha-Lissberg E, et al. Injuries to the tarsometatarsal joint. Incidence, classification and treatment. J Bone Joint Surg [Br] 1982;64:349–56.

[40] Quenu E, Kuss E. Etude sur les luxations du metatarse [Study on dislocations of the metatarsals]. Rev Chir 1909;39:281–336.

[41] Mills WJ. Lisfranc injuries. In: Sangeorzan BJ, editor. The traumatized foot. An American Academy of Orthopedic Surgeons monograph series. Rosemont, Illinois: American Academy of Orthopedic Surgeons; 2001. p. 31–9.

[42] Vuori J, Aro H. Lisfranc joint injuries. Trauma mechanisms and associated injuries. J Trauma 1993;35:40–5.

[43] Coiney R, Connell D, Nicholls D. CT evaluation of tarsometatarsal fracture-dislocations injuries. AJR Am J Roentgenol 1985;145:985–91.

[44] Blanco RP, Rodríguez-Merchán EC, Canosa R, et al. Tarsometatarsal fractures and dislocations. J Orthop Trauma 1988;2:188–94.

[45] Trevino SG, Kodros S. Controversies in tarsometatarsal injuries. Orthop Clin North Am 1995; 26:229–38.

[46] Myerson M. Injuries to the forefoot and toes. In: Jahss M, editor. Disorders of the foot and ankle: medical and surgical management. 2nd edition. Philadelphia: WB Saunders; 1991. p. 2240–6.

[47] Myerson MS. The diagnosis and treatment of injuries to the Lisfranc joint complex. Orthop Clin North Am 1989;20:655–64.

[48] Buzzard BM, Briggs PJ. Surgical management of acute tarsometatarsal fracture dislocation in the adult. Clin Orthop 1998;353:125–33.

[49] Richter M, Wippermann B, Krettek C, et al. Fracture and fracture-dislocations of the midfoot: occurrence, causes and long-term results. Foot Ankle Int 2001;22:392–8.

[50] Treadwell J, Kahn M. Lisfranc arthrodesis for chronic pain: a cannulated screw technique. J Foot Ankle Surg 1998;37:28–36.

[51] Brunnet JA, Wiley JJ. The late results of tarsometatarsal joint injuries. J Bone Joint Surg 1987;69B:437–40.

[52] Heckman JD. Fractures and dislocations of the foot. Injuries of the tarsometatarsal (Lisfranc's) joints. In: Rockwood Jr CA, Green DP, editors. 2nd edition. Fractures in adults, vol. 2. Philadelphia: JB Lippincott; 1984. p. 796–1806.

CLINICS IN
PODIATRIC
MEDICINE AND
SURGERY

ELSEVIER
SAUNDERS

Clin Podiatr Med Surg
23 (2006) 343–353

The Use of Ilizarov Technique and Other Types of External Fixation for the Treatment of Intra-Articular Calcaneal Fractures

Thomas Zgonis, DPM[a],*, Thomas S. Roukis, DPM[b],
Vasilios D. Polyzois, MD, PhD[c]

[a]Division of Podiatry, Department of Orthopaedics, University of Texas Health Science Center at
San Antonio, 7773 Floyd Curl Drive, San Antonio, TX 78229, USA
[b]Department of Vascular Surgery MCHJ-SOP, Madigan Army Medical Center,
9040-A Fitzsimmons Avenue, Tacoma, WA 98431, USA
[c]Department of Orthopaedic Traumatology, KAT Hospital, University of Athens Medical School,
Athens, Greece

Since Garongeot first described the calcaneal "smash fracture" in 1720 [1], myriad conservative and surgical methods of treating this complicated injury have been described. To date, however, no formal consensus exists regarding the optimal treatment of displaced intra-articular calcaneal fractures [2–12]. Although the exact means of intervention remains highly controversial, it is universally accepted that restoration of normal anatomic alignment of the calcaneus with regards to its height, length, width, and axis, as well as complete reduction of the subtalar joint posterior articular facet, reduces the complexity of any subsequent surgical intervention as opposed to a malunited calcaneus with an impacted articular surface [9,13]. There is even greater controversy regarding the long-term benefit of open primary operative intervention because of the fairly high incidence of posttraumatic osteoarthritis of the subtalar joint, symptomatic hindfoot stiffness (especially when fixed in varus), wound dehiscence, and potential for the development of osteomyelitis because of the extensive soft tissue trauma inherent with these injuries [2–15]. For these reasons, closed treatment techniques using minimally invasive reduction techniques with application of

---

* Corresponding author.
E-mail address: zgonis@uthscsa.edu (T. Zgonis).

0891-8422/06/$ – see front matter © 2006 Elsevier Inc. All rights reserved.
doi:10.1016/j.cpm.2006.01.011 *podiatric.theclinics.com*

ring-type fine-wire external fixation, although not entirely novel, have recently gained popularity [12,16].

External fixation: literature review

In 1931, Böhler [17] described the use of a clamp to squeeze the calcaneal body to restore its width and height. This process was followed by application of either a transfixion pin through the calcaneal tuber through which continuous skeletal traction was applied or a transfixion pin through both the calcaneal tuber and distal tibia with subsequent application of a total-contact plaster cast to maintain the reduction.

In 1943, Shaar and Kreuz [18] described the application of two transfixion pins through the distal tibia connected to each other with a clamp and a single transfixion pin placed through the calcaneal tuber attached to a U-shaped bar. A pair of distraction bars attached between the tibial clamps and the calcaneal U-shaped bar medially and laterally was used to restore calcaneal height and axial alignment, with manual compression used to restore calcaneal width. The authors presented the short-term results of nine cases (eight patients), none of whom required further surgical intervention or developed deep infection.

In 1987, Lutz and colleagues [19] described the application of a triangular tube-to-bar external fixation system with centrally threaded transfixion Schanz screws placed through the distal tibia, calcaneal tuber, and talar neck and connected by metallic bars. Under direct image intensification, reduction of the calcaneal fracture was performed through manual distraction and angulation. The authors presented the results of 22 cases (17 patients) and stated that anatomic reduction (as determined by restoration of Böhler's angle) was achieved in each case, with return to activities of daily living and work-related endeavors.

In 1990, Bosacco and colleagues [20] described the application of a triangular external fixation system with centrally threaded transfixion pins placed through the distal tibia, calcaneal tuber, and metatarsal region which were all connected using carbon fiber rods. Reduction of the calcaneal fracture was performed under direct image intensification through distraction and angulation. The authors presented the results of 11 cases (10 patients) by comparing postoperative Böhler's angle and calcaneal width with the contralateral calcaneus or historical controls. There was anatomical reduction of the calcaneal fracture in all but one case, which involved an open calcaneal fracture.

In 1993, Forgon [21] described the application of a triangular external fixation system with centrally threaded transfixion pins placed through the talar body, calcaneal tuber, and cuboid and connected through distraction rods. Calcaneal height was restored under direct image intensification through distraction of the anterior and posterior pins; the width and axial alignment of the calcaneus was restored through application of a metal clamp, similar to Böhler's device. The depressed posterior articular facet was reduced with the use of a percutaneous pin that manipulated the fragment into proper alignment under direct image intensification followed by stabilization with percutaneous screws. Using this approach, the authors presented "good" or "excellent" results in 90% of their series of 265 displaced intra-articular calcaneal fractures.

In 1993, Paley and Fischgrund [22] presented a retrospective review of seven displaced intra-articular calcaneal fractures (seven patients) treated with application of a ring-type fine-wire external fixation system, followed by arthrodiastasis of the subtalar joint and a limited lateral incision for percutaneous image intensification–assisted reduction of the posterior facet, followed by early guarded weight bearing. Over a follow-up period between 2 and 4 years, no secondary subtalar arthrodesis procedures were required, although one patient developed a loss of reduction of the posterior facet. The authors attributed the subtalar joint range of motion (>50% compared with the contralateral side) to the arthrodiastasis effect across the subtalar joint. They attributed the lack of plantar heel pain to early assisted weight bearing, which they theorized helped desensitize the heel pad.

In 2003, McGarvey and colleagues [16] presented a retrospective review of 32 displaced intra-articular calcaneal fractures (30 patients) treated with a limited plantar incision for percutaneous image intensification–assisted posterior facet reduction and application of a ring-type fine-wire external fixation system to achieve calcaneal alignment. Although pin-site irritation and infection were common in their series, only one patient developed a deep infection even though eight patients initially presented with open fractures. Over a follow-up period lasting between 3 months and 4 years, no secondary subtalar arthrodesis procedures were required, and at the time of final follow-up all patients were described as being weight bearing to tolerance.

In 2004, Talarico and colleagues [12] presented a retrospective review of 25 displaced intra-articular calcaneal fractures (23 patients) treated with initial calcaneal transfixion pin traction to achieve restoration of calcaneal alignment and limited lateral-incision percutaneous image intensification–assisted reduction of the posterior facet. This treatment was followed by application of a ring-type external fixation system with the subtalar joint held in a distracted position and immediate guarded weight bearing, similar to the technique previously de-scribed by Paley and Fischgrund [22]. In their series, pin-site irritation and infection were common occurrences, but no deep infections occurred. During a follow-up period of 2 to 7 years, no secondary subtalar arthrodesis procedures were required. Subtalar joint range of motion was greater than 50% (compared with the contralateral side) in 21 feet (84%). All patients were ambulating in normal shoe gear, with the majority finding benefit from in-shoe orthoses.

In 2005, Roukis and colleagues [23] presented the long-term follow-up of the triangular tube-to-bar external fixation system technique described by Lutz and colleagues [19] involving 66 displaced intra-articular calcaneal fractures in 62 patients treated between 1982 and 2000. The authors achieved good, very good, or excellent clinical results in 51 patients (82%). Each radiographic mea-surement obtained revealed a significant difference between the preoperative and immediate postoperative and between preoperative and final follow-up measurements ($P \leq .05$) but no significant difference between the immediate postoperative and final follow-up measurements. Therefore the authors showed that use of this technique allows radiographic correction in the normally accepted ranges even though an open reduction of the articular surface of the posterior facet of the subtalar joint and bone grafting were not performed. Through manual manipulation and distraction of the calcaneus the authors were able to restore the height, length, width, and axial alignment of the calcaneus with no significant loss of correction over time. Overall, one patient required a subtalar joint arthrodesis (1.6%), and two patients (3.2%) required adjustment of the external fixation device during the treatment period. The authors concluded that this technique should be used with caution in patients who have Essex-Lopresti [24] joint depression and comminuted fracture patterns and in patients who have experienced polytrauma, because poorer clinical results, less anatomic radiographic reduction, and a greater incidence of complications occurred.

Operative technique: ring-type fine-wire external fixation

Under general or spinal anesthesia, the patient is positioned on the operating room table in the supine position with the entire affected lower extremity draped free to afford unlimited access to the entire foot, ankle, and lower extremity. The patient is placed on a traction table, and under sterile techniques a calcaneal pin is inserted posteriorly and attached to a half ring on the traction device (Fig. 1). Under direct image intensification, the subtalar joint is distracted and manipulated to the desired position. A limited incision is placed underneath the subtalar joint, and a Freer elevator or a small osteotome is used to elevate and realign the subtalar joint, making sure the peroneal tendons and sural nerve are retracted appropriately. Bone graft material is used to maintain the alignment of the subtalar joint and fill in the space from the comminuted fracture fragments (Fig. 2). The lateral wall is then reduced by placing two olive wires from lateral to medial direction and tensioning from the medial side of the calcaneus (Fig. 3, A–C). A third olive wire is placed in the midfoot to counteract the forces applied in the rearfoot. The ring-type fine-wire external fixator can be prebuilt for the surgeon and applied in a static fashion. The traction on the calcaneus as well as the initial calcaneal pin is removed at the end of the procedure. Patients are allowed to bear weight with an assistance device as early as the first postoperative week. A bottom ring can also be applied to the U-shaped footplate to protect the plantar aspect of the foot during the early postoperative period (Fig. 4).

The circular fixation device is removed as an outpatient procedure under local anesthesia with intravenous sedation. A weight-bearing removable cast is applied, and aggressive physical therapy is initiated to obtain as much motion as possible through the subtalar and midfoot articulations. Over the course of the ensuing 4 to 6 weeks the patient gradually progresses to full, unassisted weight

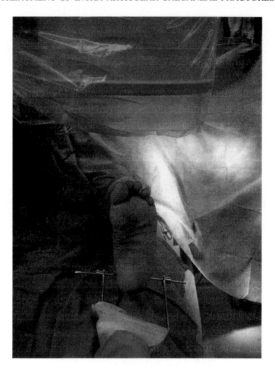

Fig. 1. Intraoperative picture of the initial calcaneal pin and distraction.

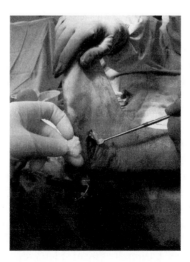

Fig. 2. Intraoperative picture of the skin incision and bone-grafting technique.

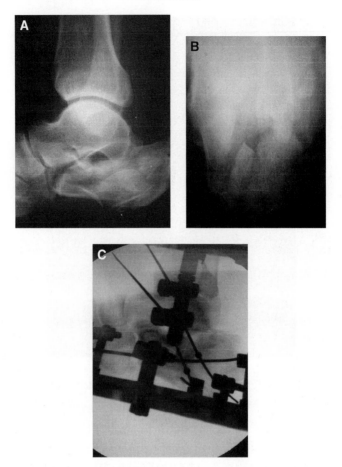

Fig. 3. (*A*) Preoperative lateral, (*B*) calcaneal axial, and (*C*) postoperative lateral views showing the placement of olive wires and fracture reduction.

bearing in sturdy shoe gear, most commonly with an in-shoe orthoses for support and shock absorption.

Operative technique: tube-to-bar external fixation

Under general or spinal anesthesia, the patient is positioned on the operating room table in the supine position with the entire affected lower extremity draped free to afford unlimited access to the entire foot, ankle, and lower extremity. The tube-to-bar components from any of the proprietary company's large external fixator systems are used for the procedure, with each step being performed under image intensification. First, a centrally threaded large-diameter pin is passed from lateral to medial at the level of the dense posterior-inferior calcaneal tuber in the

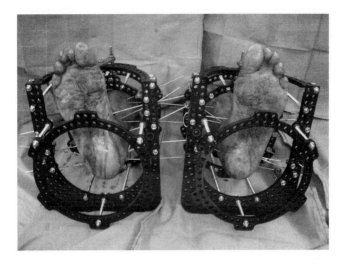

Fig. 4. Immediate postoperative picture of the Ilizarov technique in a bilateral comminuted calcaneal fracture reduction.

plane of the axial deformity of the posterior calcaneal fragment. Next, a second pin is passed from lateral to medial through the dense talar neck parallel to the ankle joint. Finally, a third pin is passed from medial to lateral at the anterior-posterior midpoint of the distal tibia approximately 15 cm proximal to and parallel with the ankle joint (Fig. 5). Next, two steel or carbon fiber rods are attached to the medial and lateral aspects of the tibial and talar pins with adjustable clamps. Similarly, two steel or carbon fiber rods are attached to the medial and lateral aspects of the tibial and calcaneal screws with adjustable clamps (Fig. 6). With the knee flexed to relieve tension from the Achilles tendon, the calcaneal pin (ie, calcaneal fragment) is manually manipulated into an orientation parallel with the tibial and talar screws to correct the varus axial

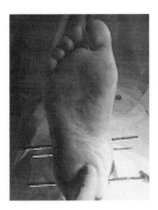

Fig. 5. Intraoperative plantar view demonstrating the location and alignment of the transfixion pins through the tibia, talus, and calcaneus.

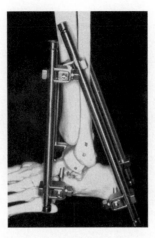

Fig. 6. Lateral view of a triangular tube-to-bar external fixator on a saw-bone model.

malalignment, then is laterally translated to correct the medial displacement, and finally is distracted distally to correct the loss of calcaneal height and provide distraction across the ankle and subtalar joints. Once satisfactory anatomic alignment is achieved, the adjustable clamps are terminally tightened between the tibial and calcaneal pins and rods. Finally, manual traction is placed between the tibial and talar pins to rotate the talar head and neck plantarly to restore the talocalcaneal angle. Once satisfactory distraction and alignment have been verified, the adjustable clamps are tightened between the tibial and talar screws and rods. The final reduction is considered satisfactory if the calcaneal malalignment is fully restored, the posterior facet is reduced, the ankle and subtalar joints are

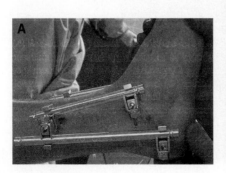
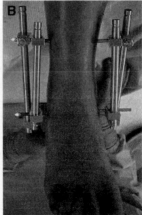

Fig. 7. (A) Lateral and (B) antero-posterior views after application of the triangular tube-to-bar external fixation device.

distracted, and all three Schanz screws are aligned parallel to one another based upon intraoperative clinical and image-intensification evaluation (Fig. 7).

The tube-to-bar external fixation device is removed as an outpatient procedure under local anesthesia with intravenous sedation. A non–weight-bearing removable cast is applied, and aggressive physical therapy is initiated to obtain as much motion as possible through the subtalar and midfoot articulations. Over the course of the ensuing 4 to 6 weeks the patient progresses gradually to full, unassisted weight bearing in sturdy shoe gear, most commonly with an in-shoe orthosis for support and shock absorption.

Discussion

The ideal treatment of displaced intra-articular fractures of the calcaneus remains elusive at best, especially in patients who have bilateral involvement [2–12,16–30]. Myriad factors that might influence the clinical results of calcaneal fracture treatment have been reported, and anatomic reduction of the articular surface of the posterior facet of the subtalar joint does not guarantee an improved clinical outcome [2–12,31–35]. It is clear, however, that incision breakdown and deep infection after extensile open surgical approaches are potentially devastating complications that cannot be easily resolved. Furthermore, restoration of normal calcaneal morphology seems to afford less complex secondary surgical intervention than a malunited calcaneus, regardless of what type of conservative or surgical management is employed [9,11,13–15].

Although not directly measured in any of the previously discussed studies evaluating the use of external fixation, the arthrodiastasis obtained across the ankle and subtalar joints with this technique may aid in limiting postoperative hindfoot and ankle stiffness and the late development of osteoarthrosis [12,26,36]. van Valberg and colleagues [37] have demonstrated reparative activity within traumatized articular cartilage in the absence of shear stresses following arthrodiastasis with a ring-type external fixation system. Unfortunately, these authors have not presented any long-term data, and the concept remains a matter for conjecture at this time.

Summary

Although the treatment of displaced intra-articular calcaneal fractures using either a ring-type fine-wire or tube-to-bar external fixation system is conceptually simple, in practice it is fairly complex to perform. Attention to detail is mandatory to avoid nerve-related injuries and structural malalignment. As with any external fixation, proper care of the screw-pin site is necessary to avoid deep wound infection and osteomyelitis. The techniques described in this article may be used as an alternative in patients who have a severe comminuted intra-articular calcaneal fracture and soft tissue compromise.

References

[1] Garengeot RJ. Traites des operations. 2nd edition. Paris: 1790.

[2] Järvholm U, Körner L, Thorén O, et al. Fractures of the calcaneus. A comparison of open and closed treatment. Acta Orthop Scand 1984;55:652–6.

[3] Bunckley RE, Meek RN. Comparison of open versus closed reduction of intra-articular calcaneal fractures: a matched cohort in workmen. J Orthop Trauma 1992;6:216–22.

[4] Parmar HV, Triffitt PD, Gregg PJ. Intra-articular fractures of the calcaneum treated operatively or conservatively. A prospective study. J Bone Joint Surg [Br] 1993;75:932–7.

[5] Leung KS, Yuen KM, Chan WS. Operative treatment of displaced intra-articular fractures of the calcaneum. Medium-term results. J Bone Joint Surg [Br] 1993;75:196–201.

[6] Thordarson DB, Krieger LE. Operative versus non-operative treatment of intra-articular fractures of the calcaneus: a prospective randomized trial. Foot Ankle Int 1996;17:2–9.

[7] Eastwood DM, Phipp L. Intra-articular fractures of the calcaneum: why such controversy? Injury 1997;28:247–59.

[8] Randle JA, Kreder HJ, Stephens D, et al. Should calcaneal fractures be treated surgically? A meta-analysis. Clin Orthop 2000;377:217–27.

[9] Sanders R. Current concept review: displaced intra-articular fractures of the calcaneus. J Bone Joint Surg [Am] 2000;82:225–50.

[10] Tennet TD, Calder PR, Salisbury RD, et al. The operative management of displaced intra-articular fractures of the calcaneum: a two-centre study using a defined protocol. Injury 2001; 32:491–6.

[11] Harvey EJ, Grujic L, Early JS, et al. Morbidity associated with ORIF of intra-articular calcaneus fractures using a lateral approach. Foot Ankle Int 2001;22:868–73.

[12] Talarico LM, Vito GR, Zyryanov SY. Management of displaced intra-articular calcaneal fractures by using external ring fixation, minimally invasive open reduction, and early weightbearing. J Foot Ankle Surg 2004;43:43–50.

[13] Stephens HM, Sanders R. Calcaneal mal-unions: results of a prognostic computed tomography classification system. Foot Ankle Int 1996;17:395–401.

[14] Levin LS, Nunley JA. The management of soft-tissue problems associated with calcaneal fractures. Clin Orthop Rel Res 1993;290:151–6.

[15] Heier KA, Ingante AF, Walling AK, et al. Open fractures of the calcaneus: soft-tissue injury determines outcome. J Bone Joint Surg [Am] 2003;85:2276–82.

[16] McGarvey WC, Burris MW, Clanton TO. Treatment of displaced intra-articular calcaneus fractures with indirect reduction and small wire ring external fixation. Presented at the American Orthopaedic Foot and Ankle Society summer meeting. Hilton Head, SC, June 27, 2003.

[17] Böhler L. Diagnosis, pathology, and treatment of fractures of the os calcis. J Bone Joint Surg 1931;13:75–89.

[18] Shaar CM, Kreuz Jr FP. Fractures of the os calcis. In: Manual of fractures: treatment by external skeletal fixation. Philadelphia: W.B. Saunders; 1943. p. 137–57.

[19] Lutz HP, Ohmer M, Kirschner P. Aufrichtung von Fersenbeintrümmerbrüchen mit dem Fixateur externe: methode, erfahrungen und ergebnisse 1982 bis 1986. Presented at the fifth annual German-Austrian, Switzerland Traumatologic Meeting. Berlin, November 3, 1987.

[20] Bosacco SJ, Berman AT, Connolly TC, et al. Treatment of calcaneal fractures with carbon fiber external fixation. Presented at the meeting of the American Academy of Orthopaedic Surgeons. San Francisco, February 21, 1990.

[21] Forgon M. Closed reduction and percutaneous osteosynthesis: technique and results in 265 calcaneal fractures. In: Tscherne H, Schatzker J, editors. Major fractures of the pilon, talus, and the calcaneus. Berlin: Springer-Verlag; 1993. p. 207–13.

[22] Paley D, Fischgrund J. Open reduction and circular external fixation of intra-articular calcaneal fractures. Clin Orthop 1993;290:125–31.

[23] Roukis TS, Wuenschel M, Lutz HP, et al. Treatment of displaced intra-articular calcaneal fractures with triangular tube-to-bar external fixation: long-term clinical follow-up and

radiographic analysis. Presented at the American College of Foot and Ankle Surgeons 63rd Annual Scientific Conference. New Orleans, March 12, 2005.

[24] Essex-Lopresti P. The mechanism, reduction technique, and results in fractures of the os calcis. Br J Surg 1952;39:395–419.

[25] Gupta A, Ghalambor N, Nihal A, et al. The modified Palmer lateral approach for calcaneal fractures: wound healing and post-operative computed tomographic evaluation of fracture reduction. Foot Ankle Int 2003;24:744–53.

[26] Paley D, Hall H. Intra-articular fractures of the calcaneus. A critical analysis of results and prognostic factors. J Bone Joint Surg [Am] 1993;75:342–54.

[27] Kurozumi T, Jinno Y, Sato T, et al. Open reduction for intra-articular calcaneal fractures: evaluation using computed tomography. Foot Ankle Int 2003;24:942–8.

[28] Omoto H, Nakamura K. Method for manual reduction of displaced intra-articular fracture of the calcaneus: technique, indications, and limitations. Foot Ankle Int 2001;22:874–9.

[29] Aktuglu K, Aydogan U. The functional outcome of displaced intra-articular calcaneal fractures: a comparison between isolated and polytrauma patients. Foot Ankle Int 2002;23:314–8.

[30] Dooley P, Buckley R, Tough S, et al. Bilateral calcaneal fractures: operative versus non-operative treatment. Foot Ankle Int 2004;25:47–52.

[31] Prasartritha T, Sethavanitch C. Three-dimensional and two-dimensional computerized tomographic demonstration of calcaneal fractures. Foot Ankle Int 2004;25:262–73.

[32] Thordarson D, Latteier M. Open reduction and internal fixation of calcaneal fractures with a low profile titanium calcaneal perimeter plate. Foot Ankle Int 2003;24:217–21.

[33] Gavlik JM, Rammelt S, Zwipp H. The use of subtalar arthroscopy in open reduction and internal fixation of intra-articular calcaneal fractures. Injury 2002;33:63–71.

[34] Rammelt S, Gavlik JM, Barthel S, et al. The value of subtalar arthroscopy in the management of intra-articular calcaneus fractures. Foot Ankle Int 2002;23:906–16.

[35] Davies MB, Betts RP, Scott IR. Optical plantar pressure analysis following internal fixation for displaced intra-articular os calcis fractures. Foot Ankle Int 2003;24:851–6.

[36] van Valburg AA, van Roermund PM, Marijnissen AC, et al. Joint distraction in treatment of osteoarthritis: a two-year follow-up of the ankle. Osteoarthritis Cartilage 1999;7:474–9.

[37] van Valburg AA, van Roermund PM, Marijnissen AC, et al. Joint distraction in treatment of osteoarthritis (II): effects on cartilage in a canine model. Osteoarthritis Cartilage 2000;8:1–8.

CLINICS IN
PODIATRIC
MEDICINE AND
SURGERY

Clin Podiatr Med Surg
23 (2006) 355–374

Treatment of Late Complications of Intra-Articular Calcaneal Fractures

Pier Carlo Pisani, MD[a], Enrico Parino, MD[a],*,
Paola Acquaro, MD[b]

[a]Center for Foot Surgery, Casa di Cura Fornaca di Sessant, Corso Vittorio Emanuele II 91,
10128 Torino, Italy
[b]Casa di Cura "Villa dei Gerani", Via A. Manzoni, 83 91016 Sant'erice, Trapani, Italy

The late complications of intra-articular calcaneal fractures are related to the possible degeneration of the subtalar joint and to the entire complex deformation produced at the moment of the injury. The acute treatment therefore must minimize the possibility of secondary problems, and reconstruction must re-establish the overall shape of the calcaneus bone.

The most relevant problem inherent in calcaneus fractures is the axial deviation of the calcaneus on its frontal, horizontal, and (less frequently recognized) sagittal planes. The sagittal deviation contributes to the functional limitation of the tibiotalar joint and can cause the painful syndrome of distal tibiofibular syndesmosis.

Other possible secondary problems are nerve branch compression (tibialis or sural nerves), fibulo-calcaneal bone impingement, plantar osseous protrusion, and toe retraction.

All these problems, in isolation, combination, or in association with painful rigidity of the subtalar joint, were seen in varying degrees in the patients for whom data are presented in this article.

Surgical treatment of late complications of calcaneal fractures represents a problem with highly uncertain results, although the surgical stabilization of the subtalar joint, in absence of other problems, is easy to establish.

* Corresponding author.
E-mail address: info@chirurgiapiede-pisani.it (E. Parino).

Therefore the authors believe that it is important to take into consideration the entire complex deformation produced by the trauma, not merely the damage to the subtalar joint that compromises the thalamus.

Calcaneus fractures account for 60% of the important traumatic pathology of the tarsus and involve a high degree of associated morbidity. These fractures have an enormous social impact, often occurring in men of working age; 20% of cases result in a period of disability lasting up to 3 years and partial residual disability lasting as long as 5 years.

The treatment of transthalamic fractures, in particular, remains an issue of debate among the supporters of conservative treatment [1–13] and those who advocate open reduction with various types of synthesis [14–25]. Therefore the approach to this condition is controversial. In the past, the opposition to surgical treatment of the calcaneus fractures may have seemed justified by the relative technical difficulty of surgical treatment, by the limited ability—before the advent of the CT scan—to assess the pathologic anatomy of the lesion, by the problems caused by stabilization and synthesis, and by the fear of complications to the soft tissues.

On the other hand, ever since the beginning of the twentieth century, some have chosen to treat these fractures surgically. The sporadic reports in the first decades were followed by the work of Lerich [26] and Palmer [27] regarding the methods of fixation and the use of autologous grafts to sustain the elevated and reduced thalamic fragment. Essex-LoPresti [28] demonstrated the possibility of reduction and stabilization of the calcaneus fracture with results definitely superior to those obtained by conservative treatment.

There has been a gradual change in practice, from conservative care without open reduction to increasing use of reduction and the re-establishment of the overall form of the calcaneus (both through open surgery and through conservative methods). Reports by Copin [29], Vigroux and Goutallier [30], Stephenson [31], Burdeaux [32], Letournel [33], Monsey and Levine [34], Paley and Hall [35], Sanders and Fortin [36], Zwipp and Tscherne [37], and many other authors have documented this change.

More recently the three-dimensional analysis of the fracture morphology provided by CT scan [38–42] (with the resulting capability for improved surgical planning), the development of the internal synthesis, and the availability of cutaneous vascularized grafts have facilitated surgical care, which is desirable in all articular fractures. Surgery allows the re-establishment of the surface geometry, insofar as possible, correction of axial defects, and early mobilization of the contiguous joints to avoid osteodystrophy.

The authors believe a strong argument in favor of surgical reduction is made by the late sequelae of conservatively treated or poorly reduced fractures. Only recently has attention been given to the problems that are secondary to the outcomes of the fracture event and that go beyond the favorable outcomes of the subtalar joint.

This article focuses on transthalamic fractures and does not discuss extra-articular fractures, which are simpler to treat and have a more favorable outcome.

In transthalamic fractures, treatment is closely related to the anatomy of the lesion and hence to the surgical techniques necessary for the reduction. An overview of the anatomy and pathology of the lesion shows alterations and deformities produced by the fracture that may be summarized as follows (Fig. 1):

- Reduction of the overall height of the calcaneus
- Superior dislocation of various entity of the posterior tuberosity (followed by the functional loss of tibiotalar sagittal angle)
- Increase in the transverse diameter of the calcaneus body
- Dislocation, most frequently in varus, of the posterior tuberosity (which is not always clinically identifiable, because it is masked by edema and widening of the heel, which is well demonstrated in axial radiographic views or in coronal CT scans)
- Subversion of the posterior subtalar joint
- Primitive involvement of the calcaneocuboid joint caused by the propagation of the sagittal fracture line to the anterior process of the calcaneus, caused by the destabilization of the antero-lateral fragment. The latter, being integral with the cuboid, is isolated from the rest of the calcaneus (four-part fracture, Fig. 2)

This pathologic anatomy indicates that the initial injuries, when not treated, lead to the late sequelae of the fracture. Therefore treatment must be chosen according to its potential for remedying the damage caused by the injury.

Anatomic reductions cannot be obtained through external maneuvers or with distractions using percutaneous screws (ie, by conservative methods). It makes no sense to reserve surgical reduction for only highly dislocated fractures: an articular fracture, whatever the degree of dislocation, must be reduced (a concept affirmed by Judet in 1954, but always been known).

At first glance, data seem to suggest equivalent outcomes for conservative and surgical treatment, with perhaps slightly better outcomes in surgically treated

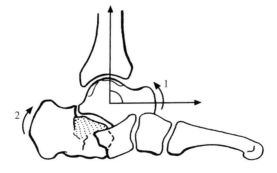

Fig. 1. The various calcaneus deformities caused by the fracture: the reduction of the overall height of the calcaneus, elevation of the posterior tuberosity, and subversion of the posterior subtalar joint caused by thalamic depression. 1, talus dorsiflexion; 2, elevation of posterior tuberosity.

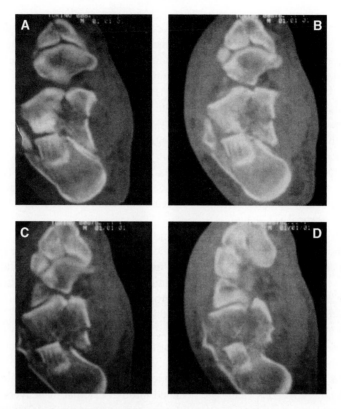

Fig. 2. Coronal CT scan showing the delimitation of the four fragments, the axial deviation of the posterolateral fragment, the increase in the transverse diameter of the calcaneus, and the involvement of the calcaneocuboid joint. (*A*) Axial deviation of the posterolateral fragment. (*B*) Increase in the transverse diameter of calcaneus. (*C*–*D*) Involvement of the calcaneo-cuboid joint.

cases. A closer analysis of the possible adverse sequelae, however, shows that reports favoring conservative treatment fail to take later-developing problems into consideration. These sequelae can be prevented only by treatment in the acute phase directed towards restoring the morphologic characteristics of the calcaneus and its contiguous structures.

In this article the authors discuss the late sequelae secondary to the outcomes of the fracture: axial defects of the hindfoot, plantar bony prominences, alterations of the tarsal mechanics, canalicular syndromes, limitation of the toe flexion, subtalar syndrome, and painful stiffness of the subtalar joint.

Axial defects of the hindfoot

The axial defects of the hindfoot must be evaluated in all three planes: frontal, horizontal, and sagittal. In the frontal and horizontal planes, malunion of the posterior fragment dislocated posteriorly in varus, valgus, or intrarotation in horizontal

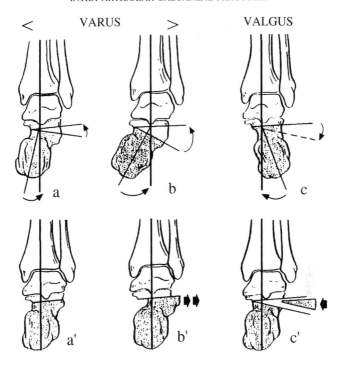

Fig. 3. Corrective calcaneus osteotomy scheme for axial defects on the frontal planes: subthalamic joint valgus increasing osteotomy (*a, b*), lateral open-wedge valgus reduction osteotomy (*c, c'*), lateral translation osteotomy (*a', b'*).

plane inevitably causes secondary imbalance of the tibiotarsal joint and deformity of the hindfoot, leading to biomechanical alterations caused by an anomalous load distribution to the astragalic and calcaneus foot, with the possibility of metatarsalgia as well as stress fractures.

The deformities in the frontal and horizontal planes therefore require directional osteotomies that distribute the weight on the physiologic axis (Fig. 3): subthalamic valgus osteotomy according to Pisani [43] to correct the calcaneal

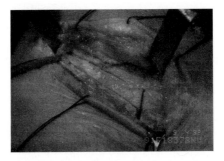

Fig. 4. Subthalamic horizontal varus reducing osteotomy: layout of the osteotomic lines.

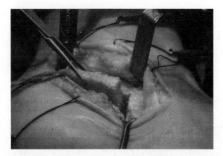

Fig. 5. Subthalamic horizontal varus reducing osteotomy: removal of the bone wedge with lateral base (whose width corresponds in degrees to the degree of correction obtained).

varus; Dwyer's [44] oblique osteotomy in cases of calcaneus curvature. To correct the valgus, medial closed-wedge osteotomy or lateral open-wedge osteotomy is used, although, as with all open-wedge osteotomies, one must always be aware of the possibility of deterioration and thus the loss of correction over time. These osteotomies can be performed when the entire volume of the calcaneus has not been reduced (eg, because a large fragment does not allow reduction). Otherwise such techniques are difficult to apply, and it is necessary to use translational osteotomy of the posterior tuberosity, without bone-wedge subtraction.

In general, correction of the calcaneal varus (a real deformity on the frontal plane) is more economically obtained by a horizontal subthalamic osteotomy (Figs. 4–7), in which the degree of bone subtraction corresponds exactly to the degree of correction because the osteotomy plane is perpendicular to the plane of the deformity. Dwyer's oblique osteotomy is more correctly and economically used to correct the curvature of the heel bone.

The osteotomies are performed to correct the axial defects, with the assumption that the subtalar joint is both injury free and pain free. Such cases are unusual. If the subtalar joint has been injured, the axial defect must be corrected simultaneously with resection-arthrodesis of the subtalar joint [46].

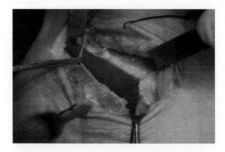

Fig. 6. Subthalamic horizontal varus reducing osteotomy: the breach in the calcaneal body after removal of the bone wedge.

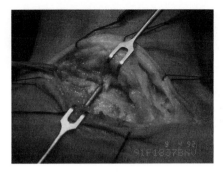

Fig. 7. Subthalamic horizontal varus reducing osteotomy: closure of the breach and stabilization with staples.

The deformities in the sagittal plane, ranging from a flat calcaneus to a rocker-bottom calcaneus (a consequence of the inflection between the posterior fragment and the anterior fragment, with plantar apex), result in the loss of tibiotalar-sagittal angle anatomically or functionally (Fig. 8) [45]. The results are

1. A loss in dorsiflexion of the tibiotarsal joint proportional to the degree of loss of tibiotalar-sagittal angle
2. Anterior impingement of the tibia and the talar neck with the possible formation of marginal osteophytes of the tibia and talar neck
3. The painful syndrome of the distal tibiofibular syndesmosis

In the acute phase, the loss in the range of motion in dorsiflexion of the tibiotarsal joint is caused by the reduction of the tibiotalar angle. The tibiotalar angle may be reduced from its normal 120° to less than 90°. To evaluate the angle reduction correctly, the radiograph must be done under load-bearing conditions (Fig. 9). Even with good clinical and radiologic results, painful symptomatology may develop over time. Such pain is generically referred to the ankle and often is hastily attributed to the tibiotarsal joint.

A careful and attentive examination in which the patient is asked to identify the location of the pain reveals that the pain is clearly presyndesmotic, is

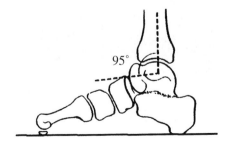

Fig. 8. Reduction of the anterior inclination of the talus following horizontal plane of the calcaneus.

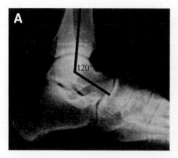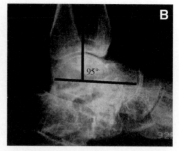

Fig. 9. (*A*) In the lateral radiographic views of the foot, the tibio-talar angle is normally about 120°. (*B*) The evaluation of reduction of the anterior inclination of the talus requires roentgenograms under load-bearing conditions.

worsened by forced dorsiflexion of the foot, and is induced by specific palpation. Limitation of dorsiflexion and the reduction of the tibiotalar angle are the clinical and radiologic proofs (under load-bearing conditions) (Fig. 10).

This syndrome described Pisani [47] is anatomically explained by the geometry of the talar pulley that is larger in its anterior portion and is under continuous strain in the tibioperoneal mortise, where the point of minor resistance is represented by the distal syndesmosis stabilized by its relative ligaments and characterized by very little elasticity.

As Le Coeur [48] emphasized, the elastic movement of the mortise cannot be attributed to the elasticity of the tibiofibular ligaments, which are basically nonextendible and are unable to withstand the high pressures of the talus during ambulation.

The elevation of the fibula during dorsiflexion, its internal rotation and lateral dislocation, and the inverse movements during the plantarflexion are caused by the oblique direction of the ligaments.

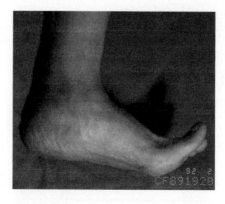

Fig. 10. Limitation of the dorsal range of motion of the tibio-tarsal joint caused by the reduction of the anterior inclination of the talus.

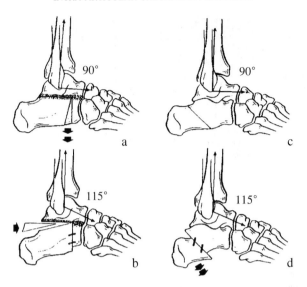

Fig. 11. Desialization osteotomy of the calcaneal posterior process. (*a–b*) Posterior bone wedge insert. (*c–d*) Desialization osteotomy of the calcaneal posterior process.

The muscles active during dorsiflexion, except for common extensor digitorum, insert on the tibia. Therefore the fibula is not involved in this movement, and it may passively mobilize in lateral elevation. On the other hand, the muscles active in plantarflexion, except for the common flexor digitorum, insert on the fibula, and their contraction leads to lowering and locking proportional to the muscular force applied.

The sum of the components of this clench accounts for about five eighths of the muscular force employed (eg, standing on the tips of the toes produces a clench force of about 2000 kg).

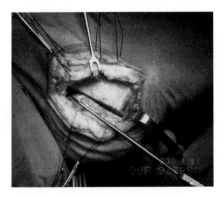

Fig. 12. Desialization osteotomy of the calcaneal posterior process: once the osteotomy has been performed, the posterior fragment is tractioned toward the bottom.

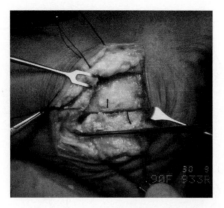

Fig. 13. Desialization osteotomy of the calcaneal posterior process: two linear traces to highlight the degree of dislocation.

Also, the fibula may rotate about 20° on its proper longitudinal axis, thus adapting itself to the external profile of the talar trochlea. The axis of rotation is at the level of the anterior tibiofibular ligaments.

The clinical picture of pain caused by the syndesmosis and the radiologic appearance of osteophytes resulting from the impingement caused by reduction of the tibiotalar angle requires surgical realignment of the hindfoot to improve the congruent tibiotalar relation.

The realignment is obtained by desialization osteotomy of the posterior process of the calcaneus (Fig. 11) or by posterior open-wedge osteotomy.

Desialization osteotomy of the posterior process of the calcaneus

With access to the lateral wall of the calcaneus, sparing the sural nerve, the osteotomy has an oblique direction in plantar-distal sense, performed at the limit between the body and posterior process (Figs. 12, 13). With the foot in equinus and through recoil of the osteotomic fragment of about 1 cm (Fig. 14),

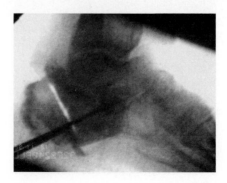

Fig. 14. Desialization osteotomy of the calcaneal posterior process: intraoperative ampliscopic control of the obtained displacement.

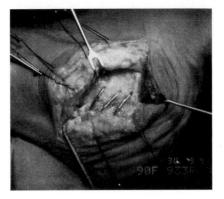

Fig. 15. Fistulization osteotomy of the calcaneal posterior process: the stabilization of the osteotomy with stables carried over in the distal-plantar direction, in opposition to the traction of the triceps over the fragment that has undergone osteotomy.

the focus is stabilized with staples stretched in the distal and anterior direction to eliminate the pressure of the Achilles tendon on the posterior fragment (Fig. 15).

Posterior open-wedge osteotomy

The posterior open-wedge osteotomy has a two-fold purpose: arthrodesis of the subtalar joint, if it is painful, and correcting the loss in anterior inclination of the talus, the tibiotalar-sagittal angle (Fig. 16). Excellent access is obtained

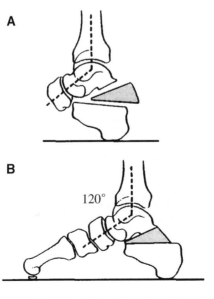

Fig. 16. (*A–B*) Osteoarthrotomy of the posterior subtalar joint with addition of a posterior wedge bone transplant to limit the reduction of the anterior inclination of the talus.

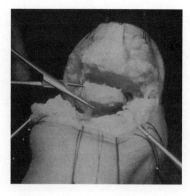

Fig. 17. Osteo-arthroresection of the subtalar joint through the trans-Achilles tendon approach and placement of an appropriately shaped posterior wedge bone graft.

with a posterior and lateral approach, after isolation and protection of the saphenous bundle and the sural nerve, Achilles tenotomy, and retraction of the peroneal and hallux long flexor tendons. The resection of the subtalar joint is performed by the posterior approach. It is mobilized in aperture and maintained through the use of an appropriate iliac tricortical wedge-shaped transplant with a posterior base (Fig. 17). Rarely, it is possible to obtain the bone for transplantation from the superior portion of the posterior process of the calcaneus displaced superiorly.

Peroneal-calcaneal Impingement

In addition to tibiotalar impingement, a common problem resulting from a fracture is a mechanical one that results from the functional limitation, pain, and tenovaginitis of the peroneal muscles at the level of the apex of the peroneal malleolus and the fragment of the lateral wall that is expelled and defectively

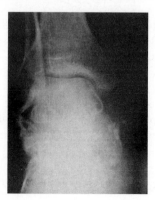

Fig. 18. In the anteroposterior radiographic view, the fibular impingement with the unreduced and malunion of the parietal calcaneal fragment.

consolidated (Fig. 18) [49]. Weight-bearing radiographs in anteroposterior views and coronal CT scans can identify the protruded fragment. Sometimes the fragment may be a posterior lateral fragment lateralized and in valgus under the fibula. At other times, fragments or a good portion of the calcaneal wall are seen. The excessive calcaneal valgus increases the impingement.

In any case, a subcortical resection of the excessive bony mass is necessary. The loose piece of the lateral wall initially removed must be also replaced, so that there is no residual rough parietal surface along the span of the peroneal tendons.

Plantar bony protrusions

Plantar bony protrusions, even outside the rocker-bottom calcaneus, cause pain because of localized overload after progressive sectional damage to of the fibro-adipose subcalcaneal pad, with possible cutaneous manifestations of painful hyperkeratosis or even ulceration.

Canalicular syndromes

Canalicular syndromes caused by irritation or compression may be observed and may be either sensitive in type, caused by the involvement of the sural nerve, or motor or mixed in type, caused by the involvement of the posterior tibial nerve at the tarsal tunnel. Involvement of the posterior tibial nerve may lead to damage of the intrinsic muscles and the appearance of claw toes. The irritation or frank compression of the nerve branches results from posttraumatic edema and from stretching and compression caused by unreduced bone fragments.

Alterations of the tarsal mechanics

Alterations of tarsal mechanics at the tibiotarsal joint after reduction of the anterior inclination of the talus caused by the loss of the range of motion in dorsiflexion have already been mentioned [50].

The subversion of the subtalar joint leads to various complex cases of insufficiency or of painful stiffness caused by alterations in the articular structure and axial defects of consolidation of the posterior fragment.

The talar-calcaneus-scaphoid joint (coxa pedis) is the enarthrosic structure in which the lines of force and weight are translated from the frontal plane to the horizontal plane, and vice versa. Because of the functional interdependence of the components of this joint, the possible alterations resulting from a calcaneal fracture (calcaneal varus-valgus, the reduction of the tibiotalar sagittal angle) can translate into significant functional damage.

The calcaneo-cuboid joint may be involved if the anterior process of the calcaneus is involved by the extension of the line of fracture (the bone fragment usually remains connected with the cuboid) or by the articular subversion with stiffness secondary to the plurifragmentation of the fracture of the anterior process of the calcaneus [51].

Claw toes

Claw toes may be observed both with reduction and with a structured proximal interphalangeal articulation and may be related to the retraction or incorporation in scar of the long flexors or to possible vague compartmental syndromes. Lengthening surgery of the retromalleous flexors (flexor digitorum longus and flexor hallucis longus), dorsal transposition of F1 of the short flexors, or resection-arthrodesis of the PIF should be considered, depending on the indications.

Subtalar joint syndrome

Subtalar joint syndrome may manifest in a complex clinical situation in which, in addition to varying degrees of stiffness, instability of the hindfoot is caused by the loss of three components of stability in the joint: structural, active, and passive [52,53].

Pathologic aspects of inversion in the calcaneal varus lead to the loss of structural stability. The loss of passive stability is associated with ligamentous lesions or is secondary to skeletal trauma, mainly involving the interosseous ligament and the lateral and medial calcaneocuboid ligament. Associated with the loss of passive stability is the loss of active stability caused by alterations of the proprioceptive system, with subsequent reflex alterations in the neuromuscular control.

In addition to insufficiency of the subtalar joint, for which pathologic movements must be present, a classic long-term problem of the calcaneus is painful stiffness, referred to as "posttraumatic arthrosis of the subtalar joint." The authors will return later to the topic of residual pain following fractures of the calcaneus caused by damage to the subtalar joint, although one must remember that the residual pain is not the only or the most relevant concern.

Patient data collection

In the foot surgery center, Centro Chirurgia del Piede Prof. G. Pisani, 306 patients (193 men and 113 women) complaining of problems resulting from past calcaneus fractures were seen between January 1989 and April 2000. Most of the patients were in the third to sixth decade of life (Fig. 19); there was a male predominance. Of these patients, 101 underwent surgery. The patients who underwent surgery were in the same age range, but the gender distribution was more equal.

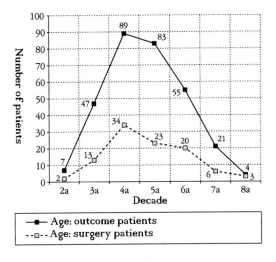

Fig. 19. Age distribution of patients who had late complications of calcaneus fractures.

The problems encountered surgically are listed in Table 1. Often multiple problems were seen in individual patients. This collection of patient data demonstrates the necessity for surgical intervention in an already painful sub-ankylotic subtalar joint. This finding is in accordance with reports in the literature. Relevant findings are the percentage of problems related to the deformity of the hindfoot in the frontal as well as the sagittal plane, and the painful symptoms caused by skeletal impingement (tibiotarsal, peroneal-calcaneus) and by the entrapment of nerve branches (tibial nerve).

Table 1
Fractures of the calcaneus (1989–2000)*

Problem	Number of patients (%)
Subtalar joint pain	59 (58.41)
Axial defects	
Frontal plane	
hindfoot valgus	16 (15.84)
hindfoot varus	28 (27.72)
Sagittal plane	
reduction of the anterior inclination of the talus	27 (26.73)
10° limited dorsiflexion	32 (31.68)
syndrome of distal tibio-peroneal syndesmosis	9 (8.91)
subtalar syndrome	6 (5.94)
Tibialis nerve syndrome	19 (18.81)
Calcaneal-fibular impingement	14 (13.86)
Claw toes	8 (7.92)
Bony plantar protrusions	4 (3.96)
Sural nerve syndrome	3 (2.97)

  * Results of 101 patients (54 male, 47 female) operated for one or more problems secondary to the outcomes of the fracture.

It is also evident that in many cases the patient's discomfort is caused by the totality of the separate problems (eg, a painful subtalar joint plus a painful calcaneofibular conflict and tibialis at the tarsal tunnel, or a paresthetic sensation of the sural nerve in calcaneal varus plus a painful external overload of the foot and tenderness of the tibiotarsal and subtalar joints). To these problems may be added a painful contracture of the toes or a painful plantar bony protrusion. Such developments make obvious the importance of repairing in the acute phase all the deformations that may later cause such problems.

In the authors' series, only six patients had arthrodesis of the subtalar joint with the calcaneus in correct axis. In all the other cases it was necessary to correct axial defects in the frontal (varus deviations prevail over valgus deviations) and sagittal planes.

The subtalar joint pain associated with axial deviations in the sagittal plane is the most difficult problem to resolve. The reduction of the anterior inclination of the talus resulting from the flatness of the calcaneus is often seen when the subtalar joint is highly disordered and the calcaneus is considerably shortened. The need simultaneously to resolve the pain resulting from the residual articulation and to correct the reduction of the anterior inclination of the talus leads to often difficult osteo-arthroresections with bone wedge addition. The same is true for the resolution of distal tibio-peroneal syndesmosis.

Summary

The authors believe it is important to underline the problems associated with the late sequelae of the calcaneus fractures to emphasize the importance of surgical treatment. In the past, emphasis was placed avoiding osteoarthritis of the posterior-subtalar joint; the other sequelae that often cause of severe functional disabilities were disregarded.

It now has been ascertained that the restoration of the mobility of the subtalar joint is always partial and is limited to 50% of the cases treated, regardless of the method of treatment.

According to Claustre [53], posttraumatic arthritic manifestations of this joint occur in 50% of thalamic fractures (independent of type of fracture and treatment approach). According to Roncalli and colleagues [54], this incidence is instead always present.

According to Senis [55] osteoarthritis occurs in 50% of the fractures surgically treated. Slatis and Coll [56] report that this outcome is observed in 74% of the patients who have had a calcaneus fracture (similar to the 75% reported by Lance [57]); this percentage rises to 80% in thalamic fractures with depression. Frankel and colleagues [58] report frequent involvement of the subtalar joint, even in minimal and correctly treated fractures.

Wagner and colleagues [59] have demonstrated through experimental studies how functional alterations of the subtalar joint caused by changes in the direction of the forces may occur as the result of even minimal persisting movements, consequent to articular calcaneus fractures or traumatic chondral lesions. Ischemia that occurs in the acute phase, even after reconstruction, could cause secondary degenerative arthrosis.

On the other hand, if the joint is in the intermediate functional position, the nonpainful stiffness of the subtalar joint leads to a good functional compensation without damage to the body structures or to the hindfoot and without secondary biomechanical metatarsalgia.

Surgical treatment does not guarantee absence of residual incongruence of the thalamic surface, nor does it repair the cartilage damage (the source of secondary arthrosis and functional mobility limitation), but it allows the relationship between the talus and calcaneus to be re-established in the various planes. Nonpainful subanchylosis of the subtalar joint may be an expected and satisfactory result.

On the other hand, because the causes of pain and functional alterations over a long period of time do not depend solely on the thalamic factor, it is evident that treatment must not be limited to trying to re-establish the congruence of the subtalar joint. Instead, treatment must aim at correcting, insofar as possible, all potential factors that may cause secondary problems. Therefore, one must take into consideration

Re-establishing calcaneal height

Reducing the widening deformities

Reducing the lateral and plantar protrusions

Re-establishing the correct axis of the posterior external fragment in the frontal plane (controlling the final varus-valgus)

Possible lysis of the tarsal tunnel

Hence, in a complex fracture, the critical factor seems to be re-establishing the overall form of the calcaneus in all three planes and restoring the relations in the three poles: the anterior process, the thalamus, and the posterior tuberosity, with as correct as possible an orientation of the articular facets in the body in relation to the bone.

There are biologic injuries caused by the trauma—cartilage damage, crushing or blunt trauma of the adipose subcalcaneal pad, fibrosis of the plantar structures—that may not be corrected by surgery and may influence the final functional result.

The goal therefore is to try to correct as much damage as possible in the acute phase to avoid deferring to the later phase of stabilized lesions a surgical procedure that would essentially be a salvage procedure, often difficult to perform and with uncertain results.

Arthrodesis of the subtalar joint alone does not present particular difficulties if it is performed as a later procedure in a calcaneus that has been normalized, with the hindfoot aligned and in the absence of any associated problems (which would have already been dealt with in the acute phase). Arthrodesis may be easily performed through a contained access, trans-senotarsic by simple decortication, and stable intraoperative synthesis to avoid the use of a plaster cast and to allow rapid recovery.

Among the complications are the algodystrophic syndromes that are reported in varying but significant percentages in all patient series. The authors are convinced that the eventual development of the algodystrophy is closely related to the persistence of pain and to prolonged, rigid immobilization of the foot.

Pain may be relieved or attenuated in the immediate postfracture period by early intervention. Posttraumatic edema, deep hematomas, osseous disorder, and the stretching of the nerve branches are all pain-causing elements that benefit from early care. The hematomas are drained, the dislocated fragments (especially the articular ones) are recomposed, and the nerve branches are relaxed.

Delaying the operation in the hope of spontaneous reduction of the swelling or, even worse, conservative treatment after possibly insufficient reductions, with the foot immobilized in a plaster cast in which the intense pain is unrelieved, are conditions that favor the development of the worst algodystrophic syndromes.

The second element, the reduction of foot movement through the use of rigid orthosis, is overcome by obtaining stable intraoperative synthesis, using metallic fixation methods appropriate to the individual case.

What the foot poorly tolerates is not the absence of weight bearing but immobilization: the syntheses that are surgically obtained must allow the active mobilization of all the joints within a brief period of time (ie, 15 days after the operation). A simple below-knee splint is used for protection only during ambulation (without weight bearing), which should be permitted on the second day after the operation.

The authors' have found that, in the acute-phase treatment of all displaced fractures of the calcaneus, independent of the type of soft tissue involvement, the incidence of severe algodystrophic syndromes is statistically insignificant.

Stable synthesis, early mobilization, and ambulation with crutches without weight bearing also offer the best prevention against vascular problems such as phlebitis, thrombophlebitis, and deep vein thrombosis.

References

[1] Dragonetti M. Nuovo metodo di cura incruenta delle fratture del calcagno. Bollettino della Società Medico Chirurgica di Pavia 1945;4:1–19.

[2] Macioce D. Sul trattamento incruento delle fratture talamiche calcaneali. Archivo di Ortopedia Istituto per la diffusione di Opere Scientifiche, Milano 1961;74:486–99.

[3] Dragonetti L. A proposito del trattamento incruento delle fratture di calcagno. Arch Ortop 1969;82:381–94.

[4] Roncalli-Benedetti L, Scaraglio C. Risultati a distanza nel trattamento incruento delle fratture calamiche di calcagno. Minerva Ortop 1973;24:534–7.

[5] Piccoli E, Barelli M. Un metodo di riduzione incruenta delle fratture talamiche di calcagno. Bollettino e Memorie della Società Tosco Umbra di Chirurgia 1975;36:3–12.

[6] Jacchia GE, Bardelli M, Gusso MI, et al. Il trattamento incruento nelle fratture talamiche di calcagno. Chirurgia del Piede 1983;7:181–8.

[7] Capozzi A, Semeraro F, Ghirelli D, et al. Il trattamento funzionale nelle fratture di calcagno. Chirurgia del Piede 1982;6:215–8.

[8] Costanzo D, Pisano L. Revisione clinica di pazienti con fratture talamiche di calcagno scomposte trattate incruentemente. Chirurgia del Piede 1983;7:335–8.

[9] Maiotti A, Battaglia A, Barbaro V. Il trattamento incruento e funzionale delle fratture di calcagno. Chirurgia del Piede 1984;8:79–84.

[10] Hanam SR, Dale SJ. Conservative treatment of calcaneal fractures: a preliminary report. J Foot Surg 1985;24:127–30.

[11] Martinelli B, Lubrano G, Frausin L, et al. Il trattamento incruento delle fratture di calcagno. Atti Congr "Fratture del calcagno. SIMCP Bologna: Aulo Gaggi 1994;3:81–8.

[12] Manes E, Barbato M, Sodano R. Le fratture di calcagno: trattamento funzionale. Atti Congr. "Fratture del calcagno. SIMCP Bologna: Aulo Gaggi 1994;3:99–104.

[13] Scarfì G, Leonardo P, Liotta P. Il trattamento incruento nelle fratture di calcagno. Chirurgia del Piede 1994;18:199–202.

[14] Senis G. La riduzione cruenta delle fratture del calcagno con infossamento talamico: esiti a distanza. Atti e Memorie della SOTIMI 1996;13:353–9.

[15] Pisani G. Considerazioni sul trattamento delle fratture talamiche di calcagno. Chirurgia del Piede 1978;2:9–16.

[16] Lanzetta A, Meani E. Indicazione operatoria nelle fratture del calcagno. Problemi di riduzione ed osteosintesi. Ital J Orthop Traumatol 1978;4:31–6.

[17] Rosa G, Bova A, Coppola D, et al. Il trattamento chirurgico delle fratture del calcagno. Chirurgia del Piede 1986;10:35–9.

[18] Paparoni E, Delfanti M. Trattamento chirurgico delle fratture calamiche con infossamento del calcagno. Chirurgia del Piede 1989;13:101–5.

[19] De Simon PA, Pecchia P, Bonetti E, et al. -Il trapianto cortico-spongioso massivo nel trattamento delle fratture talamiche di calcagno. Annuali Società Ortopedia e Traumatologia Italia Centrale 1991;4:145–52.

[20] Andreasi A. Trattamento chirurgico delle fratture del calcagno. Chirurgia del Piede 1992;16:273–6.

[21] Zwipp H, Tscherne H, Thermann H, et al. Osteosynthesis of displaced intraarticular fractures of the calcaneus. Clin Orthop Rel Res 1993;290:76–86.

[22] Frankel JP, Anderson CD. The use of a calcaneal reconstruction plate in intraarticular calcaneal fractures. J Foot Ankle Surg 1996;35:318–30.

[23] Copin G, De Smedt M. L'osteosynthése stable des fractures thalamiques du calcanéus par la plaque multitrous Greco. Med Chir Pied 1999;15:42–6.

[24] Milano L, Chiacchio C, Grippi M, et al. La reconstruction du thalamus enfancé par fracture. Chirurgia del Piede 1981;5:235–6.

[25] Pisani G. Il trapianto sostitutivo del calcagno nel trattamento delle fratture talamiche. Minerva Ortop 1981;32:271–6.

[26] Leriche R. A propos des fractures du calcaneus. 44ᵉ Congrès Franc De Chir. In: Masson, editor. Paris: Livre de Congrès; 1935. p. 680–3.

[27] Palmer I. The mechanism and treatment of fractures of the calcaneus: open reduction of the use of cancellous grafts. J Bone Joint Surg [Am] 1948;30:28–31.

[28] Essex L, Presti P. The mechanism reduction technique and results in fractures of the os calcis. Br J Surg 1952;39:395–419.

[29] Copin G. -Les fractures du calcanéum. Chirurgia del Piede 1981;5:219–27.

[30] Vigroux JP, Goutallier D. Influence des resultats anatomique final sur le resultai fonctionnelle des fractures thalamiques du calcanéum. Rev Chir Orthop Reparatrice Appar Mot 1989;(Suppl 75): 99–105.

[31] Stephenson J. Displaced fractures of the os calcis involving the subtalar joint: the key rode of the superomedial fragment. Foot Ankle 1983;2:91–101.

[32] Burdeaux Jr BD. The medial approach for calcaneal fractures. Clin Orthop 1989;3(290):96–7.

[33] Letournel E. Open treatment of acute calcaneal fractures. Clin Orthop 1993;290:60–7.

[34] Monsey RD, Levine BP. Operative treatment of acute displaced intra-articular calcaneus fractures. Foot Ankle 1995;l6(2):57–63.

[35] Paley D, Hall H. Intra-articular fractures of the calcaneus. J Bone J Surg [Am] 1993;75:342–54.

[36] Sanders R, Fortin P. Operative treatment in 120 displaced intra-articular calcaneal fractures. Results using a prognostic CT scan classification. Clin Orthop 1993;290:87–95.

[37] Zwipp H, Tscherne H. Ostheosyntesis of displaced intra-articular fractures of the calcaneus. Clin Orthop 1993;290:76–86.

[38] Sartoris D, Resnick D. Diagnostic imaging approach to calcaneal fractures. J Foot Surg 1987; 26:524–9.

[39] Grandi A, Querin F, Neri M. La TC nelle fratture calcaneari. In: Martinelli B, editor. Riunione Internazionale in Medicina e Chirurgia del Piede. Trieste: Libreria Goliardica; 1989. p. 27–38.

[40] Neri M, Querin F. La TC nelle fratture di calcagno. Ital J Orthop Traumatol 1990;l6:137–42.

[41] Magnan B, Montanari M, Bragantini A, et al. A system for prognostic evaluation of CT imaging of heel fractures: the score analysis Verona (SAVE). Foot Dis 1994;2:19–25.

[42] Ebraheim NA, Biyani A, Padanilam T, et al. A pitfall of coronal computed tomographic imaging in evaluation to calcaneal fractures. Foot Ankle 1996;17:503–5.

[43] Pisani G, Milano L. Le osteotomie correttive del calcagno in esiti di frattura. Fratture del calcagno. Bologna. Aulo Gaggi 1994;3:207–12.

[44] Dwyer FC. Osteotomy of the calcaneum for pes cavus. J Bone Joint Surg [Br] 1959;41(1):80–6.

[45] Pisani G. La talizzazione dell'astragalo negli esiti di frattura del calcagno. Chirurgia del Piede 1992;16:289–93.

[46] Carr JB, Hansens T, Bernischke SR. Subtalar distraction bone block fusion for late complications of os calcis fractures. Foot Ankle 1981;5(2):81–6.

[47] Pisani G. La sindrome della sindesmosi tibio-peroneale distale. Chirurgia del Piede 1985;9:179–80.

[48] Le Coeur P. -La pince malléolaire. Atti College International de Charleroi du CIP. Paris: Brd De Fontaine; 1976.

[49] Andreasi A. La sindrome da conflitto calcaneale fibulare negli esiti di frattura del calcagno. Chirurgia del Piede 1996;20:33–8.

[50] Milano L. -Artropatia di tibia-carsica nelle fratture malconsolidate di calcagno. Comunicaz XXIII Congr Soc It Med Chirurgia del Piede. Montegrotto Tenne, May 31, 1990.

[51] Ebraheim NA, Biyani A, Padanilam T, et al. Calcaneocuboid joint in involvement in calcaneal fractures. Foot Ankle 1996;17:563–5.

[52] Piccolo P, Sanfilippo A, Corsello C, et al. La sindrome seno-tarsica in esiti a fratture di calcagno. Chirurgia del Piede 1988;12:87–91.

[53] Claustre J, Simon L. Le traitement médical des sèquelles de fractures de calcanéum. Rhumatologie 1979;31:17–9.

[54] Roncalli-Benedetti L, Straglio C. Risultati a distanza nel trattamento incruento delle fratture talamiche di calcagno. Minerva Ortop 1973;24:534–7.

[55] Senis G. La riduzione cruenta delle fratture di calcagno con infossamento talamico; esiti a distanza. Atti e Memorie SOTIMI 1966;13:353–9.

[56] Slatis P, Kiviluoto A, Santavirta S. Fractures of the calcaneus. Acta Ortop Scand 1979;50:361–7.

[57] Lance EM, Care FJJ, Wade PA. Fractures of the os calcis: treatment by early mobilizatio-. Clin Orthop 1963;30:76–90.

[58] Frankel J, Turf R, Miller G. -Cult fractures of the talus. J Foot Surg 1992;31:538–43.

[59] Wagner UA, Ananthakrishnan D, Sangeorzan BJ, et al. Influence of talar neck and intraarticular calcaneal fractures on subtalar joint mechanics. Foot Ankle Surgery (ESFAS) 1996;2:19–26.

ELSEVIER
SAUNDERS

Clin Podiatr Med Surg
23 (2006) 375–422

CLINICS IN
PODIATRIC
MEDICINE AND
SURGERY

Ankle Fractures

Denise M. Mandi, DPM[a,b,*], W. Ashton Nickles, DPM[a],
Vincent J. Mandracchia, DPM, MS[a,b],
Jennifer B. Halligan, DPM[a], Patris A. Toney, DPM, MPH[a]

[a]Division of Podiatric Surgery, Department of Surgery, Broadlawns Medical Center,
1801 Hickman Road, Des Moines, IA 50314, USA
[b]College of Podiatric Medicine and Surgery, Des Moines University, 3200 Grand Avenue,
Des Moines, IA 50312-4198, USA

Injuries to the ankle are an extremely common occurrence, accounting for more than 1 million visits to the physician's office and emergency room yearly [1,2]. Although most of these injuries are diagnosed as sprains, fractures must be ruled out [3]. It is estimated that 260,00 ankle fractures occur each year in the United States. Twenty-five percent undergo surgical intervention [4]. Injuries to the ankle involve both soft tissue and bone (Fig. 1A and B). Both components must be addressed to limit short- and long-term disability. The ultimate goal is to restore normal anatomy and function. This restoration can be accomplished only with a proper and thorough understanding of the anatomy, biomechanical function, mechanisms of injury, the principles of fracture healing, and fixation techniques.

As Bohler [5] stated, "the joints that are no longer congruent are therefore abraded. With time, the greater the displacement, the more pronounced the arthritic changes. The ankle joint remains permanently painful." The function of the ankle joint relies on its exact congruity. Any malalignment must be recognized and restored to avoid complications.

The ankle joint is not an inherently stable joint. Intrinsic and extrinsic musculature, as well as its own osseous architecture, provides stability [6,7]. During ambulation, the ankle joint must withstand 1.25 to 5.5 times the normal

* Corresponding author. 1791 Hickman Road, Des Moines, IA 50314.
  E-mail address: dmandi@broadlawns.org (D.M. Mandi).

0891-8422/06/$ – see front matter © 2006 Elsevier Inc. All rights reserved.
doi:10.1016/j.cpm.2006.02.001

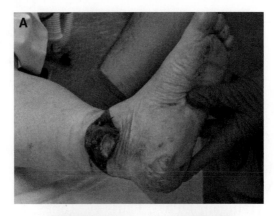

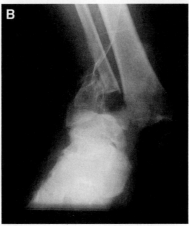

Fig. 1. (*A*, *B*) Significant open fracture dislocation of the ankle with exposed distal tibia.

body weight, depending on the activity [8]. Its motion involves dorsiflexion and plantarflexion and internal and external rotation. It also must accommodate inversion and eversion because of its proximity to the subtalar joint.

Management of ankle injuries requires a thorough knowledge of the anatomic structures involved and a thorough evaluation of the damage severity [9,10]. These injuries may involve bone, articular surfaces, ligaments, tendon, nerves, and blood vessels. The skin must not be overlooked or discounted, because as it can create further complications [11]. Systemic illness must also be taken into account, especially with the rise in the diabetic population and the increased morbidity and complications caused by that disease [12]. Once evaluation and identification are performed, results are relatively predictable. Operative treatment is fast becoming the treatment of choice over more conservative reduction and casting.

Anatomy

As mentioned previously, a thorough understanding of the anatomy and mechanics of the ankle joint is paramount for its successful treatment. The anatomy is well known and adequately reported [9,13,14]. The tibia, fibula, and talus make up the osseous components. The hinge- or mortise-type joint is formed with the talus situated between the tibial and fibular malleoli in a structural arrangement known as the malleolar fork [9,15].

The major load-bearing area of the ankle joint is formed between the tibia and talus. The tibial plafond is concave to match the talar dome with the anterior and posterior aspects projecting more distally. The anterior aspect of the talus is approximately 25% wider than the posterior aspect, which corresponds to the tibial plafond [9]. Inman [6] quantifies this difference as 2.4 ± 1.3 mm. This highly congruous surface between the pilon (tibia) and talar dome is flanked medially by the distal tibial extension and laterally by the distal fibula. These articulations form the medial and lateral gutters, respectively (Fig. 2). The medial malleolus is further divided into two projections, the anterior and posterior colliculi, with a groove between them. The lateral surface is covered with articular cartilage corresponding to the medial talus. The anterior colliculus provides the attachment for the superficial deltoid ligament. This ligament travels distally to the talus, navicular, and calcaneus but does not provide the majority of stability to the joint. The primary medial stabilizer of the ankle is the deep portion of the deltoid ligament, which attaches to the posterior colliculus and the intercollicular groove (Fig. 3). This function was proven by Harper [16] and Michelson and colleagues [17] who demonstrated talar instability only after sectioning the deep portion of the medial collateral ligament. This work indicates the type of repair necessary for restoring ligamentous stability [8].

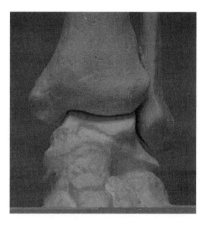

Fig. 2. Sawbones ankle model clearly demonstrating the highly congruous surface articulation between the distal tibia and superior talus. The medial and lateral gutter spaces are also noted.

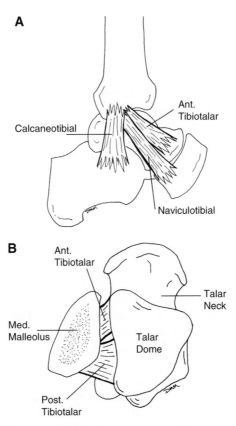

Fig. 3. (*A*, *B*) Demonstration of the deltoid ligament as the primary medial stabilizer of the ankle. (*From* Mandracchia DM, Mandracchia VJ, Buddecke DE. Malleolar fractures of the ankle. Clin Podiatr Med Surg 1999;679–723; with permission.)

The lateral tibia forms a shallow groove for its articulation with the distal fibula, the anterior portion or tubercle (Chaput's or Tillaux-Chaput's tubucle), and the smaller posterior tubercle. The triangular lateral malleolus ends with the styloid, its postero-distal projection. The three lateral collateral ligaments provide stability. First, the anterior talo-fibular ligament is an intracapsular thickening running from the anterior fibular malleoli to the talus. It prevents anterior excursion of the talus from the leg. It is the weakest and most frequently injured ligament. The calcaneo-fibular ligament is a cordlike structure extending from the distal fibula (styloid) to the lateral calcaneus and primarily prevents talar tilt. These first two ligaments form a 105° angle in the sagittal plane [6,18,19]. Injuries to these ligaments are the most common injuries incurred during ankle sprains [20]. The posterior talo-fibular ligament extends from the fossa of the lateral malleolus to the postero-lateral talus (Fig. 4).

Posteriorly, the distal tibia provides restraint to posterior dislocation/translation of the talus [21,22]. Its posterior lip of the distal plafond provides the

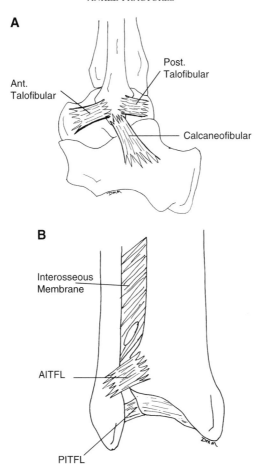

Fig. 4. (*A, B*) Diagram of the lateral collateral ankle ligaments and the syndesmosis. (*From* Mandracchia DM, Mandracchia VJ, Buddecke DE. Malleolar fractures of the ankle. Clin Podiatr Med Surg 1999;679–723; with permission.)

insertion for the posterior inferior tibiofibular syndesmotic ligament. It does not escape injury, however, especially with rotational fractures. It is the third malleolus in the well-documented trimalleolar fractures. When 50% of the articular surface of this posterior malleolus is fractured, a subsequent 35% reduction in contact pressure occurs at the distal tibio-talar articulation, which will lead to significant degenerative joint sequelae. Therefore, the literature indicates that a posterior malleolus fracture that involves 25% to 35% of the articular surface should undergo open reduction with fixation [9,21–24]. One author advocates routine fixation of all posterior malleolar fractures [25]. The authors regularly repair posterior fractures of 30% or greater, with Vassal's phenomenon providing adequate reduction with the smaller fragments.

The syndesmosis, along with the deltoid ligament, contributes to the rotational stability of the ankle joint. It is made up of three important structures, which together unite the distal fibula and tibia. First, the anterior inferior tibiofibular ligament (AITFL) runs oblique and distal from the anterolateral tubercle of the tibia (Chaput's tubercle) to the anterior portion of the lateral malleolus (Wagstaff's tubercle). Second, the posterior inferior tibiofibular ligament (PITFL) runs oblique and distal from the posterior malleolus, Volkmann's tubercle, and is distinguished from a similar fibrocartilaginous connection between the tibia and fibula, the inferior transverse tibiofibular ligament. Last, the tibiofibular interosseous membrane begins a short distance above the ankle and eventually becomes the interosseous ligament running proximally the entire length of the tibia and fibula.

The incidence of syndesmotic injury in association with ankle sprains has been estimated to be between 1% and 11% [26,27], with the AITFL being the most commonly ruptured ligament in ankle fractures [15]. If the syndesmosis fails in an ankle injury, the fibular malleolus displaces laterally, and the talus follows, losing its normal relationship with the weight-bearing surface of the tibial plafond [28–30]. This displacement usually occurs with external rotation mechanisms [31]. When combined with a deltoid ligament rupture, the area of the syndesmosis most likely to fail is 3 to 4.5 cm above the mortise. An intact deltoid contributes significantly to talar stability, helps preserve the syndesmosis, and in many cases eliminates the need for syndesmotic fixation.

Biomechanics

In the normal, healthy ankle joint, sagittal-plane motion predominates. Coronal- and transverse-plane motion also occurs, however [32,33]. It is generally accepted that 10° of dorsiflexion and 25° of plantarflexion are required for normal ambulation [34], but a much wider range has been reported [32,35–38]. There are two schools of thought regarding the axis of motion of the ankle joint. Inman [6] describes the empiric ankle joint axis, passing postero-inferior from medial to lateral just below the malleoli. The actual axis of the ankle joint is more oblique than the joint surface. The joint surface of the tibial plafond is angled in the coronal plane relative to the midline of the tibia; however, it is oriented in the opposite direction to the ankle joint, which causes an average of 3° valgus angulation of the ankle (Fig. 5A, B).

During range of motion, the ankle joint remains congruent [39,40]. This congruity is crucial because of the forces that travel through the joint during the gait cycle, especially at heel rise [41,42]. The contact area varies from 1.5 to 9.4 cm^2, depending on the load and position of the ankle [43]. This variation in contact area becomes increasingly important given the incongruities that occur in the joint after injury. Ramsey and Hamilton [29] stated that a slight lateral displacement of the talus (1 mm) causes a significant decrease (42%) in ankle joint contact-surface area. Harris and Fallat [44] presented similar findings. Other

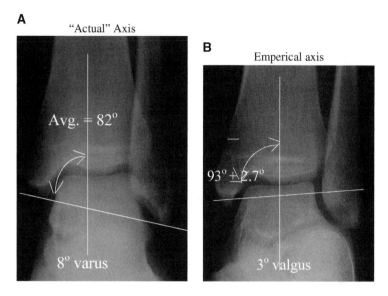

Fig. 5. (*A, B*) The actual and empirical axes of the ankle joint. With the joint surface of the tibial plafond angled in the coronal plane relative to the midline of the tibia, the empirical axis demonstrates a 3° valgus orientation of the ankle. (*From* Mandracchia DM, Mandracchia VJ, Buddecke DE. Malleolar fractures of the ankle. Clin Podiatr Med Surg 1999;679–723; with permission.)

authors have demonstrated increased stress with lateral talar shifting in the presence of a large posterior malleolar fracture fragment [23,45,46].

The joint surface has been likened to a portion of a frustum of a cone, the axis of which is the ankle's axis of motion [6]. The obliquity of the ankle joint axis produces relative medial deviation of the foot (internal rotation) with plantarflexion and relative lateral deviation (external rotation) with dorsiflexion (Fig. 6A, B) [7].

The gait cycle is divided into three stance phases. From its starting point at heel-strike in dorsiflexion, the foot will plantarflex to 18° to maximize pronation. The foot then dorsiflexes again, reaching its neutral position at midstance. The oblique axis of the ankle joint determines the relative motion of the leg [7]. Because of the structure of the ankle joint and its more medial position on the calcaneus, the leg bones will move internally or externally during the gait cycle. In other words, the foot dictates the accompanying rotation of the tibia and fibula. The anterior muscles are contracting, and the leg bones are internally rotating, allowing a compensatory pronation of the subtalar joint. Heel-rise begins with continued plantarflexion of the foot. The long flexors of the foot actively control the forward motion of the tibia on the talus. The leg bones externally rotate, coupled with subtalar supination, to create a more rigid construct. During propulsion, the ankle plantarflexes from its extreme dorsiflexed position to a little more than 10° of plantar position. The posterior musculature continues to

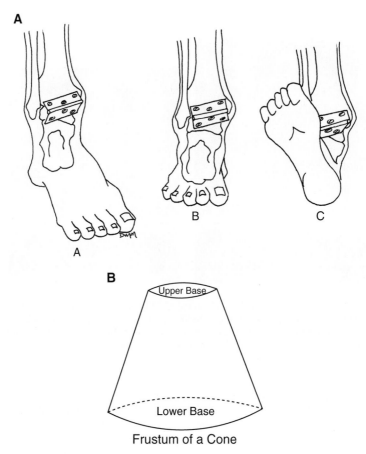

Fig. 6. The frustum of a cone design to the ankle joint surface allowing internal rotation with plantarflexion and external rotation with dorsiflexion. (*A*) Three views of ankle joint as a hinge-type joint. (*B*) Frustum. (*From* Mandracchia DM, Mandracchia VJ, Buddecke DE. Malleolar fractures of the ankle. Clin Podiatr Med Surg 1999;685; with permission.)

contract, the leg externally rotates, and the subtalar continues to supinate in preparation for toe-off.

Pathogenesis of ankle fracture

The position of the foot, forces acting upon it, and the velocity of the injury are the major players in any type of fracture, with the talus playing the major role [47]. In low-velocity injuries, the soft tissue structures have time to stretch and will avulse bone. Higher-velocity injuries cause rupture of the soft tissue structures before fracture. Using a childhood toy, "Silly Putty" helps to demonstrate this phenomenon. Moved slowly, the putty stretches; similarly, a ligament puts significant stretch on its attached bone until Young's modulus of elasticity allows failure of the bone and an avulsion fracture occurs perpendicular to the pull of the ligament. Pulling the putty apart quickly, however, results in breakage with a snap; likewise high-velocity stresses rupture the ligament structure.

The major motions of the talus include external rotation, adduction, abduction, and axial compression. These motions are usually coupled [47]. With the foot in the inverted position, the lateral structures are tight, making them more prone to injury. Conversely, with the foot everted, the medial structures are at a higher risk [48].

Classification

There are many classification schemes for ankle fracture and much literature evaluating those classification systems and their ease of use [47,49–61]. Ashhurst and Bromer [52] published the first such scheme in 1912. They based their classification on the mechanisms of injury and grouped them as external rotation, abduction, and adduction injuries. Currently, the two major schemes in use are the Danis-Weber [48] and the Lauge-Hansen systems [62–66]. As with all classification schemes, there are three main goals: to facilitate communication among treating physicians, to provide the basis for the selection of treatment options, and to predict outcomes.

Danis-Weber classification

The Danis-Weber Arbeitsgemeinschaft für osteosynthesefragen (AO) classification, also referred to as the Muller AO classification, is based on the level of the fibular fracture in relation to the ankle joint [57,67,68]. Many consider this classification to be a practical schematic basis for treatment of fibular malleolar fractures (Table 1) (Fig. 7) [69].

The type A, or infrasyndesmotic, injury occurs when the foot is supinated and an adductory force is applied. This injury begins on the lateral side, which is under tension because of foot position. Either the lateral collateral ligament is

Table 1
Danis-Weber and AO classification of ankle fractures

Type A Infrasyndesmotic	Type B Trans-syndesmotic	Type C Suprasyndesmotic
A1: isolated	B1: isolated	C1: simple diaphyseal fibular fracture
A2: with medial malleolar fracture	B2: with medial malleolar fracture or deltoid rupture	C2: complex diaphyseal fibular fracture
A3: with posteromedial fracture	B3: with medial lesion and posterolateral fracture	C3: proximal fibular fracture

From: From Mandracchia DM, Mandracchia VJ, Buddecke DE. Malleolar fractures of the ankle. Clin Podiatr Med Surg 1999;687; with permission.

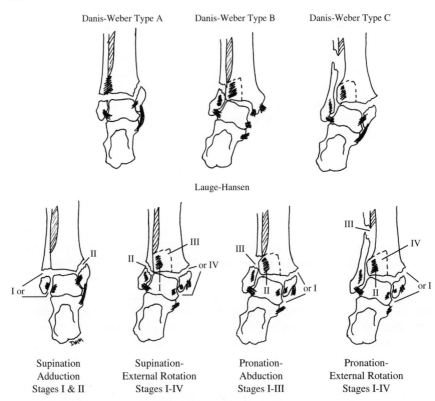

Fig. 7. Danis-Weber (top three illustrations) and Lauge-Hansen (bottom four illustrations) classification schemes. Note the correlations between Danis-Weber type A and Lauge-Hansen supination-adduction injuries, Danis-Weber type B and Lauge-Hansen supination-external rotation and pronation-abduction injuries, and Danis-Weber type C and Lauge-Hansen pronation-external rotation injuries. (*From* Mandracchia DM, Mandracchia VJ, Buddecke DE. Malleolar fractures of the ankle. Clin Podiatr Med Surg 1999;686; with permission.)

ruptured or the distal fibula is avulsed, resulting in a transverse fracture below the level of the ankle joint. If the force continues, a near-vertical fracture of the medial malleolus occurs.

The type B, or transsyndesmotic, injury is by far the most common fracture seen. The pathologic force involved is external rotation of the talus, which initially causes failure of the AITFL. The force may continue causing an oblique, spiral, fibular fracture beginning at the ankle mortise and extending proximal from anterior to posterior. Next, a rupture of the PITFL or Volkman's fracture would occur. Finally, the medial malleolus incurs a transverse fracture, or the deltoid ligament is ruptured.

The type C, or suprasyndesmotic, injury occurs when the foot is pronated, and an external rotary force is applied. This injury begins on the medial side, which is under tension because of foot position. The injury begins with either a deltoid ligament rupture or a medial malleolar avulsion fracture. The injury progresses with the talus externally rotating, causing failure of the AITFL, PITFL, and syndesmotic ligaments, resulting in an indirect fibular fracture above the ankle joint. The exact location of the fracture depends on the extent of syndesmotic rupture; fractures described by Dupuytren (mid-shaft fibula) or Maisonneuve (proximal fibula) are possible.

The Danis-Weber classification is based on the premise that the more proximal the fibular fracture, the higher the likelihood for open reduction and internal fixation (ORIF) as the treatment of choice [47].

Lauge-Hansen classification

In 1940, Lauge-Hansen [56] described a genetic classification scheme based on cadaveric studies that has become a popular and valuable aid to understanding the mechanism of ankle fracture injuries and provides a key to their reduction (Box 1) (Figs. 8–11). His classification system demonstrated a sequence of injuries, with each end point in this scheme represented by a fracture or damaged ligament.

No practical discussion of prognosis was given, because this was a cadaveric study. In fact, Lauge-Hansen [56] stated, "In this study, the mechanism of fracture was determined by fracturing, the pathologic anatomy was ascertained by dissection, the genetic roentgenologic diagnosis was established by roentgen examination, and the genetic reduction technique of the fractures was found by reduction maneuvers."

Lauge-Hansen described five different types of fractures: supination-adduction, pronation-abduction, supination-eversion (external rotation), pronation-eversion (external rotation), and pronation-dorsiflexion (pilon). In this scheme, the terms "eversion" and "external rotation" are used synonymously, which causes confusion in communication. The first part of the name of the fracture mechanism is the position of the foot at the time of injury, either pronated or supinated. The second part of the name indicates the deforming force that was applied: adduction, abduction, or external rotation. There is a correlation between the Lauge-Hansen and the Danis-Weber classification schemes. Lauge-Hansen supination-adduction injuries correspond to Danis-Weber type A, pronation-abduction and supination-external rotation injuries correspond to Danis-Weber type B, and pronation-external rotation injuries correspond to Danis-Weber type C. These categories are not absolutes, however.

Supination-external rotation injuries account for most fractures in this scheme, with Hamilton [9] reporting 40% to 75% prevalence. Supination-adduction injuries account for 10% to 20%; pronation-abduction and pronation-external rotation injuries account for 5% to 21% and 7% to 19%, respectively. In the authors' experience, 70% to 75% of all ankle fractures of the supination-external rotation type.

Christey and Tomlinson [70], in a retrospective study involving 336 ankle fractures, noted that Lauge-Hansen's supination-external rotation predominated in middle-aged women, with most injuries involving a fall at home; men were

---

Box 1. Lauge-Hansen classification of ankle fractures

Supination-adduction

> Tear of the lateral collateral ligaments or transverse avulsion-
> type fracture of the fibula below the joint level
> Near vertical fracture of the medial malleolus

Supination-external rotation

> Rupture of the AITFL
> Spiral oblique distal fibula fracture
> Rupture of the PITFL
> Avulsion fracture of the medial malleolus or deltoid
> ligament rupture

Pronation-abduction

> Transverse avulsion fracture of the medial malleolus or deltoid
> ligament rupture
> Rupture of syndesmotic ligaments or avulsion fracture of
> their insertion
> Short, oblique fracture of the fibula at or slightly above the
> joint level

Pronation-external rotation

> Transverse fracture of the medial malleolus or deltoid
> ligament rupture
> Disruption of the AITFL
> Oblique fracture of the fibula above the level of the joint
> Rupture of the PITFL or posterior lip fracture

From Mandracchia DM, Mandracchia VJ, Buddecke DE. Malleolar fractures of the ankle. Clin Podiatr Med Surg 1999;690;
with permission.

---

more likely to sustain an equal number of supination-external rotation and pronation-external rotation injuries primarily caused by sports activity.

Supination-adduction

The supination-adduction injury pattern begins on the lateral side of the ankle joint complex because of the tension created by the position of the foot.

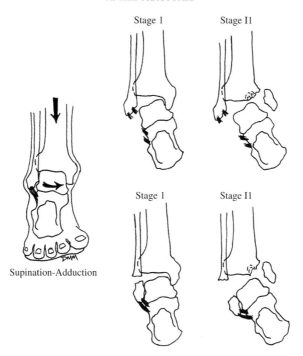

Fig. 8. Lauge-Hansen supination-adduction injury. (*From* Mandracchia DM, Mandracchia VJ, Bud-decke DE. Malleolar fractures of the ankle. Clin Podiatr Med Surg 1999;679–723; with permission.)

Supination-abduction injuries are caused by inversion with two distinct stages. Stage I is a transverse (avulsion) fracture of the distal fibula below the level of the ankle joint or a tear of the lateral collateral ligaments. This injury corresponds with a Danis-Weber type A fracture pattern (Fig. 12). Avulsion fractures are easily recognized by their transverse nature. The pull of the attached ligament or tendon is parallel to the applied force, and the fracture line occurs perpendicular to the applied force. The transverse fracture of the distal fibula is the classic finding in the supination-adduction injuries.

Following fracture or rupture of the lateral structures, the motion continues transverse plane as the talus moves medially and contacts the medial gutter at its most superior pole, causing a near-vertical fracture of the medial malleolus (Fig. 13). This near-vertical fracture is the characteristic finding in supination-adduction II injuries.

A vertical fracture of the medial malleolus may occur without a corresponding fibular fracture. With ligamentous laxity is identified, repeated lateral ankle sprains can lead to medial malleolar fracture. Giachino and Hammond [71] make a definitive distinction between a vertical and oblique fracture of the medial malleolus. Oblique fractures involve dorsiflexion and abduction, whereas vertical fractures result from avulsion rather than impact. These vertical fractures, as seen in supination-adduction II injuries, therefore are unstable.

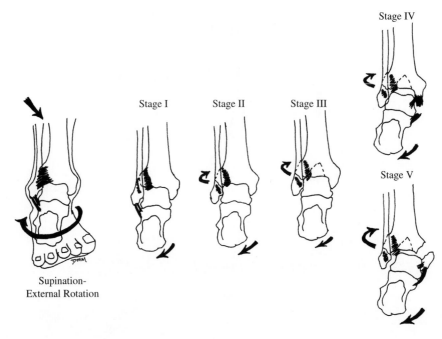

Fig. 9. Lauge-Hansen supination-external rotation injury. (*From* Mandracchia DM, Mandracchia VJ, Buddecke DE. Malleolar fractures of the ankle. Clin Podiat Med Surg 1999;689; with permission.)

Supination-external rotation

As mentioned earlier, supination-external rotation injuries account for the vast majority of ankle fractures. The spiral oblique fracture of the distal fibula beginning anterior-inferior, at the level of the joint, and extending posterior-superior is the hallmark of these injuries (Fig. 14). The fracture pattern occurs predominantly in the frontal plane, and is best observed on a lateral radiograph. The mechanism of this spiral fracture is a rotational shearing force produced by pressure on the fibula and talus while the tibia is internally rotating, usually because the body is falling to the opposite side [72].

As described by Lauge-Hansen [56], a predictable order of injury occurs during this external rotation mechanism, with subsequent failure of ligament or bone. Four stages make up the supination-external rotation scheme. Stage I involves anterior-inferior tibiofibular ligament rupture. Stage II involves the previously described fibular fracture. Continuing around the joint from lateral to medial, stage III involves rupture of the posterior-inferior tibiofibular ligament or posterior malleolar fracture (Volkmann's fracture). Finally, stage IV involves deltoid ligament rupture or avulsion fracture of the medial malleolus (Fig. 15A, B).

The AITFL is the first structure to fail as the talus separates from the tense lateral aspect of the ankle. This process is seen easily during surgical correction

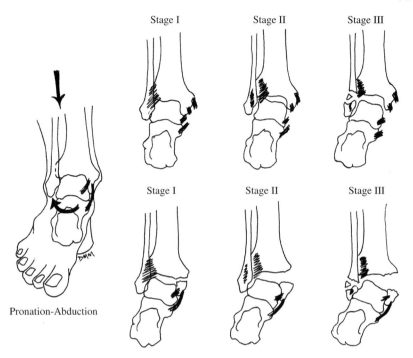

Fig. 10. Lauge-Hansen pronation-abduction injury. (*From* Mandracchia DM, Mandracchia VJ, Buddecke DE. Malleolar fractures of the ankle. Clin Podiatr Med Surg 1999;689; with permission.)

of these injuries. Avulsion fractures from Chaput's tubercle on the tibia (ie, Tilliux-Chaput fracture) or from Wagstaffe's tubercle (ie, Wagstaffe fracture) may be noticed. With the foot supinated or inverted and the lateral collateral ligaments under tension, the talus rotates externally, causing a spiral fibular fracture. With the AITFL ruptured, the anterior aspect of the distal fibula is unstable, but the PITFL remains intact. This situation allows a twisting motion to occur starting at the anterior-inferior aspect of the fibula and progressing posterior and superior as fatigue of the bone occurs. This process explains the spiral nature of the fracture and the reason for its beginning at the level of the plafond. Even with failure of the AITFL and PITFL, the proximal syndesmosis is intact and stabilizes the fibular shaft [8].

Although most supination-external rotation fractures begin at the level of the ankle joint, the same pattern does manifest regularly above the level of the joint (Fig. 16) [73], leading to confusion concerning the mechanism of injury of these fractures and whether they should be classified as supination-external rotation or pronation-external rotation. Whether supination or pronation, spiral fractures of the fibula are caused by pathologic rotational forces that must be addressed and understood at time of treatment.

Stage III of the supination-external rotation fractures involves disruption of the PITFL or fracture of the posterior malleolus, which leads to further instability.

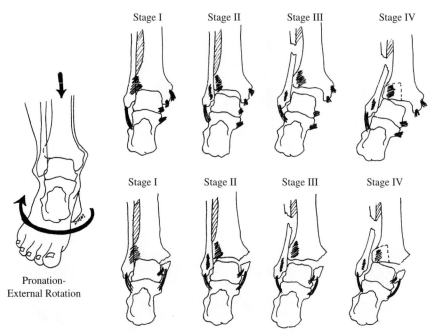

Fig. 11. Lauge-Hansen pronation-external rotation injury. (*From* Mandracchia DM, Mandracchia VJ, Buddecke DE. Malleolar fractures of the ankle. Clin Podiatr Med Surg 1999;690; with permission.)

The tibiofibular syndesmosis is under increased tension, increasing the likelihood of ankle joint dislocation in conjunction with the fracture.

The last component of supination-external rotation injuries involves the medial structures, with rupture of the deltoid apparatus or medial malleolar fracture (Fig. 17). Occasionally, a hybrid lesion is seen, with fracture of the anterior colliculus representing superficial deltoid ligament failure and rupture of the fibers of the deep deltoid ligament although the posterior colliculus remains intact [74]. The importance of evaluating the deltoid ligament in all supination-

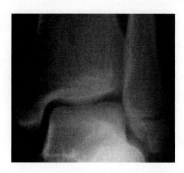

Fig. 12. Supination-adduction ankle fracture corresponding to a Danis-Weber A type injury.

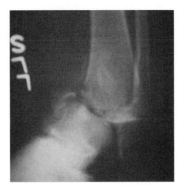

Fig. 13. Near vertical fracture of the medial malleolus.

external rotation injuries cannot be overemphasized. An apparent supination-external rotation stage II fracture of the lateral malleolus may actually be a stage III or stage IV injury with deltoid rupture (Fig. 18). The appearance of lateral talar shift, significant displacement of the fibular fracture, or a posterior lip fracture on initial radiographic examination provides evidence that more than a stage II injury is present. True supination-external rotation stage II injuries are treated well with nonoperative weight bearing [75], although some potential lateral mobility of the talus may be present [26,76–78]. On the other hand, true supination-external rotation IV injuries have a high incidence of talar subluxation, malunion, and ankle arthrosis if not treated surgically. The authors no longer surgically repair all deltoid ligaments with supination-external rotation stage IV injuries. This practice is in agreement with several authors' statements that repair of the deltoid is unnecessary if the lateral malleolus has been properly restored to its anatomic alignment and there is no evidence of the deltoid blocking reduction [16,30,79–82].

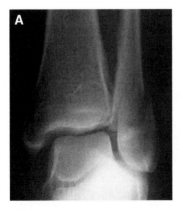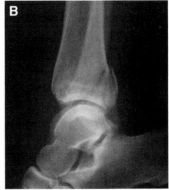

Fig. 14. (A) Anteroposterior and (B) lateral view of the classic spiral oblique fracture associated with supination-external rotation ankle injuries.

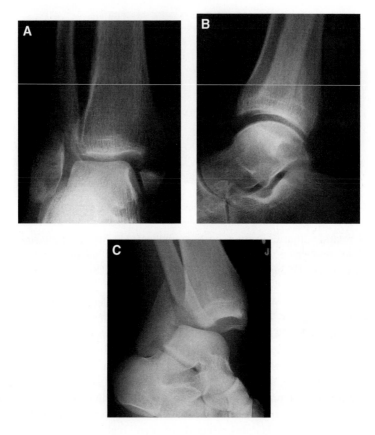

Fig. 15. (*A*, *B*, *C*) Supination external rotation ankle fractures stage IV. Note the avulsion fracture of the medial malleolus and total instability of the ankle joint.

Pronation-abduction

All pronation injuries begin on the medial side secondary to the position of the foot and the structures under tension. The mechanism of this injury is forced abduction of the pronated foot. Because of the force applied, the talus adducts and plantarflexes, positioning the head of the talus medially and placing tensions the medial collateral ligaments. This tension causes a rupture of the deltoid ligament or a transverse/avulsion fracture of the medial malleolus (stage I). As the deforming force continues, the AITFL and PITFL are ruptured simultaneously (stage II), or avulsion fractures occur at their insertions, beginning at the level of the syndesmosis. This process makes the most distal aspect of the fibula unstable, with the interosseous ligament securing the more proximal fibula, and allows a short, oblique (sometimes transverse) fibular fracture (stage III) beginning at the level of the plafond. A butterfly-shaped fragment is often seen with this type of injury, secondary to the proximal fibula being fixed while the distal fibula is free to give way to the continued abductory force (Fig. 19).

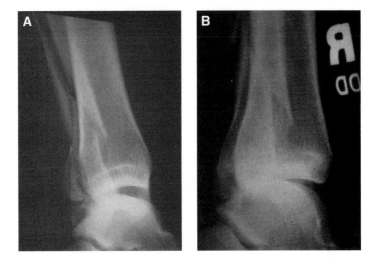

Fig. 16. (*A*, *B*) Radiographs demonstrating a high supination-external rotation fracture pattern.

Confusion may exist between diagnosis of supination-external rotation and pronation abduction injuries because these fractures occur at similar levels. The patterns of the fractures are usually readily distinguishable however. Pronation-abduction fibular fractures are usually short, oblique or transverse, and often are laterally comminuted because the bending forces applied to the fibula cause medial tension and lateral compression [8]. Some of these injuries may be hybrids, however, initiated by abduction followed by rotation about the axis of the PITFL [83]. Limbird and Aaron [84] emphasized that these injuries may have an associated impaction fracture of the lateral plafond that is analogous to the supination-external rotation pattern.

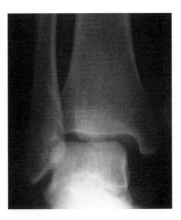

Fig. 17. Bimalleolar ankle fracture with distal fibular osseous involvement and an increase in the medial gutter space.

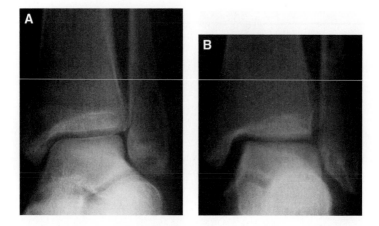

Fig. 18. (*A*, *B*) Supination-external rotation stage II or IV. The subtlety of the injury can cause confusion in the classification scheme.

Although it is not a true hybrid fracture, the authors occasionally have observed two distinct fracture lines in the distal fibula with supination-external rotation and pronation-abduction injuries. They have theorized that, as these fractures progress at the moment of injury; the patient makes a conscious attempt to reverse the deforming force (abduction or rotation) and thereby adds a further component to the orientation of the fibular fracture.

Some pronation-abduction fractures (similar to the supination-external rotation fracture), may present above the plafond level. In this case, the proximal syndesmotic architecture may not be able to stabilize the tibiofibular relationship, making intraoperative evaluation of the syndesmosis imperative.

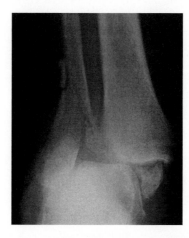

Fig. 19. Pronation ankle injury demonstrating a classic butterfly fragment of the fibula.

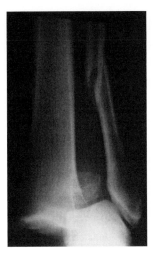

Fig. 20. Radiograph demonstrating a severe pronation-external rotation fracture dislocation of the ankle.

Pronation-external rotation

The pathognomonic fracture seen in pronation-external rotation injuries is a spiral, oblique fracture running posterior-inferior to anterior-superior (opposite of supination-external rotation) and beginning above the level of the syndesmosis (Fig. 20) [73,85]. There are four stages in the progression of these injuries, beginning medially and working their way around to the lateral side. Stage I consists of a deltoid ligament tear or avulsion fracture of the medial malleolus. Stage II involves rupture of the AITFL and leads into the classic stage III high

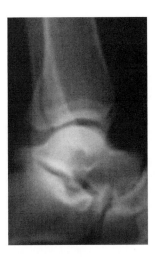

Fig. 21. Posterior malleolar (Volkman's) fracture of the tibia.

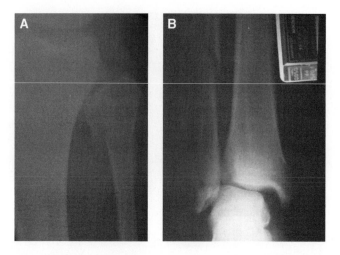

Fig. 22. (*A*) Maisonneuve fracture of the proximal fibula. (*B*) Dupuytrens' mid-shaft fibula fracture.

fibular fracture. Stage IV involves a rupture of the PITFL or a Volkmann's fracture of the posterior malleolus (Fig. 21). Confusion can exist between a high supination-external rotation fracture that can occur above the level of the syndesmosis and a pronation-external rotation fracture [73,85].

This mechanism is also responsible for higher fibular fractures involving the midshaft (Dupuytren), or fibular neck (Maisonneuve's fracture). These fractures may be isolated or involve the other malleoli (Fig. 22). Therefore, when evaluating an isolated medial or posterior malleolar fracture, the treating physician should be suspicious of a high fibular fracture [8]; because of the progression of the fracture, the syndesmosis probably will be damaged, requiring primary repair during malleolar fixation.

Evaluation

History and physical examination

Patients who have ankle fractures or witnesses of the injury usually will be able to describe the mechanism of injury for the treating physician. They will describe the position of the foot (dorsiflexed or plantarflexed) and the motion during injury (inversion or eversion). They may describe a twisting or a "popping" sensation on the medial or lateral ankle.

Timing of the injury is important when dealing with open fractures and possible contamination (Fig. 23) [86,87]. Systemic illnesses, such as diabetes, clearly affect overall patient management [12,88]. Smoking is a well-documented deterrent to wound and fracture healing [89,90].

The physical examination must be done systematically. Obvious deformity (eg, severe dislocation or an open fracture) makes diagnosis and early inter-

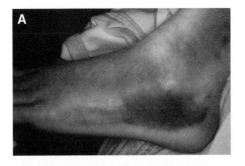

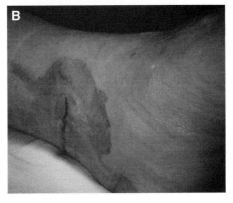

Fig. 23. (*A*) Dependent ecchymosis and edema following an acute ankle fracture. Edema must be reduced before surgical intervention. (*B*) Open ankle fracture necessitating conversion of a contaminated environment into a clean environment.

vention easier. The ankle should be inspected circumferentially and thoroughly, however. This inspection enables the examiner to go beyond the initial findings and detect on more subtle injuries that may have occurred [8].

Vascular examination of the foot is vital. Check for pulses and capillary refill time. If pulses are not easily palpable, Doppler examination must be performed. Because three major arteries cross the joint, it is unusual to sustain a limb-threatening arterial injury. Pallor may suggest ischemic changes caused by arterial impingement secondary to significant ankle dislocation or early findings of compartment syndrome [8].

As one would surmise, all ankle fractures have the potential to cause compartment syndrome. In such cases, pain may be the only complaint [91]. A neurologic examination of the foot and a functional assessment of the structures crossing the ankle should be performed. Impaired distal sensory and motor function may be an early manifestation of compartment syndrome. Compartmental pressures may be measured if the physician is still in doubt, although the authors rarely find such measurement necessary. Range-of-motion examination is usually deferred because of the severity of the injury.

Because most ankle fractures are of the inversion type, certain areas must be examined: the lateral collateral ligaments, deltoid ligament, medial and lateral malleoli, syndesmosis, talar done, anterior process of the calcaneus, and the base of the fifth metatarsal. Any area where injury is suspected requires radiographs to assess osseous pathology.

Radiographic findings

Two major indications for obtaining radiographs of the ankle are inability to bear weight and localized malleolar pain with palpation [92]. Schemes (eg, the Ottawa rules) have been developed to reduce the number of radiographs taken, but these practices are falling out of favor [93–95]. The authors agree with the statements of Lee and Hofbauer [96], who recommend obtaining routine ankle films with all lateral ankle injuries.

Routine studies include anteroposterior, mortise, and lateral views of the ankle joint. When more proximal fractures of the fibula are suspected, full-leg antero-posterior films are obtained. Because of the normal adult malleolar torsion, ranging from 13° to 18° externally rotated, the mortise is considered the true anteroposterior of the ankle. This view is taken with the leg internally rotated 15° to 20°, placng the ankle joint parallel with its empiric axis [97]. Sartoris and Resnick [98] and Weber [58] agree that the ankle mortise view is the best for visualization of the ankle joint. Geissler and colleagues [99] emphasize the importance of obtaining a mortise view before closure during ORIF of ankle fractures. Gourineni and colleagues [100] studied the capabilities of the antero-posterior and mortise views in detecting the position of hardware after surgical treatment. They prefer the anteroposterior radiograph to the mortise, stating that the medial malleolar articular surface is oriented tangentially to the x-ray beam, providing better representation of the medial gutter. The authors agree with Geissler and colleagues [99] and rely more on the mortise view for evaluating the pre- and postoperative ankle injuries; however, they routinely observe hardware placement intraoperatively with anteroposterior and mortise views and often use stress views.

In addition to the obvious fractures of the malleoli, the medial clear space and syndesmosis must be evaluated. On the anteroposterior view, the medial space is normally equal to the superior space between the talar dome and the tibial plafond. Any space greater than 4 mm is considered abnormal and indicates a lateral shift of the talus [99]. The tibiofibular overlap should be at least 10 mm. Any less overlap would lead the observer to expect syndesmotic rupture. Resnick and Niwayama [101] state that the medial gutter space is most clearly evident with the mortise view, as is tibiofibular overlap.

CT scans may be helpful in visualizing articular damage, fracture comminu-tion, the presence of osteochondral lesions of the talus and tibia, and the relationship of the fibula to the tibia and talus in the mortise [102–105]. The authors rarely incorporate CT evaluations with routine ankle fractures. These studies are reserved for cases where large posterior malleolar fragments are visualized and the amount of articular surface involved needs to be determined to provide surgical planning (Fig. 24) [106–109].

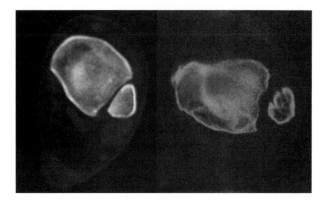

Fig. 24. Bilateral CT ankle scan confirms the presence of a syndesmotic rupture.

MRI generally is reserved for evaluation of tendon and soft tissue damage or the extent of articular surface involvement [98,104,110,111]. Bone scans may be useful in localizing stress or other occult fractures, infections, or neoplastic lesions [112–114]. The authors have found Technetium-99m bone scans to be a useful aid in the diagnosis of stress fracture in patients who have continued pain in the face of negative plain films.

The differential diagnosis of ankle fractures involves many areas that must be inspected and evaluated. The physician must avoid tunnel vision and evaluate each facet of the injury [3,115–119].

Treatment

An abundance of literature discusses the treatment of ankle fractures. Treatment methods range from reduction and splintage to ORIF to arthroscopy-guided repair [120–128]. Regardless of the modality chosen, the basic principles remain the same.

General principles

The ultimate goal in the treatment of ankle fractures is the anatomic alignment of the ankle joint itself [8,48]. The reduction of the distal fibula is usually all that is required to achieve this joint realignment [129]. When evaluating ankle fractures, the following areas should be assessed:

1. Blood supply
2. Reduction of marked dislocation or deformity
3. Care of open wounds or other soft tissue injuries
4. Precise anatomic reduction of osseous structures
5. Repair of damaged soft tissue (ie, tendons, nerves)

6. Rehabilitation

7. Prompt identification and treatment of any complications that may develop

When patients initially present with these injuries, the authors immediately evaluate the vascular status (palpation of pulses, capillary refill). If pulses are not palpable, Doppler studies are performed. If vascular compromise exists, it most commonly is caused by severe malalignment or dislocation of the ankle itself. Emergent reduction should be performed to restore vascularity and reduce tension on the soft tissues (Fig. 25). Allioto [130] described local infiltration of the ankle joint, in the form of the hematoma block, to allow comfortable reduction. The authors use this block in conjunction with a common peroneal block and conscious sedation to reduce these fracture/dislocations safely and effectively.

Open wounds require immediate surgical intervention. The principles described by Gustilo and Anderson [86,87] should be followed. These injuries usually present with extensive soft tissue damage that extends beyond the wound itself [131,132]. After anatomic alignment, surgical débridement of devitalized tissue is performed with aggressive irrigation and subsequent empirical antibiotic treatment.

Open versus closed reduction

Carr and Trafton [8] state, "The quality of the reduction is more important than whether it was achieved by open or closed techniques." Previously, Charnley had proposed that the only way to achieve both perfect anatomic alignment and freedom of joint movement was with internal fixation. The popularity

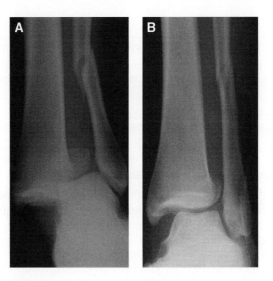

Fig. 25. (*A*) Severe fracture dislocation with compromised vascular supply. Note the widened medial gutter space. (*B*) Closed reduction to relieve tension on the tibial artery.

of internal fixation has increased with the advent of newer materials. When AO/Association for the Study of Internal Fixation (ASIF) principles and techniques are followed and applied properly, good results can be obtained in 90% of supination-external rotation injuries [81,133,134]. Although the AO group advocated rigid, internal fixation, other less rigid techniques have been described in certain scenarios [135].

Many opinions and recommendations are presently reported for the treatment of ankle fractures [136–138]. The basic guideline is to achieve the safest and most reliable restoration of normal anatomy possible [9,57,139,140]. The authors believe that any degree of fibular displacement or shortening or significant involvement of the posterior malleolus (>30%) causes direct or indirect articular damage. They therefore recommend ORIF in all supination-external rotation, pronation-abduction, and pronation-external rotation ankle fractures with associated malleolar fractures. Closed reduction of spiral or oblique fractures usually fail because of their inherent instability. Nondisplaced incomplete fractures of the malleoli can often be treated satisfactorily with short-leg walking casts.

Displaced fractures with vascular compromise or soft tissue tenting should be reduced immediately. If more than a day has elapsed since initial injury, reduction becomes more difficult [8]. Closed reduction is best achieved by recreation of the injury mechanism first, followed by distraction. Reduction of the talus brings the malleoli back into position and maintains alignment [8]. Carr and Trafton [8] believe that, although closed reduction restores the anatomic alignment of the tibiotalar relationship, it rarely reduces the lateral malleolus to its anatomic position because of the residual shortening or rotation that occurs. These cases usually require internal fixation.

Operative treatment

The authors propose that 2 to 3 mm of displacement of a malleolus warrants open reduction. A lateral shift of the talus of 2 mm or more is a general indication for operative treatment of ankle fractures [139–144]. Open repair should be performed as soon as possible. The acute injury may be repaired immediately. If delay is necessary, repair should take place within 3 weeks, because delay in treatment beyond 2 weeks decreases the likelihood of true anatomic reduction [145].

As with almost all traumatic injuries, swelling occurs and becomes the surgeons' enemy. Swelling must be controlled or reduced to prepare patients for operative intervention. A Jones compression dressing with a posterior splint, along with elevation and ice, will limit edema and decrease the time from injury to repair. Two to 3 days are usually sufficient to decrease the edema. The return of skin wrinkles is a good sign of reduction in edema.

Fracture blisters form as the result of high-energy trauma in combination with decreased soft tissue coverage (Fig. 26). Fracture blisters can occur in any area with sparse or absent sweat glands or hair follicles (structures that help anchor

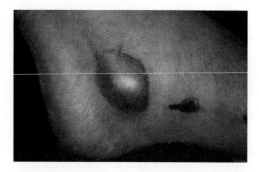

Fig. 26. Fracture blister formation following an ankle fracture caused by a high-energy traumatic event.

the epidermal-dermal junction), such as seen in the ankle region. There is controversy regarding the perioperative treatment of patients who have fracture blisters. In the authors' experience edema, and not the presence of fracture blisters, dictates the timing of surgery. If blisters occupy the incision site, the authors carry the incision through the blister. The fracture blister bed is then dressed with a moist dressing, and topical antibiotic creams are often used after the first dressing change. The most severe complication the authors have encountered from this choice of treatment is superficial wound infection with a slight delay in wound healing.

The authors regularly use prophylactic antibiotics (a first-generation cephalosporin or clindamycin) in patients who have a penicillin allergy. The use of these medications is debatable in clean orthopedic procedures [146,147]. Inpatient antibiotic therapy continues for the duration of the hospital stay; outpatients typically are sent home with a 5- to 7-day supply of oral antibiotics.

The techniques used for reduction and fixation of ankle fractures are widely published, and most follow the AO/ASIF guidelines [25,68,76,148]. Using atraumatic technique, correct anatomic alignment, rigid internal fixation, and early active range of motion are goals of the surgery. The ability to repair the fracture and protect the repair from continued deforming forces can be achieved following these principles.

Fibular fractures

The fibula and its role in weight bearing often can be overlooked when discussing biomechanics [149,150]. In ankle fractures, however, its central role must not be overlooked, because it is the primary fracture. The correct anatomic alignment and length restoration during fracture repair are key to preventing posttreatment complications. Malalignment of the distal fibula leads to widening of the mortise and can allow talar shift, even if the medial ligaments are intact [8,151].

Distal fibular fractures in the supination-external rotation and pronation-abduction patterns usually demonstrate 1 to 2 mm of gap at the fracture site. This slight displacement can result in significant shortening and resultant lateral talar displacement. According to Ramsey and Hamilton [29], there is a 42% decrease in the articulation of the talus and tibia with 1 mm of lateral shift in the fibula. With 3 mm of lateral shift, a full 60% of the articulating surface is lost. These results have been validated and built upon [44,142,152,153]. In 1979 Thordarson [154] studied the effects of fibular shortening, lateral displacement, and external rotation in regards to contact pressures of the ankle joint. The findings suggest that all three variables, especially shortening, increase contact pressures to the mid- and postero-lateral areas of the talar dome. Curtis [155] duplicated these findings and expanded the study, taking into account the importance of the deltoid ligament. A lateral malleolar fracture can have devastating effects on the ankle, even with the deltoid intact. For this reason, the authors routinely repair all complete lateral malleolar fractures.

Not all authors agree with Ramsey and Hamiltons' [29] findings. In fact, Clarke and colleagues [156], Kimizuka and colleagues [157], and Vrahas and colleagues [45] report confounding data. Pereira [158] hypothesized that an axially loaded talus would not displace laterally but rather would seek its own position of maximal congruency.

When treating supination-external rotation injuries, the treating physician must identify the subtleties that may exist. Stage IV supination-external rotation and pronation-abduction injuries are bimalleolar, and this condition necessitates ORIF. The stage II supination-external rotations are more difficult to assess, because they are unimalleolar and may seem to respond well to conservative therapy. One must always evaluate the medial gutter with spiral fractures of the fibular. These fractures, with the deltoid intact, may do well with casting [159]. If the deltoid is in question, the treating physician should err on the side of caution and internally fixate these fractures (Fig. 27).

Fixation of the fibula is performed under thigh tourniquet, with a sandbag under the ipsilateral hip, so the affected leg is internally rotated. A longitudinal

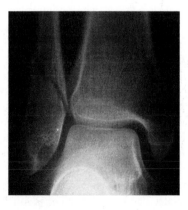

Fig. 27. Although only the fibular is fractured, with an increase in the medial gutter space, this is an unstable bi-malleolar fracture presentation.

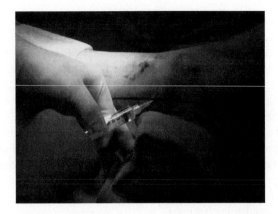

Fig. 28. Preemptive analgesia with infiltration of bupivicaine before incision placement. Besides the obvious benefits of the local anesthetic, the needle "bouncing" off of the fibular helps confirm the planned incision.

incision is made following the distal fibula. Incision placement may be confirmed before the incision by using the needle during local infiltration to "bounce" off the fibula (Fig. 28). An anterior curve at the distal aspect of the incision will allow visualization of the syndesmosis. The primary purpose of ORIF of the fibula is to restore and reconstruct the alignment and integrity of the ankle joint. This incision allows visualization or repair of the following structures: fibular fracture, lateral gutter, AITFL and syndesmotic ligament damage, lateral collateral ligaments, tibial plafond, and talar dome. Care must be taken to extend the incision proximally to allow plate fixation and to preserve a thick layer of periosteum for covering hardware and as a source of osteoprogenitor cells.

Avulsion fractures of the distal fibula can be repaired using suture, anchors, pins, or a small screw with or without a washer [160,161]. If the piece is extremely small, the authors usually excise the avulsion and repair the lateral ligaments with or without an anchor. The authors usually fixate these larger avulsion fractures with a single intramedullary screw, although tension band wiring could also be used (Fig. 29).

Spiral oblique fractures can be treated with interfragmentary screws, one-third tubular plating, or a combination of the two. The fibula is accessed as described previously, and a bone reduction forceps is used to reduce the fracture temporarily. The clamp may be used to help with reduction and restoration of length with a simple twisting of the jaws. An interfragmentary lag screw (4.0 partially threaded) is placed, and the plate is bent to contour the lateral fibula. Every attempt should be made to insert this interfragmentary screw, because it will prevent any sliding and loss of length that may occur.

The single interfragmentary screw then is supplemented with a contoured one-third tubular or similar plate. The rule of cortices is followed with placement of screws proximal and distal to the fracture. These rules must be violated occasionally because of the distal nature of these fractures (Fig. 30). Typically, fully

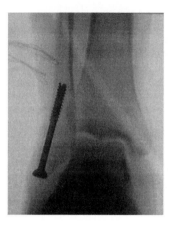

Fig. 29. Single-screw fixation of a distal fibular fracture.

threaded cancellous screws are used in the lateral malleolus. Cortical screws are used when both cortices are to be engaged. The authors usually insert two screws distal to these fractures and two to three screws proximal, in conjunction with the interfragmentary screw. In the past, they used cancellous screws proximal as well as distal to the fracture to eliminate the need to tap. With the newer self-tapping cortical screws, the authors now use cortical screws whenever both cortices are engaged.

Application of the plate has been described on the posterolateral surface of the fibula to prevent proximal gliding [162]. This technique also allows the plate to be less prominent laterally and better tolerated [163]. This technique requires a

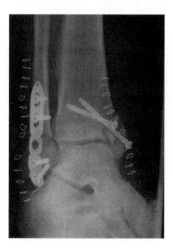

Fig. 30. The location of the fracture may occasionally necessitate violating the rule of cortices. In such cases bimalleolar fixation is obtained to stabilize the ankle regardless of Vassal's phenomenon.

posterior incision and limits visualization of the vital structures mentioned earlier, a trade-off the authors are not willing to make.

During the treatment of pronation-abduction injuries, interfragmentary compression cannot always be used. These injuries may also create a butterfly fragment, making fixation more difficult. Dynamic compression plates may be used in a buttress fashion. External fixators also may be used to regain and maintain length of the fibula [164]. In most cases, a one-third tubular plate (or equivalent) is adequate to repair these fractures.

More proximal fibular fractures, as seen in pronation-external rotation injuries, respond well to plate fixation. Again, interfragmentary compression may not be possible because of the short fracture pattern often seen [164]. Reducing these fractures accurately is not the ultimate goal of treatment; the restoration of the ankle joint restoration is key [8]. In most cases, reduction of the fibular fracture will reduce any ankle dislocation (Fig. 31). Lindsjo [134,165] reported good-to-excellent results in 217 patients who had well-reduced, originally displaced malleolar fractures and only 68% good-to-excellent results in 89 patients who had inadequate fixation. Osteoarthritis is also greater if malleolar fractures heal with significant displacement [133]. In one study, 20% of ankle fractures resulted in free cartilaginous fragments within the joint [128].

Finally, the AITFL should be repaired. This repair can be done directly or indirectly. If an avulsion fracture is present, the Wagstaffe or Chaput's fracture can be fixated, which will indirectly repair the AITFL.

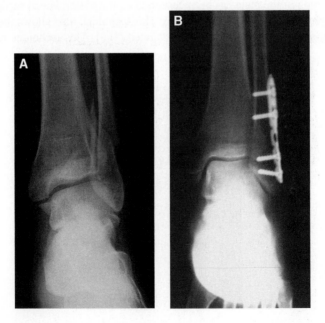

Fig. 31. (A–B) Represent Vassal phenomenon. Note the reduction of the medial malleolar fracture after the fibula is repaired.

The syndesmosis

There is much controversy about the importance of and the proper way to fixate the syndesmosis in ankle injuries. As discussed previously, the role of the syndesmosis in stabilizing the ankle mortise in paramount. As Rasmussen [31,166] demonstrated, however, sectioning of the AITFL by itself does not cause instability of the ankle.

The Cotton test may be used to evaluate the syndesmosis after fibular fixation [167]. This test is performed by laterally displacing the fibula from the tibia while observing the relationship of the two bones (Fig. 32). Repair is recommended if the talus shifts laterally 3 to 4 mm [9,83,167–170]. It has been reported that all Weber type C fractures necessitate a syndesmotic screw, but recent studies have shown that only disruption of the interosseous membrane 3.5 to 4.0 cm proximal to the ankle mortise leads to significant syndesmotic instability. These cases warrant syndesmotic repair [46,171]. Chissel and Jones [172] recommend syndesmotic repair when the deltoid ligament has been ruptured and the fibular fracture is more than 3.5 cm above the joint. Yamaguchi and colleagues [173] report fixation is not required unless the fibular fracture is more than 4.5 cm above the joint. These guidelines help predict what will be required during fixation and enable the surgeon to prepare the patient for the postoperative course, including the need for a secondary procedure for removal of any hardware spanning the syndesmosis before weight bearing.

Boden and colleagues [171] demonstrated an increase in mortise widening when the ankle was exposed to external rotation stress with syndesmotic injury and medial instability. When deltoid ligament disruption is added to syndesmotic injury, the resultant fibular diastasis is increased by 0.7 mm with a 29% decrease in tibiotalar contact and a 42% increase in intra-articular pressure [46]. With

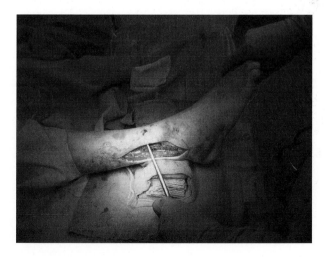

Fig. 32. Use of a bone hook to perform the Cotton test intraoperatively to access syndesmosis stability.

syndesmotic disruption, damage to the superficial deltoid ligament caused an increase in external rotation and plantarflexion of the talus. Stabilization of the fibula had no effect on this observation. With sectioning of the deep deltoid, ankle motion is altered in all planes, even with anatomic stabilization of the fibula and syndesmosis. This destabilization shows the importance of the deep deltoid in maintaining talar tracking in the mortise [17,174,175]. Medial clear space is not a reliable indicator of deep deltoid rupture, however [127]. Thus, syndesmotic injury alone may not be significant unless there is associated medial ankle derangement.

Fixation of the syndesmosis occurs from the standard lateral approach, using one or two screws 1.5 to 3.0 cm proximal to the tibial plafond. Care must be taken to angle the screw from postero-lateral to antero-medial, taking into account pseudolack of malleolar torsion, and to keep the screw parallel to the joint surface. Often the screw may be inserted through the plate used to fixate the fibula (Fig. 33). Although the AO group recommends using a fully threaded screw, it is not the only accepted form of fixation [48]. A fully threaded screw may be used to engage three or four cortices. A partially threaded screw or bioabsorbable screws may be used also [176]. The authors have recently used the Tightrope system by Arthrex to fixate the syndesmosis, thus eliminating the need for a second procedure to remove the screw (Fig. 34).

Regardless of the type of fixation, care must be taken to place the foot in a maximally dorsiflexed position during repair. Inman [6] and Grath [177] demonstrated that the fibula moves laterally approximately 2 mm with dorsiflexion of the ankle. If the syndesmotic screw engages three cortices, this normal external rotation during dorsiflexion in not affected [178]. The use of a syndesmotic screw does not alter ankle motion; thus, if the syndesmosis is stabilized in an

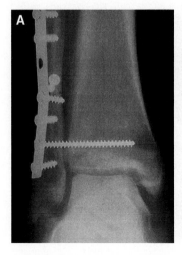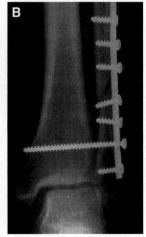

Fig. 33. (*A*) Placement of a tricortical syndesmotic screw. (*B*) Quadricortical screw placement.

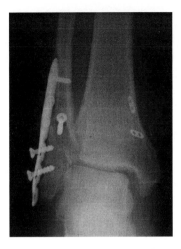

Fig. 34. The Arthrex Tightrope system to fixate the syndesmosis.

anatomic position, no limitation of ankle motion results [175]. Olerud [135,179] demonstrated a loss of 0.1° of dorsiflexion for every degree of plantarflexion of the ankle at the time of syndesmosis repair.

Successful repair of the syndesmosis requires adequate reduction and repair of the fibular fracture [8]. The lateral malleolus and lateral ligaments are the primary restraints to lateral talar shift in ankle injuries [16]. Contact pressures of the ankle consistently shifted laterally on the talus after repair of the syndesmosis [180].

Before removal of syndesmotic screws, radiographic healing of the fibular fracture should be evident [181]. Radiographic healing typically is seen at 6 weeks, at which time the screw may be removed and protected weight bearing allowed. Strict non–weight bearing is required before screw removal to prevent breakage. Scranton and colleagues [182] were able to demonstrate that the fibula pulled 2.4 mm distally during weight bearing, which may lead to breakage. Other authors, however, found no evidence of screw breakage or significant compromise in clinical outcome when full weight bearing was allowed with a syndesmotic screw in place [81,169]. Many authors do not think 6 weeks are adequate for syndesmotic repair and screw removal. In these cases, 6 weeks of strict non–weight bearing followed by 4 to 6 weeks of guarded weight bearing are used before screw removal [177,178,183,184]. In this protocol, the reported incidence of screw breakage is about 10%.

The authors usually engage all four cortices with a 3.5 cortical screw and leave it in place for at least 8 weeks. Occasionally, a 4.0 cancellous screw is used and only three are cortices engaged. The latter method allows patients to begin weight bearing earlier than the cortical fixation. With the use of the Tightrope [177] system, weight bearing is allowed even earlier, without the need for removal before full, unprotected weight bearing.

Medial malleolar fractures

As discussed previously, the deltoid ligament provides vital talar stability in the anterolateral direction and resists its external rotation, especially in plantarflexion [16,17,31,159,166,175,185]. These sources provide support for fixating these medial malleolar fractures, even though they appear to be reduced after fibular fixation. The larger the medial malleolar fragment, the more likely the deltoid is to be intact [186]. With fixation, the treating physician can avoid symptomatic non-unions and increase the ankle's overall stability. The authors have both fixated these medial malleolar fractures and allowed them to heal with immobilization. Their results in patients not undergoing primary fixation have been unsatisfactory. Therefore they fixate all but the smallest avulsion fractures (Fig. 35).

When the medial malleolar fracture is irreducible after fibular fixation, or in isolated fractures, it is important to visualize the medial soft tissue structures to prevent their interposition. The posterior tibial tendon is most commonly involved [172,187,188]. Coonrad and Bugg [189] reported three cases of irreducible fracture of the ankle secondary to entrapment of the posterior tibial tendon. This condition has become known as "Coonrad-Bugg trapping."

Fixation of these fractures depends on their orientation. Muller [190] classified these fractures into four different types. Type A is an avulsion of the tip of the malleolus. Type B is an avulsion occurring at the level of the ankle joint. Type C is an oblique fracture of the malleolus. Type D is a vertical fracture of the malleolus. Medial malleolar stress fractures may also occur [191]. Single- or double-screw fixation can be used to secure the fractured portion of the malleolus

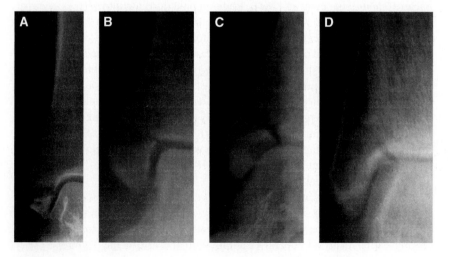

Fig. 35. The Muller classification for medial malleolar fractures. (*A*) Avulsion fracture distal to the joint. (*B*) Avulsion fracture at the joint. (*C*) Oblique fracture. (*D*) Vertical fracture.

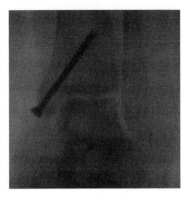

Fig. 36. Large single-screw fixation of medial malleolar fractures will prevent bending, shearing. and torsion forces.

(Fig. 36). Cannulated screws have made this repair easily manageable with the use of fluoroscopy. Care must be taken to orient these lag screws for optimal management of the type of fracture involved. Other types of fixation include the use of Kirschner wires and tension banding [192,193].

Posterior malleolar fractures

Sir Astley Cooper described the first trimalleolar fracture in 1812 [194]. In 1901, Destot termed the posterior lip of the distal end of the tibia the posterior malleolus [195]. Although isolated posterior malleolar fractures are rare (1% of all ankle fractures reported) they are seen from 7% to 44% of the time in combination with other fractures of the ankle [196,197]. Posterior malleolar fractures are most often associated with supination-external rotation and pronation-external rotation ankle fractures, however they occasionally are reported to be caused by supination-adduction or pronation-abduction mechanisms [9]. Bonin [53] described three types of posterior malleolar fractures: extra-articular (analogous to Tillaux-Chaput's anterior fracture); intra-articular (involving the posterior lateral corner of the tibia); and the posteromedial tibial margin (which may involve a large portion of the tibial plafond). These lip fractures are often hard to assess and can be especially challenging in the face of fracture dislocation until provisional reduction has been achieved [198,199]. CT scanning remains the definitive way to determine the extent of articular involvement (Fig. 37) [109].

Determining the extent of the fracture plays a crucial role in treatment and prognosis for the ankle. The posterior malleolus transmits weight-bearing loads through the articular surface and adds posterior stability to the ankle joint [198]. There is a significant decrease in tibiotalar contact when a fragment greater than 33% of the joint is present, according to the study by Gorczyca and colleagues. Posttraumatic arthritis is a known possible consequence of decreased contact in

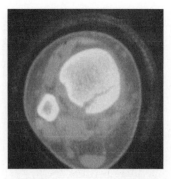

Fig. 37. CT scan demonstrating posterior malleolar fracture and acting as an aid to surgical planning.

the ankle joint [194]. According to Bauer and colleagues the incidence of significant posttraumatic arthrosis after malleolar fractures range from negligible (in supination-external rotation stage II injuries) to more than 37% in severely displaced fracture patterns [76,153]. The larger the posterior fragment the more influence the fracture has on ankle joint dynamics [194]. Macko and colleagues [23] noted a 35% loss of ankle contact with posterior malleolar fracture fragments involving 50% of the distal tibial surface. It is easy to see how the presence of a posterior lip fracture adversely affects the prognosis of ankle fractures.

Surgical fixation of the posterior malleolus was advocated as early as 1912 [198a]. Many authors agree that if more than 25% to 35% of the joint surface of the tibia is involved, the posterior fracture fragment should be reduced and stabilized with internal fixation. Mclaughlin and colleagues noted a high percentage of residual tibiotalar subluxation in posterior malleolar fractures treated conservatively [25]. In a 13-year study, DeVries and colleagues [196] demonstrated that fragments smaller than 25% did not require fixation. Harper [200] demonstrated no posterior instability with posterior fragments involving up to 40% of the distal tibia. He noted no advantage to fixation if the other components of the ankle injury were reduced and stabilized. The authors routinely fixate posterior malleolar fractures that involve more than 30% of the joint surface, but each case must be evaluated individually (Fig. 38).

The surgical approach should be guided by the location of the fragment, additional incisions required for access to associated fractures of the ankle, and the preoperative plan for fixation [25]. The anterior approach usually is performed through the same incision used for reduction of the medial malleolar fracture. Shelton and colleagues [11] described a posteromedial approach, and Henry [201] used a posterolateral incision between the peroneals and the Achilles tendon with the patient in the semilateral decubitus position. The authors prefer an anterior approach using one or two cannulated screws aided by fluoroscopy. This technique allows the screws to be placed as close to the joint as possible, affording stability but not violating the joint itself.

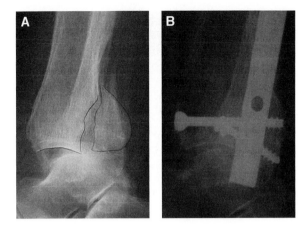

Fig. 38. Fixation of a large posterior malleolar fracture fragment. (*A*) Preoperative (*left*). (*B*) Postoperative (*right*).

Postoperative care

The authors place the patient immediately in a short-leg cast immediately after fixation of ankle fractures. Jones compression dressings with incorporated splints may also be used; both require strict non–weight bearing. With most fractures, 4 to 6 weeks of non–weight bearing are required; serial radiographs determine when patients are allowed to walk.

In isolated lateral malleolar fractures, protected weight bearing can begin as early as 2 weeks. Crutches are used as long as necessary. Range-of-motion exercises can begin at this time but are limited to motion in the sagittal plane. Physical therapy may be necessary for several months. In all cases, the patient's subjective evaluation and evidence of radiographic healing are the benchmarks for return to normal activity.

Complications

Osteoarthritis is the most common postoperative complaint after ankle fractures. The authors routinely explain this fact to patients and state their inability to predict how the patient will be affected. The more involved the fracture, the higher is the likelihood of osteoarthritis [202]. Beris and colleagues [203] reported osteoarthritis to be more common in bimalleolar fractures than in unimalleolar fractures. There was no significant difference between bi- and trimalleolar fractures. Osteoarthritis developed in 1 of 27 (3.7%) unimalleolar fractures, compared with 12 of 50 (20.7%) bimalleolar and 17 of 50 (29%) trimalleolar fractures. In addition, the size of the posterior malleolar fragment determines the incidence of osteoarthritis; for fractures comprising up to 25% of the joint surface, the reported occurrence of arthritis is 26.2%. For fragments larger than 25% of the surface, the incidence of osteoarthritis is 35%. Overall, the

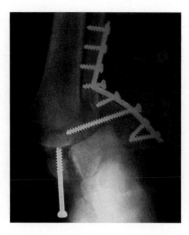

Fig. 39. A spectacular case of total hardware failure in a noncompliant patient.

incidence of osteoarthritis was significantly lower in patients who had good or excellent results than in those who had fair or poor results.

The incidence of delayed unions and non-unions in ankle fractures is relatively low, with a reported range from 0.9% to 1.9% [134]. Many factors affect the outcome of ankle fractures; most significant are the severity of the initial injury, the amount of damage to the plafond, the degree of impaction and comminution, the involvement of the posterior malleolus, and the involvement of multiple structures (Fig. 39). Anatomic reduction is the crucial determinate of outcomes.

Subjective complaints following surgical repair of ankle fractures are common and may persist many months postoperatively [204]. These symptoms tend to improve over time [153,205,206]. Removal of hardware may be required to relieve symptoms and reduce pain [207–209]. Ultimately, as Carr and Trafton state [8], "The outcome of an injury is best judged by how much it affects the patient." The authors have seen continued complaints from patients in whom exact anatomic reduction was achieved and maintained, and patients with less than desirable results have presented with no complaints.

Summary

Although ankle injuries are common, it is imperative for the treating physician to be able to identify the mechanism of injury and accurately restore the normal anatomy of the ankle joint. Attention must be given to restoring the normal alignment and length of the fibula because of its dominant role in controlling talar stability. The medial ankle must not be overlooked, with the role of the deltoid taken into consideration. With a thorough understanding of the anatomy, biomechanics, mechanism of injury, and fixation techniques, repair of the damaged ankle joint can lead to rewarding outcomes for the patient and physician.

References

[1] McCulloch PG, Holden P, Robson DJ, et al. The value of mobilization and nonsteroidal anti-inflammatory analgesia in the management of inversion injuries of the ankle. Br J Clin Pract 1985;29:69–72.

[2] Ruth CJ. The surgical treatment of injuries of the fibular collateral ligaments of the ankle. J Bone Joint Surg [Am] 1961;43:229–39.

[3] Buddecke Jr DE, Mandracchia VJ, Pendarvis JA, et al. Is this just a sprained ankle? Hosp Med 1998;12:46–52.

[4] Flynn JM, Rodriquez-del Rio F, Piza PA. Closed ankle fractures in the diabetic patient. Foot Ankle Int 2000;21:311–9.

[5] Bohler L. Diagnosis, pathology, and treatment of the os calcis. J Bone Joint Surg 1931;13:75.

[6] Inman VJ. The joints of the ankle. Baltimore (MD): Williams & Wilkins; 1976.

[7] Mann RA. Biomechanics of the fot and ankle. In: Mann RA, editor. Surgery of the foot and ankle. 5th edition. St. Louis (MO): CV Mosby; 1986. p. 3–43.

[8] Carr JB, Trafton PG. Malleolar fractures and soft-tissue injuries of the ankle. In: Browner BD, Jupiter JB, Levine AM, et al, editors. Skeletal trauma: fractures, dislocations, ligamentous injuries. 2nd edition. Philadelphia: WB Saunders; 1998. p. 2327–97.

[9] Hamilton WC. Traumatic disorders of the ankle. New York: Springer-Verlag; 1984.

[10] Segal D. Introduction. In: Yablon IG, Segal D, Leach RE, editors. Ankle injuries. New York: Churchill Livingstone; 1983. p. 21.

[11] Shelton ML, Anderson Jr RS. Complications of fractures and dislocations of the ankle. In: Epps Jr CH, editor. 2nd edition. Complications in orthopedic surgery, vol. 1. Philadelphia: JB Lippincott; 1986. p. 599–648.

[12] Ganesh SP, Pietrobon R, Cecilio WA, et al. The impact of diabetes on patient outcomes after ankle fracture. J Bone Joint Surg [Am] 2005;87(8):1712–8.

[13] Draves DJ. Anatomy of the lower extremity. Baltimore (MD): Williams & Wilkins; 1986.

[14] Sarrafian SK. Anatomy of the foot and ankle. Philadelphia: JB lippincott; 1983.

[15] Guman G. Ankle fractures. In: Scurran B, editor. Foot and ankle trauma. 2nd edition. New York: Churchill Livingstone; 1996. p. 731–86.

[16] Harper MC. An anatomical study of the short oblique fracture of the distal fibula and ankle stability. Foot Ankle 1983;4:23–9.

[17] Michelson JD, Helgemo SL, Ahn UM. Dynamic biomechanics of the normal and fractured ankle. Trans Orthop Res Soc 1994;40:253.

[18] Downing JW, Oloff LM, Jacobs AM. Radiologic diagnosis and assessment oflateral ligamentous injuries. J Foot Surg 1984;18:135–46.

[19] Klein SN, Oloff LM, Jacobs AM. Functional and surgical anatomy of the lateral ankle. J Foot Surg 1981;20:170–6.

[20] Brostrom L. Sprained ankles: anatomic lesions in recent sprains. Acta Chir Scand 1964; 128(pt1):483–95.

[21] Wilson FC. The pathogenesis and treatment of ankle fractures: historical studies. Instr Course Lect 1990;39:79–83.

[22] Wilson FC. Fractures and dislocations of the ankle. In: Rockwood DA, Green DP, editors. Fractures in adults. 2nd edition. Philadelphia: JB Lippincott; 1984. p. 1665–701.

[23] Macko VM, Matthews LS, Swerkoski P, et al. The joint contact area of the ankle: the contribution of the posterior malleolus. J Bone Joint Surg [Am] 1991;73:347–51.

[24] McDaniel WJ, Wilson FC. Trimalleolar fractures of the ankle: an end-result study. Clin Orthop 1977;122:37–45.

[25] Heim UF. Trimalleolar fractures: late results after fixation of the posterior fragment. Orthopedics 1989;12:1053–9.

[26] Cedell CA. Ankle lesions. Acta Orthop Scand 1975;46:425–45.

[27] Hopkinson WJ, St. Pierre P, Ryan JB, et al. Syndesmosis sprains of the ankle and foot. Foot Ankle 1990;10:325.

[28] Leeds GC, Ehrlich MG. Instability of the distal tibiofibular syndesmosis after bimalleolar and trimalleolar ankle fractures. J Bone Joint Surg [Am] 1984;66:490–503.

[29] Ramsey P, Hamilton W. Changes in tibiotalar area of contact caused by lateral talar shift. J Bone Joint Surg [Am] 1976;58:356–7.

[30] Yablon IG, Segal D, Leach RE. Ankle injuries. New York: Churchill Livingstone; 1983.

[31] Rasmussen O, Kromann-Andersen C. Experimental ankle injuries: analysis of the traumatology of the ankle ligaments. Acta Orthop Scand 1983;54:356–62.

[32] Lundberg A, Svensson OK, Nemeth G. The axis of rotation of the ankle joint. J Bone Joint Surg [Br] 1989;71:94–9.

[33] Linardini A. Geometry and mechanics of the human ankle complex and ankle prosthesis design. Clin Biomech (Bristol, Avon) 2001;16:706–9.

[34] Sammarco J, Burnstein AH, Frankel VH. Biomechanics of the ankle: a kinematic study. Orthop Clin North Am 1973;4:75–96.

[35] Laurin C, Mathieu J. Sagittal mobility of the normal ankle. Clin Orthop 1975;108:99–104.

[36] Locke M, Perry J, Campbell J. Ankle and subtalar motion during gait in arthritic patients. Phys Ther 1984;64:504–9.

[37] Murray MP, Drought AB, Kory RC. Walking patterns of normal men. J Bone Joint Surg [Am] 1965;46:335–60.

[38] Sammarco J. Biomechanics of the ankle: surface velocity and instant center of rotation in the sagittal plane. Am J Sports Med 1973;5:231–4.

[39] Close JR. Some applications of the functional anatomy of the ankle joint. J Bone Joint Surg [Am] 1956;38:761–81.

[40] Castro MD. Ankle biomechanics. Foot Ankle Clin 2002;7:679–93.

[41] Stauffer RN, Chao E, Brewster RC. Force and motion analysis of the normal diseased, and prosthetic ankle joint. Clin Orthop 1977;127:189–96.

[42] Michelson JD, Checcone M, Kuhn T, et al. Intra-articular load distribution in the human ankle joint during motion. Foot Ankle Int 2001;22(3):226–33.

[43] Ward KA, Soames RW. Contact patterns at the tarsal joints. Clin Biomech (Bristol, Avon) 1997;12:496–501.

[44] Harris J, Fallat L. Effects of isolated Weber B fibular fractures on tibiotalar contact area. J Foot Ankle Surg 2004;43(1):3–9.

[45] Vrahas M, Veenis B, Nudert S, et al. Intra-articular contact stress with simulated ankle malunions. Orthop Trans 1990;14:265.

[46] Burns WC, Prakash K, Adelaar RS, et al. Tibiotalar joint dynamics: indications for the syndesmotic screw: a cadaver study. Foot Ankle 1993;14:153–8.

[47] Wilson FC. Fractures of the ankle: pathogenesis and treatment. J South Orthop Assoc 1999; 9(2):105–15.

[48] Ruedi TP, Murphy WM. AO Principles of fracture management. Stuttgart (Germany): AO Publishing; 2000.

[49] Yde J. The Lauge Hansen classification of malleolar fractures. Acta Orthop Scand 1980;51: 181–92.

[50] Arimoto HK, Forrester DM. Classification of ankle fractures: an algorithm. Amer J Roentg Rad 1979;135:1057–63.

[51] Broos PL, Bisschop AP. A new and easy classification system for ankle fractures. Int Surg 1992;77:309–12.

[52] Ashurst APC, Bromer RS. Classification and mechanism of fractures of the leg bones involving the ankle. Arch Surg 1922;4:51.

[53] Bonin JG. Injuries to the ankle. London: William Heinemann; 1950. p. 248–60.

[54] Dabezies E, D'Ambrosia RD, Shoii H. Classification and treatment of ankle fractures. Orthopedics 1978;1:365–73.

[55] Henderson MS. Trimalleolar fracture of the ankle. Surg Clin North Am 1932;12:867–72.

[56] Lauge-Hansen N. Fractures of the ankle. Combined experimental-surgical and experimental-roentgenologic investigations. Arch Surg 1950;60(pt2):957–85.

[57] Weber BG. Die verletzunger des oberen sprunggellenkes: Aktuelle probleme in der chirurgie. Bern (Switzerland): Verlag Hans Huber; 1966.

[58] Weber BG. Die verletzunger des oberen sprunggellenkes: Aktuelle probleme in der chirurgie. Bern (Switzerland): Verlag Hans Huber; 1972.

[59] Brage ME, Rockett M, Vraney R, et al. Ankle fracture classification: a comparison of reliability of three x-ray views versus two. Foot Ankle Int 1998;19(8):555–62.

[60] Kennedy JG, Johnson SM, Collins AL, et al. An evaluation of the Weber classification of ankle fractures. Injury 1998;29(8):577–80.

[61] Nielsen JO, Dons-Jensen H, Sorensen HT. Lauge-Hansen classification of malleolar fractures: an assessment of the reproducibility in 118 cases. Acta Orthop Scand 1990;61(5):385–7.

[62] Lauge-Hansen N. Fractures of the ankle: analytic historic survey as the basis of new experimental, roentgenologic investigations. Arch Surg 1948;56:269–317.

[63] Lauge-Hansen N. Fractures of the ankle. Combined experimental-surgical and experimental-roentgenologic investigations. Arch Surg 1950;60(Pt 2):957–85.

[64] Lauge-Hansen N. Fractures of the ankle: III. Genetic roentgenologic diagnosis of fractures of the ankle. AJR Am J Roentgenol 1954;71:456–71.

[65] Lauge-Hansen N. Fractures of the ankle: IV. Clinical use of the genetic roentgen diagnosis and genetic reduction. AMA Arch Surg 1952;64:488–500.

[66] Lauge-Hansen N. Fractures of the ankle: V. Pronation-dorsiflexion fracture. AMA Arch Surg 1963;67:813–20.

[67] Danis R. Theorie et practigue de l"osteo-synthese. Paris: Masson & Cie; 1947.

[68] Muller ME, Allgower M, Schreider R, et al. Manual of internal fixation: techniques recommended by the AO group. 2nd edition. New York: Springer-Verlag; 1979.

[69] Lindsjo U. Classificationn of ankle fractures: the Lauge-Hansen or AO system? Clin Orthop 1985;199:12–6.

[70] Christey GR, Tomlinson M. Risk factors for ankle fracture requiring operative fixation. Aust N Z J Surg 1999;69:220–3.

[71] Giachino AA, Hammond DJ. The relationship between oblique fractures of the medial malleolus and concomitant fractures of the anterolateral aspect of the tibial plafond. J Bone Joint Surg [Am] 1987;69:381–4.

[72] Markoff KL, Schmalzried TP, Ferkel RD. Torsional strength of the ankle in vitro: the supination-external rotation injury. Clin Orthop 1989;246:266–72.

[73] Pankovich AM. Fractures of the fibula proximal to the distal tibiofibular syndesmosis. J Bone Joint Surg [Am] 1978;60:221–9.

[74] Skie M, Woldenberg L, Ebraheim N, et al. Assessment of collicular fractures of the medial malleolus. Foot Ankle 1989;10:118–23.

[75] Martin AG, Weber B. Ankle fracture: an unnecessary fracture clinic burden. Int J Care Injuries 2005;35:805–8.

[76] Bauer M, Johnell O, Redlund-Johnell I, et al. Ankle fractures. Foot Ankle 1987;8:23–5.

[77] Hoogenband CR, Moppes FI, Stapert JW. Clinical diagnosis, arthrography, stress examination, and surgical girding after inversion trauma of the ankle. Arch Orthop Trauma Surg 1984;103:115–9.

[78] Kristensen KD, Hansen T. Closed treatment of ankle fractures: stage II supination-eversion fractures followed for 20 years. Acta Orthop Scand 1985;56:107–9.

[79] Ahl T, Dalen N, Holmberg S, et al. Early weight bearing of displaced ankle fractures. Acta Orthop Scand 1987;58:535–8.

[80] Baird RA, Jackson ST. Fractures of the distal part of the fibula with associated disruption of the deltoid ligament: treatment without repair of the deltoid ligament. J Bone Joint Surg [Am] 1987;69:1346–52.

[81] DeSouza LJ, Gustillo RB, Meyer TJ. Results of operative treatment of displaced external rotation-abduction fractures of the ankle. J Bone Joint Surg [Am] 1983;65:260–2.

[82] Harper MC. The deltoid ligament: an evaluation of need for surgical repair. Clin Orthop 1988;226:156–68.

[83] Golterman AFL. Diagnosis and treatment of tibiofibular diastasis. Arch Chir Neerl 1964;
     16:185.

[84] Limbird LS, Aaron RK. Lateraly comminuted fracture dislocation of the ankle. J Bone Joint
     Surg [Am] 1987;69:881–5.

[85] Pankovich AM. Maisonneuve's fracture of the fibula. J Bone Joint Surg [Am] 1976;58:337–42.

[86] Gustilo RB. Management of open frctures and their complications. Philadelphia: WB
     Saunders; 1982.

[87] Gustilo RB, Anderson JT. Prevention of infection in the treatment of 1025 open fractures of
     the long bones: retrospective and prospective analysis. J Bone Joint Surg [Am] 1976;58:
     453–8.

[88] Clohisy DR, Thompson Jr RC. Fractures associated with neuropathic arthropathy in adults
     who have juvenile onset diabetes. J Bone Joint Surg [Am] 1988;70:1192–200.

[89] Haverstock BD, Mandracchia VJ. Cigarette smoking and bone healing: implications in foot
     and ankle surgery. J Foot Ankle Surg 1998;37:69–73.

[90] Ishikawa SN, Murphy GA, Richardson EG. The effect of cigarette smoking on hindfoot
     fusions. Foot Ankle Int 2002;23(11):996–8.

[91] Arciero RA, Shishido NS, Parr TJ. Acute anterolateral compartment syndrome secondary to
     rupture of the peroneus longus muscle. Am J Sports Med 1984;12:366–7.

[92] Stiell IG, Greenburg GH, McKnight RD, et al. A study to develop clinical decision rules for
     the use of radiography in acute ankle injuries. Ann Emer Med 1992;21:384–90.

[93] Aulely GR, Ravaud P, Giraudeau B, et al. Implementation of the Ottawa ankle rules in France.
     JAMA 1997;277:1935–9.

[94] Pigman EC, Klug RK, Sanford J, et al. Evaluation of the Ottawa clinical decision rules for
     the use of radiography in acute ankle and midfoot injuries in the emergency department.
     An independent site assessment. Ann Emerg Med 1994;24:41–5.

[95] Dancocks A, Rouse A, Hiscox J. A pilot study to assess the sensitivity and specificity of an
     intrasound device in the diagnosis of ankle fractures. Accident and Emergency Medicine 1997;
     120:230–2.

[96] Lee MS, Hofbauer MH. Evaluation and management of lateral ankle injuries. Clin Pod Med
     Surg 1999;16(4):659–78.

[97] Sgarlato TE. A compendium of podiatric biomechanics. San Francisco (CA): California
     College of Podiatric Medicine; 1971. p. 199–204.

[98] Sartoris DJ, Resnick D. Magnetic resonance imaging of tendons in the foot and ankle. J Foot
     Surg 1989;28:370–7.

[99] Geissler WB, Tsao AK, Hughes JL. Fractures and injuries of the ankle. In: Rockwood Jr CA,
     Heckman JD, Buckholtz RW, et al, editors. Fractures in adults. 7th edition. Philadelphia:
     Lippincott-Raven; 1996. p. 2219–25.

[100] Gourineni P, Knuth AE, Nuber GF. Radiographic evaluation of the position of implants in
     the medial malleolus in relation to the ankle joint space: anteroposterior compared with
     mortise radiographs. J Bone Joint Surg [Am] 1999;81:364–9.

[101] Resnick D, Niwayama G. Anatomy and individual joints. In: Resnick D, editor. Diagnosis
     of bone and joint disorders. 3rd edition. Philadelphia: WB Saunders; 1995. p. 751.

[102] Rosenberg ZS, Feldman F, Singson RD. Peroneal tendon injuries: CT analysis. Radiology 1986;
     161:743–8.

[103] Rosenberg GS, Jahss MH, Noto AM, et al. Rupture of the posterior tibial tendon: CT and
     surgical findings. Radiology 1988;167:489–93.

[104] Rosenberg GS, Jahss MH, Noto AM, et al. Rupture of the posterior tibial tendon: CT and MR
     imaging with surgical correlation. Radiology 1988;169:229–35.

[105] Szczukowski Jr M, St. Pierre RK, Flemming LL, et al. Computerized tomography in the
     evaluation of peroneal tendon dislocation. A report of two cases. Am J Sports Med 1983;
     11:444–7.

[106] Magid D, Michelson JD, Hey DR, et al. Adult ankle fractures: comparison of plain films and
     interactive two and three dimensional CT scans. AJR Am J Roentgenol 1985;154:1017–23.

[107] Mitchell MJ, Ho C, Howard BA, et al. Diagnostic imaging of trauma to the ankle and foot: fractures about the ankle. J Foot Surg 1989;28:174–9.

[108] Mitchell MJ, Ho C, Howard BA, et al. Diagnostic imaging of trauma to the ankle and foot. J Foot Surg 1989;28(pt2):266–71.

[109] Ferries JS, DeCoster TA, Firoozbakhsh KK, et al. Plain radiographic interpretation in trimalleolar ankle fractures poorly assess posterior fragment size. J Orthop Trauma 1994;8:328–31.

[110] Daffner RH, Riemer BL, Lupetin AR, et al. Magnetic resonance imaging in acute tendon ruptures. Skeletal Radiol 1986;15:619–21.

[111] Zeiss J, Saddemi SR, Ebraheim NA. MR imaging of the peroneal tunnel. J Comput Assist Tomogr 1989;13:840–4.

[112] Burkus JK, Sella EJ, Southwick WO. Occult injuries of the talus diagnosed by bone scan and tomography. Foot Ankle 1984;4:316–24.

[113] Marymont JV, Lynch MA, Henning CE. Acute ligamentous diastasis of the ankle without fracture: evaluation by radionuclide imaging. Am J Sports Med 1986;14:407–9.

[114] Maurice H, Watt I. Technetium-99m hydroxymethelene diphosphonate scanning of acute injuries to the lateral ligaments of the ankle. Br J Radiol 1989;62:31–4.

[115] Goris RJ. Irreducible subluxation of the tibiotalar joint due to a fracture of the calcaneus. Injury 1987;18:358–60.

[116] Kym MR, Worsing Jr RA. Compartment syndrome in the foot after an inversion injury to the ankle: a case report. J Bone Joint Surg [Am] 1990;72:138–9.

[117] Montane I, Zych GA. An unusual fracture of the talus associated with a bimalleolar ankle fracture: a case report and review f the literature. Clin Orthop 1986;208:278–81.

[118] Nitz AJ, Dobner JJ, Kersey D. Nerve injury and grades II and III ankle sprains. Am J Sports Med 1985;13:177–82.

[119] Whitelaw GP, Sawka MW, Wetzler M, et al. Unrecognized injuries of the lateral ligaments associated with lateral malleolar fractures of the ankle. J Bone Joint Surg [Am] 1989;71:1396–9.

[120] Banerjee R, Bradley MP, DiGiovanni CW. Use of emergency room external fixator in provisional reduction of posterior malleolar fractures. Am J Ortho 2004:581–4.

[121] Rammelt S, Endres T, Grass R, et al. The role of external fixation in acute ankle trauma. Foot Ankle Clin 2004;9:455–74.

[122] Lamontagne J, Blachut PA, Broekhuyse HM, et al. Surgical treatment of a displaced lateral malleolus fracture: the antiglide technique versus lateral plate fixation. J Orthop Trauma 2002;16(7):498–502.

[123] Tornetta III P, Creevy W. Lag screw only fixation of the lateral malleolus. J Orthop Trauma 2001;15(2):119–21.

[124] Dara AN, Esenyel CZ, Sener BT, et al. A different approach to the treatment of the lateral malleolar fractures with syndesmosis injury: The ANK nail. J Foot Ankle Surg 1999;38(6):394–402.

[125] Kim SK, Oh JK. One or two lag screws for fixation of Danis-Weber type B fractures of the ankle. J Trauma 1999;46(6):1039–44.

[126] Kinik H, Us AK, Mergen E. Self-locking tension band technique: a new perspective in tension band wiring. Arch Orthop Trauma Surg 1999;119:432–4.

[127] Schuberth JM, Collman DR, Rush SM, et al. Deltoid ligament integrity in lateral malleolar fractures: a comparative analysis of arthroscopic and radiographic assessments. J Foot Ankle Surg 2004;43(1):20–9.

[128] Ono A, Nishikawa S, Nagao A, et al. Arthroscopically assisted treatment of ankle fractures: arthroscopic findings and surgical outcomes. Journal of Arthroscopic and Related Surgery 2004;20(6):627–31.

[129] Rieunau G, Gay R. Enclouge du perone dans les fractures supramalleolaires. Lyon Chir 1956;51:594–600.

[130] Alioto RJ, Furia JP, Marquardt JD. Hematoma block for ankle fractures: a safe and efficacious technique for manipulation. J Trauma 1995;9:113–6.

[131] Collins DN, Teple SD. Open joint injuries: classification and treatment. Clin Orthop 1989;243: 48–65.

[132] Tscherne H, Gotzen L. Fractures with soft-tissue injuries. Berlin: Springer-Verlag; 1984.

[133] Hughes JL, Weber H, Willenegger H, et al. Evaluation of ankle fractures: nonoperative and operative treatment. Clin Orthop 1979;138:111–9.

[134] Lindsjo U. Operative treatment of ankle fracture-dislocations: a follow-up study of 306/321 consecutive cases. Clin Orthop 1985;199:28–38.

[135] Olerud C, Molander H. Bi- and trimalleolar ankle fractures operated with nonrigid internal fixation. Clin Orthop 1986;206:253–60.

[136] Calderone DR, Loder BG, Denny D, et al. Retrospective analysis of operative ankle fractures. J Foot Ankle Surg 1996;35(3):230–6.

[137] Federici A, Sanguineti F, Santolini F. The closed treatment of severe malleolar fractures. Acta Orthop Belg 1993;59(2):189–96.

[138] Stuart PR, Brumby C, Smith SR. Comparative study of functional bracing and plaster cast treatment of stable lateral malleolar fractures. Injury 1989;20:323–6.

[139] Cedell CA. Is closed treatment of ankle fractures advisable? [editorial]. Acta Orthop Scand 1985;56:101–2.

[140] Chapman MW. Fractures and fracture dislocations of the ankle. In: Mann RA, editor. Surgery of the foot. 5th edition. St. Louis (MO): CV Mosby; 1986. p. 568–91.

[141] Joy G, Patzakin MJ, Harvey JP. Precise evaluation of the reduction of severe ankle fractures. J Bone Joint Surg [Am] 1974;56:979–93.

[142] Mast JW, Teipner WA. A reproducible approach to internal fixation of adult ankle ractures, rationale, technique, and early results. Orthop Clin North Am 1989;11:661–79.

[143] Pettrone FA, Gail M, Pee D, et al. Quantitative criteria for prediction of the results after displaced fracture of the ankle. J Bone Joint Surg [Am] 1983;65:667–77.

[144] Phillips WA, Schwartz HS, Keller CS, et al. A prospective randomized study of the management of severe ankle fractures. J Bone Joint Surg [Am] 1985;67:67–78.

[145] Fogel GR, Morrey BF. Delayed open reduction and fixation of ankle fractures. Clin Orthop 1987;215:187–95.

[146] Paiemont GD, Renaud E, Dagenais G, et al. Double-blind, randomized prospective study of the efficacy of antibiotic prophylaxis for open reduction and internal fixation of closed ankle fractures. J Orthop Trauma 1994;8:65–6.

[147] Zgonis T, Jolly GP, Garbalosa JC. The efficacy of prophylactic intravenous antibiotics in elective foot and ankle surgery. J Foot Ankle Surg 2004;43(2):97–103.

[148] Ruedi TP, Allgower M. The operative treatment of intraarticular fractures of the lower end of the tibia. Clin Orthop 1979;138:105–10.

[149] Lambert KL. The weight-bearing function of the fibula: a strain gauge study. J Bone Joint Surg [Am] 1971;53:507–13.

[150] Takebe K, Nakagawa A, Minami H, et al. Role of the fibula in weight bearing. Clin Orthop 1984;184:289–92.

[151] Zindrick MR, Knight GS, Gogan WJ. The effect of fibular shortening and rotation on the biomechanics of the talocrural joint during various stages of stance phase. Trans Orthop Res Soc 1984;9–136.

[152] Moody ML, Koenenman J, Hettinger E, et al. The effects of fibular and talar displacement on joint contact areas about the ankle. Orthop Rev 1992;21:741–4.

[153] Bauer M, Bergstrom B, Hemborg A, et al. Malleolar fractures: nonoperative versus operative treatment: a controlled study. Clin Orthop 1985;199:17–27.

[154] Thordarson DB, Motamed S, Hedman T, et al. The effect of fibular malreduction on contact pressures in an ankle fracture malunion model. J Bone Joint Surg [Am] 1997;79:1809–15.

[155] Curtis MJ, Michelson JD, Urquhart RP, et al. Tibiotalar contact and fibular malunion in ankle fractures. Acta Orthop Scan 1992;63:326–9.

[156] Clarke HJ, Michelson J, Junnah RH. Tibiotalar stability in bimalleolar ankle fractures. A dynamic in vitro contact area study. Foot Ankle 1991;11:222–7.

[157] Kimizuka M, Kurosawa H, Fukabayashi T. Load-bearing pattern of the anklejoint: contact area and pressure distribution. Arch Orthop Trauma Surg 1980;96:45–9.

[158] Pereira DS, Koval KJ, Resnick RB, et al. Tibiotalar contact area and pressure distribution: the effect of mortise widening and syndesmotic fixation. Foot Ankle Int 1996;17:269–74.

[159] Michelson JD, Ahn UM, Helgemo SL. Motion of the ankle in a simulated supination-external rotation fracture model. J Bone Joint Surg [Am] 1996;78:1024–31.

[160] Robertson DB, Daniel DM, Biden E. Soft-tissue fixation to bone. Am J Sports Med 1986; 14:398–403.

[161] Yablon JG, Heller FG, Shouse L. The key role of lateral malleolus in displaced fractures of the ankle. J Bone Joint Surg [Am] 1977;59:169–73.

[162] Brunner DF, Weber BG. Special techniques in internal fixation. Berlin: Springer-Verlag; 1982.

[163] Schaffer JJ, Lock TR, Salcicciolo GG. Posterior tibial tendon ruptures inpronation-external rotation ankle fractures. J Trauma 1987;27:795–6.

[164] Mast JW, Jakob R, Ganz R. Planning and reduction technique in fracture surgery. New York: Springer-Verlag; 1989.

[165] Lindsjo U, Danckwardt-Lilliestrom G, Sahlstedt B. Measurement of the motion range in the loaded ankle. Clin Orthop 1985;199:68–71.

[166] Rasmussen O, Jensen IT, Hedeboe J. An analysis of the function of the posterior talofibular ligaments. Acta Scand Suppl 1985;211:1–75.

[167] Stiehl JB. Ankle fractures with diastasis. Instr Course Lect 1990;39:95–103.

[168] Katznelson A, Lin E, Militiano J. Ruptures of the ligaments about the tibiofibular syndesmosis. Injury 1983;15:170–2.

[169] Kaye RA. Stabilization of ankle syndesmosis injuries with a syndesmotic screw. Foot Ankle 1989;9:290–2.

[170] Needleman RL, Skrade DA, Stiehl JB. Effect of the syndesmotic screw on ankle motion. Foot Ankle 1989;10:17–24.

[171] Boden SD, Labropaulos PA, McGowin P, et al. Mechanical considerations for the syndesmotic screw: a cadaver study. J Bone Joint Surg [Am] 1989;71:1548–55.

[172] Chissell HR, Jones J. The influence of a diastasis screw on the outcome of Weber type C ankle fractures. J Bone Joint Surg [Br] 1995;77:435–8.

[173] Yamaguchi K, Martin CH, Boden SD, et al. Operative treatment of syndesmotic disruptions without use of a syndesmotic screw: a prospective clinical study. Foot Ankle Int 1994;15: 407–14.

[174] Michelson JD, Clarke JH, Jinnah RH. The effect of loading on tibiotalar alignment in cadaver ankles. Foot Ankle 1990;10:280–4.

[175] Michelson JD, Waldman B. An axially loaded model of the ankle after pronation external rotation injury. Clin Orthop Rel Res 1996;328:285–93.

[176] Hovis WD, Kaiser BW, Watson JT, et al. Treatment of syndesmotic disruptions of the ankle with bioabsorbable screw fixation. J Bone Joint Surg [Am] 2002;84:26–31.

[177] Grath GB. Widening of the ankle mortise: a clinical and experimental study. Acta Chir Scan Suppl 1960;263:1.

[178] Proctor P, Paul JP. Ankle joint biomechanics. J Biomech 1982;15:627–34.

[179] Olerud C. The effect of the syndesmotic screw on the extension capacity of the ankle joint. Arch Orthop Trauma Surg 1985;104:299–302.

[180] Peter RE, Harrinton RM, Henley MB. Effect of implants on the motion of the distal tibiofibular syndesmotic joint: comparison of screw versus Kirschner wire fixation of Weber type C injuries. Trans Orthop Res Soc 1992;38:264.

[181] Ebraheim NA, Mekhail AO, Gargasz SS. Ankle fractures involving the fibula proximal to the distal tibiofibular syndesmosis. Foot Ankle Int 1997;18:513–21.

[182] Scranton PE, McMaster JH, Kelly E. Dynamic fibular function: a new concept. Clin Orthop 1976;118:76–81.

[183] Farhan MJ, Smith TW. Fixation of diastasis of the inferior tibiofibular joint using the syndesmosis hook. Injury 1985;16:309–11.

[184] Hooper J. Movement of the ankle joint after driving a screw across the inferior tibiofibular joint. Injury 1983;14:493–506.

[185] Mote Jr CJ, Lee CW. Identification of human lower extremity dynamics in torsion. J Biomech 1982;15:211–22.

[186] Tornetta III P. Competence of the deltoid ligament in bimalleolar ankle fractures after medial malleolar fixation. J Bone Joint Surg [Am] 2000;82:843–8.

[187] DeZwart DE, Davidson JSA. Rupture of the posterior tibial tendon associated with fracture of the ankle. J Bone Joint Surg [Am] 1983;65:260–2.

[188] Soballe K, Kjaersgaard-Anderson P. Ruptures tibialis posterior tendon in a closed ankle fracture. Clin Orthop 1988;231:140–3.

[189] Coonrad RW, Bugg EI. Trapping of the posterior tibial tendon and interposition of soft tissue in severe fractures of the ankle joint. J Bone Joint Surg [Am] 1954;36:744–50.

[190] Muller ME, Nazarian S, Koch P, et al. Tibia/fibula. In: The comprehensive classification of fractures of the long bones. New York: Springer-Verlag; 1980. p. 190–1.

[191] Kor A, Saltzman AT, Wenpe PD. Medial malleolar stress fractures: literature review, diagnosis, and treatment. J Am Podiatr Med Assoc 2003;93:292–7.

[192] Georgiadis GM, White DB. Modified tension band wiring of medial malleolar ankle fractures. Foot Ankle Int 1995;16:64–8.

[193] Johnson BA, Fallat LM. Comparison of tension band wire and cancellous bone screw fixation for medial malleolar fractures. J Foot Ankle Surg 1997;36:284–9.

[194] Gorczyca TJ, Hartford JM, Mayor MB, et al. Tibiotalar contact area. Clin Orthop Relat Res 1995;320:182–7.

[195] Harden G, Harper MC. Posterior malleolar fractures of the ankle associated with external rotation-abduction injuries. J Bone Joint Surg [Am] 1988;70:1348–56.

[196] DeVries JS, Wijgman AJ, Siervelt IN. Long-term results of ankle fractures with a posterior malleolar fragment. J Foot Ankle Surg 2000;44:211–7.

[197] Gale BD, Nugent JF. Isolated posterior malleolar ankle fractures. J Foot Surg 1990;29:80–3.

[198] Carr JB. Fractures of the posterior malleolus. In: Adelaar RS, editor. Complex foot and ankle trauma. Philadelphia: Lippincott-Raven; 1998. p. 21–9.

[198a] McLaughlin HL, Ryder Jr CT. Open reduction and internal fixation for fractures of the tibia and ankle. Surg Clin North Am 1949;29:1523–34.

[199] Jaskulka RA, Ittner G, Schedl R. Fractures of the posterior tibial margin: their role in the prognosis of malleolar fractures. J Trauma 1989;29:1565–70.

[200] Harper MC. Posterior instability of the talus: an anatomic evaluation. Foot Ankle 1989;10: 36–9.

[201] Henry JH. Lateral ligament tears of the ankle. Orthop Rev 1983;12:31–9.

[202] Broos PL, Bisschop AP. Operative treatment of ankle fractures in adults: correlation between types of fracture and final results. Injury 1991;22:403–6.

[203] Beris AE, Kabbani KT, Xenakis TA, et al. Surgical treatment of malleolar fractures: a review of 144 patients. Clin Ortho Rel Res 1997;341:90–8.

[204] Belcher GL, Radomisli TE, Abate JA, et al. Functional outcome analysis of operatively treated malleolar fractures. J Orthop Trauma 1997;11:106–9.

[205] Bauer M, Jonsson K, Nilsson B. Thirty-year follow-up of ankle fractures. Foot Ankle 1985;8: 23–5.

[206] Lehto M, Tunturi T. Improvement 2 to 9 years after ankle fracture. Acta Orthop Scand 1990; 61:80.

[207] Jacobsen S, Honnens de Lichtenberg M, Jensen CM, et al. Removal of internal fixation: the effect on patients' complaints: a study of 66 cases of removal of internal fixation after malleolar fracture. Foot Ankle Int 1994;15:170–1.

[208] Roberts RS. Surgical treatment of displaced ankle fractures. Clin Orthop 1983;172:165–70.

[209] Brown OL, Dirschl DR, Obremskey WT. Incidence of hardware-related pain and its effect on functional outcomes after open reduction and internal fixation of ankle fractures. J Orthop Trauma 2001;15:271–4.

CLINICS IN
PODIATRIC
MEDICINE AND
SURGERY

Clin Podiatr Med Surg
23 (2006) 423–444

The Surgical Management of High- and Low-energy Tibial Plafond Fractures: A Combination of Internal and External Fixation Devices

Luis E. Marin, DPM[a], Dane K. Wukich, MD[b],
Thomas Zgonis, DPM[c],*

[a]Palmetto General Hospital, 2001 W 68th Street, Hialeah, FL 33016, USA
[b]Department of Orthopaedic Surgery, University of Pittsburgh School of Medicine,
Pittsburgh, PA, USA
[c]Division of Podiatry, Department of Orthopaedics,
The University of Texas Health Science Center at San Antonio, 7773 Floyd Curl Drive,
San Antonio, TX 78229, USA

Fractures of the distal tibial articular surface are complex injuries that can destroy the ankle joint. Tibial plafond fractures, or pilon fractures as they are commonly called, involve the tibial metaphysis and the weight-bearing portion of the distal articular surface. Many authors have credited a French radiologist named Destot for coining the term "pilon fracture" [1,2]. In 1911, he described the shape of the distal tibial articular surface as similar to that of a pharmacist's pestle, or pilon [3]. These injuries are infrequent, representing 3% to 10% of fractures of the tibia and 1% of all lower-extremity fractures. Approximately 10% to 50% of tibial plafond fractures are open [4,5].

Pilon fractures are probably the most destructive traumatic injuries involving the ankle joint. The poor prognosis and high complication rates associated with these injuries are well documented [5–8]. Many surgeons have made efforts to decrease this morbidity and achieve better outcomes through the use of new or revised surgical approaches. As a result, the literature on pilon fractures presents a variety of recommendations and a fair amount of controversy regarding the best

* Corresponding author.
E-mail address: zgonis@uthscsa.edu (T. Zgonis).

0891-8422/06/$ – see front matter © 2006 Elsevier Inc. All rights reserved.
doi:10.1016/j.cpm.2006.01.012 *podiatric.theclinics.com*

treatment method. In the authors' experience, no single technique or approach is suitable for all types of pilon fractures. The preferred method of treatment differs according to the patient, severity of injury, fracture pattern, soft tissue integrity, and fracture presentation. The Ilizarov method of external fixation has proven to be useful in most cases, however. The circular ring and small wire frame is a versatile tool that serves many different purposes, one or more of which may be appropriate for the needs of each different presentation of pilon fracture.

Mechanism of injury

Two general mechanisms of injury produce pilon fractures: rotational and axial (Figs. 1, 2) [6,9,10]. The rotational mechanism involves torsional and shearing forces at the joint, usually with external rotation and pronation. These rotational forces are less powerful and less destructive than those seen in the axial mechanism [1,8]. These injuries are often termed "low-energy pilons." The fracture pattern created is frequently spiral, extending from the articular surface through the metaphysis and diaphysis. The joint is broken into a few large pieces with little or no comminution. Sports injuries and accidents from daily activities such as stepping off a curb or walking down stairs are common causes of the low-energy pilon [11,12].

The second mechanism involves axial loading forces that compress the talus into the tibia [11]. These forces are high energy and generally are more destructive than the rotational type of pilon fracture. These high-energy pilon injuries fracture the tibial articular surface and metaphysis into multiple smaller pieces. This fracture pattern is characterized by comminution as well as impaction of the central plafond into the metaphyseal area. The most common causes of the

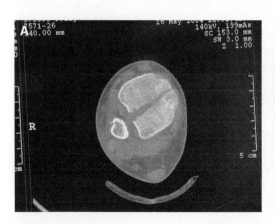
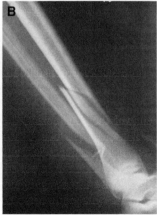

Fig. 1. CT and radiograph examples of rotational mechanism in a low-energy pilon fracture. (*A*) Coronal CT image shows one major intra-articular fracture with no comminution. (*B*) Lateral radiograph demonstrates spiral fracture extending into the ankle joint.

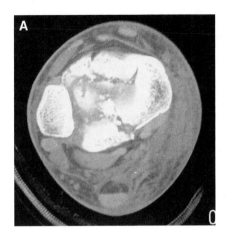
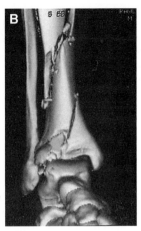

Fig. 2. CT examples of axial mechanism, high-energy pilon fracture. (*A*) Coronal CT shows comminution of the articular surface. (*B*) Three-dimensional CT reconstruction of anteroposterior view shows multiple fractures and displacement typical of the high-energy pilon.

high-energy pilon are falls from a height, industrial accidents, and motor vehicle accidents [6,12–14].

The fracture pattern may be influenced by the position of the ankle and the direction of deforming forces at the time of injury [1,15,16]. Dorsiflexion and axial loading cause fracture of the anterior lip of the tibia, whereas plantarflexion and axial loading cause fracture of the posterior malleolus. The fibula is fractured in 75% to 85% of cases [2,11,17]; fibular fracture is thought to occur when there is a valgus component to the injury [17]. It has been suggested that pilon fractures without fibular fracture result from pure axial loading of the talus into the tibia [1].

Classifications

One of the two most common classifications schemes used is the Ruedi and Allgower classification, which divides pilon fractures into three categories [13]. Type I fractures are simple fractures with little or no displacement, type II fractures are articular fractures with displacement but without comminution, and type III fractures are articular fractures with displacement and comminution [18].

The other commonly used classification system was originally created by the Arbeitsgemeinschaft fur Osteosynthesefragen (AO) group. In this scheme, type A fractures are extra-articular fractures of the metaphysis, type B fractures are articular fractures, and type C fractures are articular and metaphyseal fractures. This classification was later modified by the Orthopaedic Trauma Association (OTA) to include three subsets of each type. A1 fractures are simple metaphyseal fractures; A2 fractures are comminuted metaphyseal fractures; and A3 fractures are severely comminuted metaphyseal fractures. For B and C fractures, type 1 fractures are articular and metaphyseal fractures without comminution, type 2 fractures involve comminution of the metaphysis but not of the articular surface, and type 3 fractures involve comminution of both the articular surface and the metaphysis [19].

Ovadia and Beals [11] described five types of pilon fracture. Type I fractures are nondisplaced articular fractures. Type II fractures are minimally displaced articular fractures. Type fractures III are displaced, articular fractures with several large pieces. Type IV fractures are displaced articular fractures with multiple fragments and a metaphyseal defect. Type V fractures are displaced articular fractures with severe comminution.

Kellam and Waddell [6] categorized fractures as either type A, minimal or noncomminuted fractures with large fragments and a fibular fracture at the level of the plafond, or type B, comminuted fractures with multiple fragments and superior migration of the talus.

Lauge-Hansen [9] added a pronation-dorsiflexion category to his ankle fracture classification to include the pilon fracture. In a cadaveric study he examined the position of the foot and the direction of forces that produced fractures of the tibial plafond. He describes stage I as an oblique or transverse medial malleolar fracture, stage II as an anterior lip fracture, stage III as a fibular fracture above the level of the syndesmosis, and stage IV as a fracture of the posterior tibia.

Destot categorized pilons into four basic types: the posterior malleolar fracture, the anterior margin fracture, the explosion fracture, and the tibial fracture extending into the joint [2].

There has been some question concerning the interobserver reliability of these classification schemes. In three separate but similarly designed studies, individual surgeons independently evaluated radiographs of patients who had pilon fractures and classified them according to either the Ruedi and Allgower or the AO/OTA system. Good interobserver reliability was found using either of these systems [20,21], but interobserver agreement was poor using the AO/OTA system that breaks down the type of pilon further into groups. Using only the designation of fracture type (A, B, or C) was recommended [22].

History of treatment

Before the introduction of the AO guidelines for the surgical treatment of pilon fractures in 1969, operative care of these injuries was discouraged [23]. Nonsurgical techniques were preferred over attempts at surgical reconstruction of the joint because these surgeries were associated with a high rate of postoperative complications and a low rate of successful outcomes [24]. Casting intra-articular pilons also produced poor results and fracture displacement, however [5,11]. Inadequate reduction the articular surface has been cited as a reliable cause of posttraumatic arthrosis [6,11,25,26]. Most authors suggest that nonoperative treatment should be reserved for nondisplaced pilons and for cases that are so severely comminuted that primary arthrodesis is indicated [3,4,27].

Ruedi and Allgower published unprecedented research on distal tibial intra-articular fractures that were treated with open anatomic reduction and internal fixation (ORIF) [13]. They found that 75 cases had good or excellent late results as compared to those treated by closed reduction in a 6 year post-operative follow-up. They attributed their impressive outcomes to a surgical protocol that includes four operative principles: restoration of fibular length, anatomic reduction and internal fixation of the tibia, application of iliac crest bone graft into the metaphysis to support the articular reduction, and placement of a medial tibial buttress plate. These four guidelines became the mainstay of many authors' surgical technique for several years.

Subsequent studies, however, could not duplicate Ruedi and Allgower's successful results. Teeny and Wiss [7] used the AO guidelines in the treatment of 60 Ruedi and Allgower type I, II, and III pilon fractures. Outcomes were disappointing, with 50% poor, 25% fair, and only 25% good results. They concluded that surgical treatment is fraught with difficulty and complications. Dillin and colleagues [8] admitted to disastrous results using ORIF on 9 of 11 severely comminuted pilons, concluding that aggressive internal fixation of high-energy, comminuted pilons results in a high rate of complications.

Comparison between the Ruedi and Allgower study and subsequent studies revealed important differences in type of pilon fracture and severity of injury [13]. The former contained patients who had rotational, low-energy fractures that resulted from sporting injuries; the later, less successful studies contained mainly compressive, high-energy fractures caused by industrial accidents or motor vehicle accidents. The use of ORIF on high-energy pilon fractures with compromised soft tissues was thought to be responsible for the many wound complications and poor outcomes. Several separate research papers found that ORIF worked well on low-energy fractures but failed when used on the more severe pilons [5,6,11,28,29].

The importance of properly handling the soft tissue envelope became evident. Rommens and colleagues [30] found many complications in their study of openly reduced and internally fixated C2 and C3 pilons and concluded, "soft tissue management is as important as the bony reconstruction."

A renewed respect for the soft tissue envelope led many surgeons to use external fixation and minimally invasive surgery. Several publications in the 1990s addressed hybrid external fixation and limited internal fixation. Critics of this approach argued that minimally invasive surgery does not achieve the same level of anatomic articular reduction as ORIF [13]. One study compared the two techniques and found lower clinical scores and a higher complication rate when hybrid fixators were used [31]. Helfet and colleagues [16] delayed definitive surgical treatment (either ORIF or external fixation with fibular plating) for an average of 7.3 days. They found excellent or adequate results in 76.9% of Ruedi type II and 62.5% of Ruedi type III fractures.

Most studies comparing minimally invasive techniques and ORIF, however, found the former method to be superior [25,32–37]. Wyrsch [38] conducted a randomized, prospective study comparing 18 pilons treated with ORIF and

20 pilons that were treated with external fixation with or without limited internal fixation. At the 2-year follow-up, no statistical difference in clinical score was found between the two groups, but the ORIF group had a greater number of severe complications, three of which led to amputation [38]. Watson and colleagues [39] treated 107 pilon fractures in a staged protocol, first applying calcaneal traction followed by ORIF for Tscherne grade 0 or grade I injuries or limited open reduction and stabilization using small-wire external fixators for grade II and grade III injuries. At the average 4.9-year follow-up, 75% of the patients treated with ORIF and 81% of the patients treated with external fixation had good or excellent results. The authors concluded that "soft tissue related complications are markedly decreased when using these external fixation techniques."

More recently, a two-staged procedure has been introduced to provide initial stabilization and recovery time for the soft tissue injury. In three different studies, ORIF of the fibula and application of a medial spanning external fixator was followed an average of 12.7, 17, and 24 days later with ORIF of the tibia. These investigators concluded that this staged protocol provides acceptable results that compare favorably with other techniques [40–42].

Author's approach to pilon fractures

Initial management

The first step taken upon arrival at the emergency department for consultation is an evaluation of the lower-extremity neurovascular status. Nonpalpable pulses are common. Usually edema and the patient's intolerance for palpation of a broken ankle are responsible. In these cases capillary refill testing and a Doppler scan can be used to verify adequate blood supply and patent vascular channels to the foot. When there is obvious dislocation of the ankle in conjunction with nonpalpable pulses and a pale extremity, compression of the anterior neurovascular bundle is suspected. The most common presentation is for the talus and foot to hang posteriorly from the tibia, stretching and choking the anterior tibial artery (Fig. 3). An immediate closed reduction under conscious sedation is performed in this situation.

Evaluation for compartment syndrome is done at the initial examination, and observation continues for the next 36 hours. Any suspicion of a developing compartment syndrome during this time is confirmed or denied with intracompartmental measurements. These measurements are taken with the use of an intracompartmental pressure monitor system (Fig. 4).

Radiographs include three views of the ankle, two views of the leg, and two views of the foot when appropriate. Once a fracture of the distal tibial plafond is seen on radiograph, and the fracture is stabilized, a CT scan is ordered. The CT provides a more detailed picture of the orientation and displacement of the fracture pieces. This information is valuable preoperatively, particularly for deter-

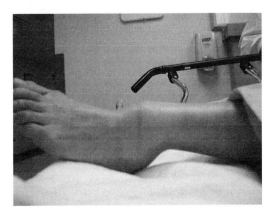

Fig. 3. Dislocation of the ankle. The foot and talus often displace posteriorly and proximally, placing tension on the anterior neurovascular bundle.

mining proper screw size, thread length, and screw alignment to achieve both fracture reduction and protection of important soft tissue structures (Fig. 5). In 1996 Tornetta and Gorup [43] published a paper that emphasized the importance of CT in preoperative planning of pilon fractures. In a prospective study over a period of 2 years, the authors evaluated the radiographs of 22 closed pilon fractures and documented the fracture classification and treatment plan based on this information. The CT scans for each patient were then reviewed to re-evaluate the fracture and treatment plan. They found that the information from the CT scan provided a better understanding of the fracture pattern in 82% of the patients and changed the surgical plan in 64% of the patients. Subjectively, they felt that having a CT shortened operative time for 77% of patients.

After the history and physical examination is complete, displaced fractures are closed, reduced, and splinted, usually after the patient has received pain

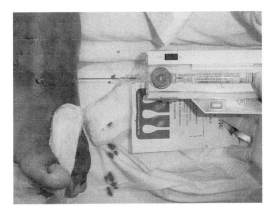

Fig. 4. Intracompartmental pressure system used to evaluate the foot.

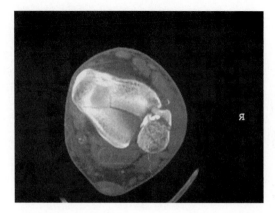

Fig. 5. CT scan of an AO type B pilon fracture just above the ankle joint. This view is used to plan the angle and location for the percutaneous screw.

medication or conscious sedation with midazolam when necessary. Special attention is given to the care of soft tissues. Proper dressings are used for abrasions and wounds. The extremity is elevated, and ice is placed under the knee. A compression dressing applied in the emergency room soon after the original injury can effectively reduce edema and the emergence of fracture blisters. Three layers of cast padding plus extra padding to the posterior heel are wrapped around the lower leg with a light stretch, followed by a layer of elastic bandage, one or two more layers of cast padding, a short-leg posterior splint, and a final layer of elastic bandage. Patients are normally brought to the operating room as soon as they are medically clear. Pilon fractures are treated as emergencies that need immediate skeletal and soft tissue stabilization. In the author's experience, the sooner the fracture is brought to the operating room, the better the healing will be for both the soft tissue and the bony components.

Surgical indications

For most tibial plafond fractures, some form of surgical treatment or attempt at reconstruction of the ankle joint is needed. The authors agree with previous reports that deem conservative care acceptable for nondisplaced fractures, but a nondisplaced fracture of the distal tibial plafond is rare. Because a CT scan is routinely done for all pilon fractures, a displacement of at least 2 mm is frequently found. Although others have suggested that severely comminuted fractures should be casted when articular reconstruction is not possible, the authors believe that application of an external fixator to correct any angular deformity and regain limb length should be done for the benefit of a future arthrodesis. Therefore, conservative care is reserved for a select group of patients, usually those who are not medically stable for surgery.

Surgical goals

Goals of surgical treatment include anatomic reduction of the articular surface, re-establishing the length of the tibia and fibula, re-establishing the normal alignment of the foot, ankle, and leg, and providing stable fracture fixation.
Because pilon fractures have different presentations, the authors' method of treatment can vary depending on the type of fracture, the amount of joint destruction,
the level of soft tissue injury, and the patient's healing potential.

Limited open reduction and Ilizarov external fixation in the treatment of low- and high-energy tibial plafond fractures

Operative technique—low-energy pilon

A low-energy pilon fracture usually contains a few large pieces that can be
reduced by closed methods. Reduction of the articular surface is addressed first.
Patients are brought to the operating room where closed reduction under general
anesthesia is attempted. Distraction is applied to the calcaneus, pulling down the
articular pieces of the tibia to anatomic length using ligamentotaxis. This
distraction could be performed many ways but is most commonly done with a
smooth wire through the calcaneus tensioned to a half-ring. Another option is to
apply the footplate as shown in Fig. 6. The half-ring or footplate is then attached
to the weighted table distractor system with sterile rope. When the medial and
lateral ankle ligaments are essentially intact, this distraction will realign the
contour of the articular surface. An imaging intensifier is used to visualize reduction of the step-off, or vertical displacement. The gap between these articular
pieces is then closed with one or more percutaneous partially threaded 4.0-mm

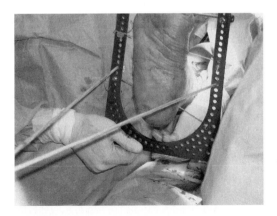

Fig. 6. The footplate is attached to the foot with tensioned smooth wires. Sterile white rope is tied to
the frame and attached to a weighted distraction system.

screws. In some fracture configurations, opposing olive wires might be used instead of screws to compress the fracture. The anatomic constraints of the posterior ankle usually prevent the use of this technique. For frontal plane fractures of the distal tibia, cannulated 4.0-mm screws are strongly recommended.

If distraction alone does not reduce the fracture, large reduction forceps are used percutaneously. If this measure is also unsuccessful, the ankle must be opened. After the major articular fracture is reduced, a prebuilt circular ring frame is properly attached to the foot and leg with reference wires. The frame consists of three full rings and a footplate held together with connecting rods (Fig. 7). Part of the presurgical preparation includes prebuilding the frame to fit the patient so that the distal/reduction ring is located just above the ankle joint. After the frame is locked onto the leg, olive wires are used to reduce remaining fractures. The nuts on the connecting rods are turned to compress or distract and correct any varus/valgus angulation, to distract any metaphyseal comminution, and to distract the fibula fracture.

Low-energy pilon fractures are not always as straightforward as they seem to be on the preoperative radiographs and CT, however. Surgeons who treat pilon fractures with the circular ring fixator must also be proficient with the use of ORIF, because unexpected intraoperative changes in the surgical plan may be needed. The following brief case presentation illustrates this point. A 43-year-old man presented to the emergency room with a closed pilon fracture after a moped accident. The radiographs and CT scan showed a fracture producing an anterolateral fragment, a medial malleolar fracture, and no fibular fracture (Fig. 8). The surgical plan was to close reduce the fracture with distraction and reduction forceps and then fixate the fractures with percutaneous screws, olive wire, and a frame. The patient's ankle was distracted under general anesthesia in the manner described previously. Under C-Arm imaging, a step-off could still be seen. Repeated attempts to reduce the fracture with manual distraction and percutaneous reduction forceps failed. At this point open reduction of the fracture was

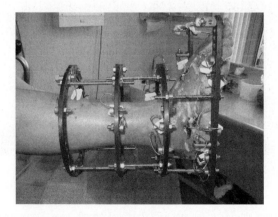

Fig. 7. Pilon frame construct: three full rings and a footplate connected with threaded rods.

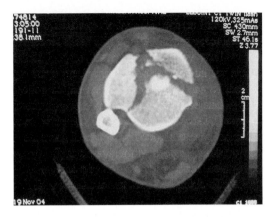

Fig. 8. Preoperative CT of a pilon fracture on which closed reduction failed. Open reduction revealed the anterior neurovascular bundle was caught between the anterolateral piece and the posterior tibia.

necessary. Two incisions were made, one over the medial malleolus and the other over the anterolateral ankle, leaving approximately 8 cm between incisions. Dissection of the anterolateral incision revealed that the anterior neurovascular bundle was caught in the fracture, between the anterolateral piece and the posterior tibia. The fractures were reduced and fixated with screws. A small-wire ring fixator was applied to add stability, provide easy access to wound care, and allow earlier weight bearing (Fig. 9).

Operative technique—the high-energy pilon

The surgical goals and postoperative expectations for high-energy pilon fractures can differ widely, depending on the presentation. For pilons with severe

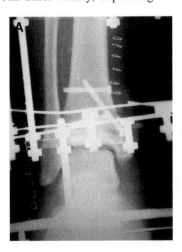
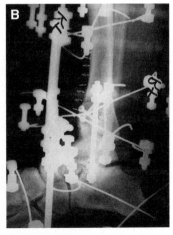

Fig. 9. Post-operative antero-posterior (*A*) and lateral (*B*) radiographs of combined internal and external fixation methods.

articular comminution that is not reconstructable, the immediate goal may be to distract the fracture and re-establish limb length with external fixation. An ankle arthrodesis would be anticipated once there is some fracture consolidation and the soft tissue injuries have resolved. An ankle fusion can significantly reduce a patient's gait and activity level. Therefore an attempt at reducing the articular surface is usually made, even when there is only a slight chance of reconstructing the plafond. The frame construct described previously for the low-energy pilon is used to obtain most of the correction. After the frame is locked on the foot and leg with proper technique, the ankle joint is distracted to regain tibial length by adjusting the screws on the connecting rods between the footplate and the distal ring. Metaphyseal comminution and angulation are corrected on the rods, distracting and shortening as appropriate. The pilon frame is applied and used as described previously to distract and correct for malalignment. The articular fractures are then addressed with percutaneous screws or wires. Many presentations of the high-energy pilon demonstrate impaction of the central portion of the plafond into the metaphysis. The surrounding articular cortical pieces are fractured as well. With distraction of the ankle joint, these pieces anatomically align when their ligamentous and capsular attachments are intact. A C-arm image taken after this distraction is misleading, because the normal contour of the ankle joint can be seen. The central, impacted piece, however, has no ligamentous attachments and will not reduce with distraction alone. It must be dislodged from the metaphysis and brought down into place, along with any other cortical pieces that may not have reduced with distraction.

The reduction of this central, impacted piece is similar in many ways to the reduction of a calcaneal fracture with a depressed posterior facet. In a subtalar joint depression calcaneal fracture, the posterior facet is impacted into the calcaneus; in many of the high-energy pilons fractures, the central plafond piece is impacted into the tibial metaphysis. Just as in the calcaneal fracture that "blows out" and fractures the lateral wall into a delicate thin piece of bone, the axial loading pilon injury frequently creates a thin cortical piece of the anterior tibia. In the calcaneal fracture, this lateral wall is removed to gain exposure of the posterior facet. In ORIF of the pilon fracture, this anterior fracture is similarly lifted away to gain access to the central plafond piece. Just as the posterior facet is lifted up with a small key elevator and temporarily held in place with a Kirschner wire, the central plafond piece is brought down to the level of the ankle and held with a wire.

Full open exposure and extensive dissection of the already compromised tissue is avoided. Instead, a small incision is made over the anterior medial tibia at the site of this fracture. A small key elevator is inserted through the fracture line or is punched through the cortical shell, aiming superiorly toward the impacted piece. The elevator is used to push the piece down to the level of the ankle as seen on the C-Arm. A guide wire or smooth wire is placed across the fragment to hold it in place relative to the other periarticular fractures. A cannulated screw may be placed over this wire to secure the reduction.

The fibula fracture in either of these two general categories of pilon fractures is also addressed with different methods of treatment depending on its presentation. The methods used to fixate the fibula include a Steinman pin placed through the fibula medullary canal, opposing olive wires, or a one-third tubular plate. The choice of method is based on many factors and has been a matter of controversy.

Most reports on the use of external fixation with pilon fractures involve the use of a monolateral or other hybrid external fixator that is placed on the medial side of the foot and leg and a plate placed on the fibula. Most of these articles do not specifically discuss the purpose of fibular plating, but those that do cite its use in establishing length and reducing the fracture of the anterolateral tibia. Williams and colleagues [44] studied the advantages and disadvantages of plating the fibula in a retrospective clinical review. All patients were treated with a monolateral fixator. One group had fibular plate fixation; the other did not. They found no statistical difference in the outcome or clinical ankle score and concluded that good clinical results may be obtained without fixing the fibula.

The circumferential construct of the Ilizarov frame stabilizes the medial and lateral sides of the ankle equally so that a fibular plate is not necessarily needed for lateral support. An intramedullary rod will keep the fibula aligned and is preferred for high fibular fractures with little comminution. This method allows frame adjustments (compression, distraction) to be made. Opposing olive wires can be effective for reducing a simple oblique fibular fracture. Fibular is plating is not routinely done but may be necessary in some cases. When the fibular fracture involves the syndesmosis, an interfragmental screw and plate may be the best way to restore the anatomic alignment of the distal fibula to achieve normal articulation between the distal fibula, tibia, and talus.

Intra-articular fractures of the tibial plafond treated with a staged combination of internal and external fixation devices

Operative technique

Upon presentation to the emergency room, complex fractures with displacement should be reduced and maintained in a well-padded splint to prevent further soft tissue injury. Figs. 10 and 11 illustrate an intra-articular fracture of the distal tibia. This type of fracture is often misdiagnosed as a bimalleolar fracture. As soon as medically feasible, the patient is taken to the operating room. The proposed operative incisions are made for the distal fibula and for the future anteromedial approach to the distal tibia. The incision for the fibula should be as posterior and lateral as possible to allow the largest skin bridge between the two incisions. At a minimum, 7 cm of skin bridge is recommended. Traditional techniques for ORIF of the fibula are used, typically using plates and screws. One-third tubular plates, reconstruction plates, or dynamic compression plates can be used at the surgeon's discretion. Once the fibula is stabilized, and the wound is

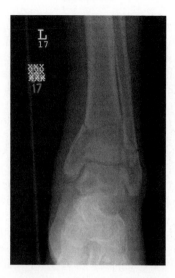

Fig. 10. Anteroposterior radiograph demonstrating an intra-articular fracture of the distal tibia.

closed, external fixation is performed. The authors use two half pins in the tibia and a centrally threaded 5.0-mm transfixion pin in the calcaneal tuberosity [45]. A delta frame is created (Fig. 12). It is important at this time to plan the placement of the pins carefully. The proximal two pins should be well out of the future operative field. The calcaneal pin should be placed inferiorly and posteriorly in a medial-to-lateral direction to avoid the neurovascular bundles. Using manual traction, maximal distraction is achieved, and the fixator is

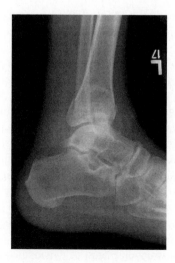

Fig. 11. Lateral radiograph of intra-articular fracture of the distal tibia.

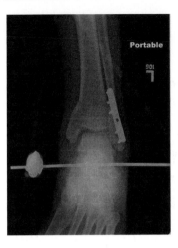

Fig. 12. Anteroposterior radiograph after stage I (ORIF of the distal fibula and application of delta frame).

tightened. If the medical condition permits, the patient usually can be discharged from the hospital within a day or two after this procedure and followed as an outpatient. Once the soft tissue conditions permit, the second stage is performed.

After the patient is brought to the operating room, the external fixator is removed. The half-pins and the transfixion pin are left in and are prepared and draped into the operative field. The external fixator is sterilized. The sterilized external fixator can be used intraoperatively for distraction, or a femoral distractor can be used as well. The distal tibia is accessed through an anteromedial approach [2]. This incision begins approximately 1 cm lateral to the tibial crest and proceeds distally just medial to the tibialis anterior tendon. The extensor retinaculum is incised. The authors try to leave the tibialis anterior tendon and its peritenon undisturbed. Full-thickness skin flaps are raised with care to avoid the saphenous vein medially. Biplanar fluoroscopy is used. Traction is applied to the external fixator or the distractor, and the articular fragments are reduced first. They can be stabilized temporarily with Kirschner wires or with pointed reduction forceps. Definitive stabilization usually includes 3.5-mm cortical screws placed in a lag fashion or 4.0-mm partially threaded cancellous screws. Once the articular surface is reduced anatomically, attention is directed to the metaphyseal extension. The metaphysis is then reduced and stabilized with a low-profile medial plate. A metaphyseal bone defect is common after reduction of the fracture is achieved. These defects should be grafted with either autogenous bone or allograft. The medial low-profile plate functions as a buttress plate connecting the articular fragment to the diaphysis (Figs. 13, 14). After thorough irrigation, the use of a drain is left to the discretion of the operating surgeon. The subcutaneous tissue is reapproximated with 2-0 polyglactin, and the skin is closed with a 3-0 permanent stitch such as nylon or polypropylene. The patient is treated

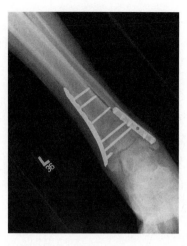

Fig. 13. Anteroposterior radiograph after stage II (ORIF of the distal tibia with less invasive skeletal stabilization).

with parenteral antibiotics for 48 hours postoperatively. If stable fixation is achieved intraoperatively, the external fixator is removed. If there is any question about the stability of the construct, the external fixation can be left on for several weeks postoperatively. The patient is seen in approximately 1 week postoperatively. If the wound is healed at that point, early range of motion can be started if the external fixator has been removed. The authors' preference is to keep the patient non–weight bearing until the fracture is healed, which is typically between 8 and 12 weeks. Sutures are usually removed between the second and third postoperative week. If patient compliance is a potential problem, application

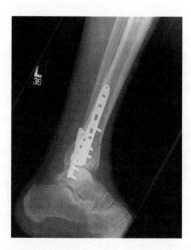

Fig. 14. Lateral radiograph after ORIF of distal tibia fracture.

of a short-leg non–weight-bearing cast is appropriate. A stiff ankle with healed soft tissues is better than an ankle with hardware failure and an open wound. By 12 weeks, most patients can be fully weight bearing in a removable boot walker. Although weight bearing is restricted until the fracture has healed, formal physical therapy may begin much sooner, when the wound has healed.

Alternatives to formal ORIF include percutaneous cannulated screw techniques and minimally invasive plating [46,47]. The percutaneous technique can be used in fractures with minimal intra-articular incongruity. If significant incongruity is present, percutaneous techniques generally are not as successful as open techniques in restoring the anatomy. Minimally invasive plating has become popular in recent years. The articular fragments are reduced percutaneously using fluoroscopy and a pointed reduction forceps. An incision is made approximately 2 to 3 cm over the anteromedial aspect of the tibia just proximal to the fracture. The plate is then placed subcutaneously both proximally and distally through tunnels created with the use of blunt dissection. A Kelly clamp is often useful for this technique. The plate is extraperiosteal, and therefore soft tissue dissection over the fracture site is minimal. Because the periosteum has not been violated, not every screw hole needs to be filled with this technique. Essentially, this plate becomes an "internal" external fixator. As in external fixation, the screws should be placed on both sides of the fracture, and subsequent screws should be placed as far away from the initial screws as possible. Because the screws are much closer to bone, the construction has more stability than a traditional external fixator in which the connecting rods are several centimeters from the bone. The key to the minimally invasive plating technique is to achieve an anatomic reduction without opening the fracture site. If an anatomic reduction is not achieved, formal open reduction is indicated.

Postoperative management

For all patients, wound care and attention to the healing of any incisions, wounds, and pin sites is given. Pin sites are cleaned in the office with saline and dressed with a small amount of antibiotic ointment, gauze, and compressive sponge. The patients are kept non–weight bearing for 6 weeks, at which time radiographs are taken. If evidence of healing across the fractures is seen, the footplate is removed, and the patient begins partial weight bearing. A continuous passive motion machine is used to put the foot and ankle through a triplanar range of motion. The speed and range of motion can be gradually increased as the patient's condition improves. Over the next 4 weeks, the patient also gradually increases the amount of weight bearing. The frame is dynamized by loosening the screws on the connecting rods between the proximal and distal fixation blocks. After 2 weeks the frame is removed if the patient has no pain. If the patient does have pain, the frame is tightened for 2 weeks, after which the dynamization process is repeated. The patient is sent to physical therapy and uses an ankle walker-boot for 4 weeks, after which regular shoe wear is usually allowed.

Prognosis

Little research on the intermediate or long-term outcome of pilon fractures is available. Ruedi and Allgower published two separate studies on the outcome of the patients in their original report on pilon fractures at 4 [13] and 9 years [48] follow-up. They found good or excellent results in 74% of patients 4 years later. Of the 54 patients available for follow-up at 9 years, 12 reported general improvement in their condition, 5 reported aggravation of their symptoms, and 37 reported no change in their status. Overall, a trend toward continued improvement in patients' functional results was shown. Etter and Ganz [29] also reported on the long-term results of low-velocity pilon fractures treated with ORIF. They found good results in 66% of patients.

Marsh and colleagues [49] studied the outcome of 33 pilon fractures treated with a transarticular external fixator coupled with screw fixation of the articular surface at an average of 6.6 years postoperatively. They reported good or excellent results in 25 of the ankles (71%). Results of the Short Form-36 and Ankle Osteoarthritis Scale, however, showed that the pilon fractures created an overall negative effect on patients' general health, ankle function, work, recreation, and health-related quality of life. Fourteen of the patients changed jobs because of their ankle injury. The presence of arthrosis had only weak correlations with clinical outcome. Patients' conditions improved for an average of 2.4 years.

Complications

The complexity of this articular fracture, the destructive nature of the injury, and the paucity of supportive soft tissue structures to the anterior medial ankle predisposes the pilon fracture to many complications. The overall published complication rates are between 13.4% and 55% [7,8,11,26,28–30,32]. The most common complications are wound problems, including skin slough, wound dehiscence, and superficial infection. The highest rates of wound complications have been associated with pilon fractures treated with ORIF. The use of external fixation has been reported to decrease the rate of wound complications when compared with ORIF [4,33,36,38,39,50]. Superficial infections and pin site infections are treated with oral antibiotics. Wound dehiscence and skin slough are treated with wound care.

Deep infection and osteomyelitis are common to almost all reports on pilon fractures and have rates of occurrence between 2.4% to 37% in older studies [7,11,16,29]. More recent studies on the use of spanning external fixation and delayed ORIF claim a much lower incidence, between 0% and 6% [40,41]. Watson and colleagues [39] compared ORIF and external fixation of pilon fractures. Deep infection was seen in 5% of the patients treated with ORIF but in none of the patients treated with external fixation. Deep infection requires more aggressive treatment, including intravenous antibiotics, débridement, and removal of hardware. Other complications associated with pilon fractures are malunion, delayed union, amputation, neuropraxia, reflex sympathetic dystrophy syndrome, and arthrosis.

Summary

Proper handling of the soft tissue has been shown to be paramount for achieving the best possible results with pilon fractures. Review of the literature has shown that the poor results and high complication rates seen in the past with ORIF of high-energy pilons can be reduced with some combination of external fixation, delayed ORIF, or limited incision and internal fixation. The authors prefer the Ilizarov method of external fixation to treat or augment the surgical techniques for most pilon fractures. The circular ring and small wire frame gives the surgeon the ability to distract the ankle, realign angular deformity, stabilize the ankle, and reduce fracture pieces with minimal or no disruption of the soft tissue. The construct is sturdy and allows early weight bearing. Many surgeons justly argue that in many presentations of pilon fracture the most accurate articular reduction is achieved with ORIF. The overall best results for long-term functional outcome and patient satisfaction may be achieved when minimal incision techniques are used, however [25,32–37].

Many studies have shown little or no correlation between radiographic arthrosis and clinical outcome[22,29,38,39]. DeCoster and colleagues [51] studied 25 pilon fractures that were treated with external fixation and limited internal fixation to investigate two generally accepted assumptions: that quality of articular reduction predicts the quality of the outcome, and that the severity of injury correlates with the inferiority of outcome. They found that neither measure correlated with clinical ankle score.

Delaying definitive surgery has been shown to be an effective method of reducing the amount of soft tissue complications in pilon fractures [16,52], but the approaches to pilon fractures described in this article involve immediate surgical attention. As previously discussed, the authors believe that the best reduction and repair occur with early intervention. The author's preference to provide definitive treatment at the initial surgery is based mainly on an understanding of the biology of fracture repair. Between 2 days and 2 weeks after the initial injury, undifferentiated mesenchymal cells migrate to the fracture site and have the ability to form cells that in turn form cartilage, bone, or fibrous tissue. The fracture hematoma is organized, fibroblasts and chondroblasts appear between the bone ends, and cartilage (type II collagen) is formed [53]. Surgery performed within the first 48 hours or as soon as possible after the injury can provide rigid immobilization of properly aligned fracture pieces before fibrous tissue or cartilage has begun to form.

The described approaches to different types of pilon fracture that emphasize the use of the Ilizarov method of external fixation have subjectively proven to be effective during the past 2 years. Formal research measuring the accuracy of articular reduction, the associated complications, and patient's functional outcomes is necessary and in progress.

References

[1] Brumback RJ, McGarvey WC. Fractures of the tibial plafond. Evolving treatment concepts for the pilon fracture. Orthop Clin North Am 1995;26(2):273–85.
[2] Carr JB. Surgical techniques useful in the treatment of complex periarticular fractures of the lower extremity. Orthop Clin North Am 1994;25(4):613–24.
[3] Egol KA, Wolinsky P, Koval KJ. Open reduction and internal fixation of tibial pilon fractures. Foot Ankle Clin 2000;5(4):873–85.
[4] Bone LB. Fractures of the tibial plafond. The pilon fracture. Orthop Clin North Am 1987; 18(1):95–104.
[5] Bourne RB, Rorabeck CH, Macnab J. Intra-articular fractures of the distal tibia: the pilon fracture. J Trauma 1983;23(7):591–6.
[6] Kellam JF, Waddell JP. Fractures of the distal tibial metaphysis with intra-articular extension— the distal tibial explosion fracture. J Trauma 1979;19(8):593–601.
[7] Teeny SM, Wiss DA. Open reduction and internal fixation of tibial plafond fractures. Variables contributing to poor results and complications. Clin Orthop Relat Res 1993;292:108–17.
[8] Dillin L, Slabaugh P. Delayed wound healing, infection, and nonunion following open reduction and internal fixation of tibial plafond fractures. J Trauma 1986;26(12):1116–9.
[9] Lauge-Hansen N. Fractures of the ankle. V. Pronation-dorsiflexion fracture. AMA Arch Surg 1953;67(6):813–20.
[10] Mast JW, Spiegel PG, Pappas JN. Fractures of the tibial pilon. Clin Orthop Relat Res 1988; 230:68–82.
[11] Ovadia DN, Beals RK. Fractures of the tibial plafond. J Bone Joint Surg [Am] 1986;68(4): 543–51.
[12] Wilson Jr LS, Mizel MS, Michelson JD. Foot and ankle injuries in motor vehicle accidents. Foot Ankle Int 2001;22(8):649–52 [erratum in: Foot Ankle Int 2001;22(9):705].
[13] Ruedi TP, Allgower M. The operative treatment of intra-articular fractures of the lower end of the tibia. Clin Orthop 1979;13:105–10.
[14] Ruwe PA, Randall RL, Baumgaertner MR. Pilon fractures of the distal tibia. Orthop Rev 1993; 22(9):987–96.
[15] French B, Tornetta III P. Hybrid external fixation of tibial pilon fractures. Foot Ankle Clin 2000;5(4):853–71.
[16] Helfet DL, Koval K, Pappas J, et al. Intraarticular "pilon" fracture of the tibia. Clin Orthop Relat Res 1994;298:221–8.
[17] Mandracchia VJ, Evans RD, Nelson SC, et al. Pilon fractures of the distal tibia. Clin Podiatr Med Surg 1999;16(4):743–67.
[18] Mueller ME, Allgower M, Schneider R, et al. Manual of internal fixation. 2nd edition. Berlin: Springer-Verlag; 1979.
[19] Muller ME, Nazarian S, Koch P, et al. The comprehensive classification of fractures of long bones. New York: Springer-Verlag; 1990. p. 37, 41, 45.
[20] Dirschl DR, Adams GL. A critical assessment of factors influencing reliability in the classification of fractures, using fractures of the tibial plafond as a model. J Orthop Trauma 1997; 11(7):471–6.
[21] Swiontkowski MF, Sands AK, Agel J, et al. Interobserver variation in the AO/OTA fracture classification system for pilon fractures: is there a problem? J Orthop Trauma 1997;11(7): 467–70.
[22] Martin JS, Marsh JL, Bonar SK, et al. Assessment of the AO/ASIF fracture classification for the distal tibia. J Orthop Trauma 1997;11(7):477–83.

[23] Anderson LD. In: Campbell's operative orthopaedics. Volume 1, Sixth edition. CV Mosby Company; 1980. p. 477–691.
[24] Jergeson F. Open reduction of fractures and dislocations of the ankle. Am J Surg 1959;98: 136–43.
[25] Marsh JL, Bonar S, Nepola JV, et al. Use of an articulated external fixator for fractures of the tibial plafond. J Bone Joint Surg [Am] 1995;77(10):1498–509.
[26] Babis GC, Vayanos ED, Papaioannou N, et al. Results of surgical treatment of tibial plafond fractures. Clin Orthop Relat Res 1997;341:99–105.
[27] Gumann G. Pilon fractures. In: Gumann G, editor. Fractures of the foot and ankle. Philadelphia: Elsevier; 2004.
[28] McFerran MA, Smith SW, Boulas HJ, et al. Complications encountered in the treatment of pilon fractures. J Orthop Trauma 1992;6(2):195–200.
[29] Etter C, Ganz R. Long-term results of tibial plafond fractures treated with open reduction and internal fixation. Arch Orthop Trauma Surg 1991;110(6):277–83.
[30] Rommens PM, Claes P, Broos PL. Therapeutic strategy in pilon fractures type C2 and C3: soft tissue damage changes treatment protocol. Acta Chir Belg 1996;96(2):85–92.
[31] Anglen JO. Early outcome of hybrid external fixation for fracture of the distal tibia. J Orthop Trauma 1999;13(2):92–7.
[32] Barbieri R, Schenk R, Koval K, et al. Hybrid external fixation in the treatment of tibial plafond fractures. Clin Orthop Relat Res 1996;332:16–22.
[33] Tornetta III P, Weiner L, Bergman M, et al. Pilon fractures: treatment with combined internal and external fixation. J Orthop Trauma 1993;7(6):489–96.
[34] Gaudinez RF, Mallik AR, Szporn M. Hybrid external fixation in tibial plafond fractures. Clin Orthop Relat Res 1996;329:223–32.
[35] Mitkovic MB, Bumbasirevic MZ, Lesic A, et al. Dynamic external fixation of comminuted intra-articular fractures of the distal tibia (type C pilon fractures). Acta Orthop Belg 2002;68(5): 508–14.
[36] Bonar SK, Marsh JL. Unilateral external fixation for severe pilon fractures. Foot Ankle 1993; 14(2):57–64.
[37] Syed AA, Agarwal M, Boome R. Dynamic external fixator for pilon fractures of the proximal interphalangeal joints: a simple fixator for a complex fracture. J Hand Surg [Br] 2003;28(2): 137–41.
[38] Wyrsch B, McFerran MA, McAndrew M, et al. Operative treatment of fractures of the tibial plafond. A randomized, prospective study. J Bone Joint Surg [Am] 1996;78(11):1646–57.
[39] Watson JT, Moed BR, Karges DE, et al. Pilon fractures. Treatment protocol based on severity of soft tissue injury. Clin Orthop Relat Res 2000;375:78–90.
[40] Patterson MJ, Cole JD. Two-staged delayed open reduction and internal fixation of severe pilon fractures. J Orthop Trauma 1999;13(2):85–91.
[41] Sirkin M, Sanders R, DiPasquale T, et al. A staged protocol for soft tissue management in the treatment of complex pilon fractures. J Orthop Trauma 1999;13(2):78–84.
[42] Blauth M, Bastian L, Krettek C, et al. Surgical options for the treatment of severe tibial pilon fractures: a study of three techniques. J Orthop Trauma 2001;15(3):153–60.
[43] Tornetta III P, Gorup J. Axial computed tomography of pilon fractures. Clin Orthop Relat Res 1996;323:273–6.
[44] Williams TM, Marsh JL, Nepola JV, et al. External fixation of tibial plafond fractures: is routine plating of the fibula necessary? J Orthop Trauma 1998;12(1):16–20.
[45] Haidukewych GJ. Temporary external fixation for the management of complex intra- and periarticular fractures of the lower extremity. J Orthop Trauma 2002;16:678–85.
[46] Syed MA, Panchbhavi UK. Fixation of tibial pilon fractures with percutaneous cannulated screws. Injury 2004;35:284–9.
[47] Borg T, Larrson S, Lindsjo U. Percutaneous plating of distal tibial fractures. Preliminary results in 21 patients. Injury 2004;35:608–14.
[48] Ruedi T. Fractures of the lower end of the tibia into the ankle joint: results 9 years after open reduction and internal fixation. Injury 1973;5(2):130–4.

[49] Marsh JL, Weigel DP, Dirschl DR. Tibial plafond fractures. How do these ankles function over time? J Bone Joint Surg [Am] 2003;85(2):287–95.

[50] Saleh M, Shanahan MD, Fern ED. Intra-articular fractures of the distal tibia: surgical management by limited internal fixation and articulated distraction. Injury 1993;24(1):37–40.

[51] DeCoster TA, Willis MC, Marsh JL, et al. Rank order analysis of tibial plafond fractures: does injury or reduction predict outcome? Foot Ankle Int 1999;20(1):44–9.

[52] Dickson KF, Montgomery S, Field J. High energy plafond fractures treated by a spanning external fixator initially and followed by a second stage open reduction internal fixation of the articular surface–preliminary report. Injury 2001;32(Suppl 4):SD92–8.

[53] McKibbin B. The biology of fracture healing in long bones. J Bone Joint Surg [Br] 1978;60(2): 150–62.

ELSEVIER
SAUNDERS

Clin Podiatr Med Surg
23 (2006) 445–453

CLINICS IN
PODIATRIC
MEDICINE AND
SURGERY

Current Concepts in Delayed Bone Union and Non-Union

Vasilios D. Polyzois, MD, PhD[a], Ioannis Papakostas, MD[a],
Emmanouil D. Stamatis, MD[b], Thomas Zgonis, DPM[c,*],
Alexandros E. Beris, MD[d]

[a]KAT Hospital, 2 Nikis str, 14561, Kifisia, Athens, Greece
[b]401 General Army Hospital, 138 Mesogion Avenue, Athens, Greece
[c]Division of Podiatry, Department of Orthopaedics,
University of Texas Health Science Center at San Antonio, 7773 Floyd Curl Drive,
San Antonio, TX 78229, USA
[d]Department of Orthopaedics and Traumatology, University of Ioannina Medical School,
PO Box 1186, 451 10 Ioannina, Greece

Healing of a fracture is a continuous process that involves various types of histologic regeneration at different sites. The processes of intramembranous ossification, endochondral ossification, and osteonal remodeling take place at the fracture site (endosteal, periosteal, and cortical) with different functional proportions according to the mechanical and biologic environment [1].

Fracture repair requires the sequential activation of four events to promote healing. The first process is the transportation of systemic undifferentiated mesenchymal osteoprogenitor cells to the fracture site. These cells, through their interrelation with the local population, are stimulated to differentiate into osteoblasts. This second process is osteoinduction. The third event is the activation of this cell population. The final process is the osteoconduction in which collagen and hydroxyapatite surfaces direct bone regeneration.

Because bone healing is a continuous process, clinical, radiologic, or biomechanical criteria must be set to define delayed union or non-union [2,3].

* Corresponding author.
E-mail address: zgonis@uthscsa.edu (T. Zgonis).

Another factor is that union depends also on the chosen method of treatment. Primary bone healing after internal fixation with compression will not show any sign of callus on the radiologic examination because union takes place with osteonal remodeling. With this type of fixation the endpoint of union is the disappearance of the fracture line with no callus formation. With other types of fixation, such as intramedullary nailing, union depends on the formation of external callus visible on the radiograph.

Radiologic examination is a crude way of defining the progress of union. Other techniques, such as the quantitative CT, single-photon absorptiometry, and dual-photon x-ray absorptiometry correlate well with the actual stiffness and biomechanical properties of the fracture site. A stiffness limit in the sagittal dimension has been found to correlate well with the strength of the union [4,5]. A level of 15 N-M/degree is the clinical threshold of union.

One useful definition of non-union is when 9 months has elapsed since the traumatic event, and there have been no visible signs of progressive healing for a minimum of 3 months. Numerous classification systems of non-union have been proposed based on

- Biologic activity
- Presence or absence of infection
- Clinical appearance
- Radiographic criteria
- Location
- Shape

Non-unions can be classified according to the following factors:

1. The presence or absence of infection
2. The amount of motion at the non-union site
3. The presence or absence of bone loss
4. The presence or absence of deformity

The various imaging studies available in nuclear medicine can be helpful in detecting the presence of synovial pseudoarthrosis at the site of the non-union. Three main types of technetium scintigraphic patterns have been described for non-union. The first has uniform increased uptake at the fracture site, the second has a cleft with decreased uptake between two areas of increased uptake, and the third has an intermediary pattern. Excluding the possibility of sepsis at the site of the non-union is of utmost importance because sepsis requires a different treatment strategy [6,7]. Clinical examinations, blood indices, iridium-labeled leukocyte scintigraphy, and MRI are all helpful in defining the presence of sepsis. The criterion standard for evaluating infection in treatment of non-union is tissue biopsy. The technique of obtaining samples should be thorough, with many specimens analyzed.

Management of non-union

Treatment of non-union should address the following issues:

- Mechanical stabilization
- Biologic stimulation
- Deformity
- Bone loss
- Infection
- Soft tissue loss

Conservative and minimally invasive modalities

There is a spectrum of various treatment modalities, and each has a place in the management of non-union [8]. One method without surgical intervention is simple weight bearing in a functional cast or brace as described by Sarmiento and Latta [7]. Weight bearing promotes healing because the intermittent cyclic loading induces the healing process. The theoretical basis of this treatment is that fractures of the skeletal system, without medical intervention, can heal despite motion. Cyclic strain induces the necessary biochemical signals to promote osteoblastic activity. This method can be enhanced with partial fibulectomy. Usually after a fracture of both the tibia and fibula, the fibula unites first, and this union may shield the tibia from the axial strain necessary to induce callus. Furthermore fibular union may result in varus malalignment at the tibial fracture site. This method is useful if there are no signs of pseudoarthrosis formation at the fracture site and if the varus deformity is beyond 15°. This technique involves the removal of 2 cm of fibula above or below the tibial non-union and at least 10 cm of the distal end of the fibula to prevent ankle instability. After the procedure the surgeon manipulates the fracture to correct alignment. Postoperatively it is of utmost importance that the patient bear weight in the plaster cast.

Biologic and biophysical modalities

Many biophysical and biologic modalities can be used to promote healing of non-union with or without other interventions. Percutaneous bone marrow injection is a safe and useful technique with or without use of autogenic bone graft [9]. With this technique a large number of pluripotent stem cells can be harvested and injected under fluoroscopic control at the site of the non-union. The patient to have the benefit of union without donor-site morbidity and the risk involved in surgical implantation of an autogenous bone graft. The usual site for marrow injection is the posterolateral aspect of the tibia, a well-vascularized area. The use of bone morphogenetic proteins is currently under investigation in the treatment of non-union as an adjuvant to internal or external fixation [10–14]. Recombinant human osteogenic protein-1 with a type I collagen carrier has been demonstrated to be an effective and safe alternative; results are comparable with those achieved with bone autograft but without donor-site morbidity [15,16].

Biophysical modalities have also a place in the treatment of non-union. Normally bone shows piezoelectric activity. Small currents generated in response to axial loads have an effect on osteoblastic and osteoclastic activity. There are invasive, semi-invasive and noninvasive techniques for applying electric current across a fracture non-union [17]. Noninvasive techniques that apply pulsed electromagnetic fields are widely accepted. Its safety and the ease of application make bioelectric stimulation useful.

Internal fixation methods

Internal fixation of non-union has an established role in clinical practice. There are two basic types of internal fixation: plate fixation and intramedullary fixation.

Plate fixation is indicated when there is no septic inflammation, the bone is not osteoporotic (thus allowing good screw anchorage), and the fragments are large enough to allow adequate screw purchase [18]. Plate fixation can be combined with cancellous bone grafting, and the surgical technique should result in interfragmentary compression [19]. In hypertrophic non-unions the excess fibrous tissue should not be resected because it will ossify under the proper mechanical conditions, promoting union. Cancellous bone grafting has a place in atrophic non-union when the bone ends are sclerotic or when there is a bone defect caused by the correction of a deformity. Plate fixation is a minimally invasive surgical technique with indirect reduction methods preserving the blood supply of the fragments [20]. The use of plate fixation has declined as newer techniques have developed. Non-unions in the metaphyseal areas of bones continue to be an indication for plate fixation. The use of broad, wide plates is usually advocated to withstand the cyclic loading and prevent fatigue failure.

Intramedullary fixation can be done as a closed or open and as a reamed or unreamed procedure [21]. Intramedullary fixation is a splinting method depending upon the formation of external callus [22]. It is preferable for the fixation to be done in a closed fashion, leaving the blood supply to the site of the non-union undisturbed and minimizing the possibility of infection [23]. In stiff deformities a minimally invasive open technique should be used. Reaming may temporarily disturb the endosteal circulation but also may induce a periosteal reaction that enhances union. With intramedullary techniques it is important to exclude the possibility of sepsis at the site of the non-union, because septic inflammation of the entire intramedullary cavity may result. Because of the possibility of this complication, intramedullary fixation after external fixator removal is not advised. In open reduction to repair a deformity, multiple tissue samples should be examined (by culture and sensitivity testing) to exclude the presence of occult sepsis at the site of non-union.

Intramedullary nailing techniques may address the problem of deformity but cannot adequately address bone defects or shortening. In sclerotic deformities nailing presents many intraoperative difficulties. Before embarking in intra-medullary nailing it is prudent to evaluate the site of non-union radiographically for intramedullary callus or step-off deformity that necessitates open reduction for nail passage. In open reductions the surgeon should use adjuvant measures such as autogenic bone grafting to ensure union.

The posterolateral bone grafting technique involves the formation of an osseous bridge between the fibula and tibia above and below the tibial defect [24]. This technique may be useful in cases of septic non-union with tibial defects. Other bone grafting techniques include the use of vascularized fibula autograft or various structural allografts [25]. These methods have been largely superseded by the evolution of external fixation and especially the circular ring fixator of Ilizarov [13,23].

External fixation methods

External fixation methods have distinct advantages for the treatment of non-unions, especially in infected cases [26]. External fixation using monolateral frames with ball joints or rails with swiveling clamps can be applied successfully to correct deformities, shortening, or infection. The diversity in the application of circular frames as described by Ilizarov achieving compression, distraction, bone transport, and correction of various angular deformities make this as the preferred technique for non-union [13,23].

Transosseous osteosynthesis is adequate for immediate functional use of the limb and promotes osteogenesis [27–32]. In atrophic non-unions corticotomy is a powerful stimulus to increase the blood supply to the limb with neo-vascularization. Infected non-unions can be treated with wide débridement and bone transport. This method has also the advantage of promoting histogenesis, as well as bone regeneration, thus achieving soft tissue coverage in difficult cases.

Clinically stiff non-unions are usually hypertrophic. Blood supply is adequate, but the interposed fibrocartilage cannot mineralize because of mechanical factors. Ilizarov showed that, with progressive compression and distraction and concomitant axial alignment, stiff non-unions can heal reliably without the need for additional bone grafting [13,23,32]. Shear loads at the fracture site should be completely eliminated, because this type of loading is detrimental in the union process.

Mobile non-unions are usually atrophic with devascularization of the segments. Mobile unions need biologic stimulation to promote healing. According to Ilizarov, corticotomy with distraction induces neovascularization and promotes the mechanical environment necessary for union [32–38]. This technique involves creating a corticotomy away of the site of the non-union and then distracting the corticotomy while applying compression at the site of the non-union. With mobile non-unions bone-grafting procedures may be needed at the site of the non-union.

In mobile atrophic non-union without sepsis, there is deficiency of both mechanical and biologic factors. Mobile non-unions require added mechanical stability with four rings and a corticotomy or the use of bone grafts to induce healing. Applying distraction at the site of the corticotomy and compression at the site of the non-union results in healing provided there is adequate frame stability.

In stiff hypertrophic non-union without deformity and without the presence of sepsis, treatment is based on progressive distraction followed by compression at the fracture site. Ilizarov advocated a preliminary phase of compression, then distraction, and finally compression to achieve union [32–38]. In these stiff non-unions the fibrous zone that lies between the fragments resembles the relatively avascular central fibrous zone of the regenerated bone. Thus distraction stimulates this fibrous tissue to promote healing. Again the construct with four rings and olive wires according to the morphology of the non-union is adequate. For successful healing it is prudent to achieve interfragmentary compression with proper placing of olive wires in oblique patterns. It is important the bone segments are congruent, in good position, and sufficiently stable.

Stiff non-union with deformity but without bone loss requires adequate preoperative planning. There are various constructs that can address deformity. Four-ring constructs with olive wires properly placed (according to the four-bending principle) and the use of hinges can restore deformity. The placement of hinges in the construct depends on the morphologic characteristics of the deformity and requires trigonometric planning for accurate corrections. Another useful construct is with transverse wires and two half-rings at the convex side, but this construct requires careful preoperative planning because transverse wires cannot be placed safely in certain fracture configurations. For stiff non-unions with severe angulation, the most mechanically rigid construct is the combined construct. With this construct, the four rings are connected at the convex side with a long connecting plate and at the concave side with a telescopic rod.

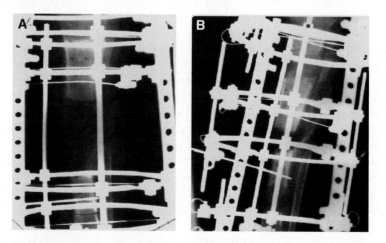

Fig. 1. (A–B) Antero-posterior and lateral radiographic views of bone transportation.

Bone defects pose different problems that require appropriate strategies [33–36]. Bone defects may be combined with preservation or loss of the overall length of the limb, or there may be a loss of limb length with segments in contact. Ilizarov's methods can treat these defects adequately with limb lengthening and bone transportation (Fig. 1) [34–38]. Various techniques are used depending on the amount of bone loss and the presence of deformity. Bone grafting may be needed at the docking site to achieve union. Monofocal bone transportation involves the placement of the rings to achieve distraction osteogenesis through a properly placed corticotomy to gap the defect and then interfragmentary compression at the docking site. In large defects bifocal transportation or extensive bone transportation with longitudinally placed olive wires may be needed.

There are special procedures to address specific problems [37]. In a subtotal tibial defect with atrophic segments, half of the bone can be transported toward the tibial defect using a longitudinal osteotomy of the fibula. A similar method used after bifocal corticotomy is the transportation of a whole fibular segment toward the posterolateral aspect of the tibia with olive wires and an appropriate frame. At the end of transportation, transverse compression is instituted. Other techniques involve the transportation of a segment of the cortex to fill partial tibial defects.

Ilizarov methods are the treatment of choice in cases of infected non-unions [37–43]. The first stage of treatment is the appropriate débridement of all necrotic infected material or foreign bodies. With débridement the surgeon imposes a stimulatory effect for promotion of the reparative process. Transosseous wire stabilization away from the inflamed site safely provides the stability necessary to promote healing. Sinus or wound dehiscence generally heals spontaneously after appropriate treatment of the internal osseous infection. The débridement of the two segments should result in viable bone ends that are congruent for future docking. The bone defect is addressed with the various bone transportation techniques described previously.

References

[1] Müller ME, Allgower M, Schneider R, et al. Manual of internal fixation techniques recommended by the AO-ASIF Group. Berlin: Springer-Verlag; 1991.

[2] Hadjiargyrou M, McLeod K, Ryaby JP, et al. Enhancement of fracture healing by low intensity ultrasound. Clin Orthop 1998;355:216–29.

[3] Reimer BL, Sagiv S, Butterfield SL, et al. Tibial diaphyseal nonunions after external fixation treated with nonreamed solid core nails. Orthopedics 1996;19:109–16.

[4] Jupiter JB, First K, Gallico GG, et al. The role of external fixation in the treatment of posttraumatic osteomyelitis. J Orthop Trauma 1988;2:79–93.

[5] Perren SM. The concept of biological plating using the limited contact dynamic compression plate (LC-DCP): scientific background, design and application. Injury 1991;22:1–41.

[6] Green SA. Skeletal defects: a comparison of bone grafting and bone transport for segmental skeletal defects. Clin Orthop 1994;301:111–7.

[7] Sarmiento A, Burkhalter WE, Latta LL. Functional bracing in the treatment of delayed union and nonunion of the tibia. Int Orthop 2003;27:26–9.

452   POLYZOIS et al

[8] Gustilo RB, Anderson JT. Prevention of infection in the treatment of one thousand and twenty-five open fractures of the long bones: retrospective and prospective analysis. J Bone Joint Surg [Am] 1976;58:453–8.
[9] Friedlaender GE, Perry CR, Cole JD, et al. Osteogenic protein-1 (bone morphogenetic protein-7) in the treatment of tibial nonunions. J Bone Joint Surg [Am] 2001;83(Suppl 1):S151–8.
[10] Brownlow HC, Reed A, Simpson AH. Growth factor expression during the development of atrophic non-union. Injury 2001;32:519–24.
[11] Klein MP, Rahn BA, Frigg R, et al. Reaming versus non-reaming in medullary nailing: interference with cortical circulation of the canine tibia. Arch Orthop Trauma Surg 1990;109: 314–6.
[12] Lamerigts NM, Buma P, Aspenberg P, et al. Role of growth factors in the incorporation of unloaded bone allografts in the goat. Clin Orthop 1999;368:260–70.
[13] Paley D, Catagni MA, Argnani F, et al. Ilizarov treatment of tibial nonunions with bone loss. Clin Orthop 1989;241:146–65.
[14] Sowa DT, Weiland AJ. Clinical applications of vascularized bone autografts. Orthop Clin North Am 1987;18:257–73.
[15] Christian EP, Bosse MJ, Robb G. Reconstruction of large diaphyseal defects, without free fibular transfer, in grade IIIB tibial fractures. J Bone Joint Surg [Am] 1989;71:994–1004.
[16] Cook SD, Baffes GC, Wolfe MW, et al. The effect of recombinant human osteogenic protein-1 on healing of large segmental bone defects. J Bone Joint Surg [Am] 1994;76:827–38.
[17] Bray TJ. A prospective, double-blind trial of electrical capacitive coupling in the treatment of non-union of long bones. J Bone Joint Surg [Am] 1994;76:820–6.
[18] Menon DK, Dougali TW, Pool RD, et al. Augmentative Ilizarov external fixation after failure of diaphyseal union with intramedullary nailing. J Orthop Trauma 2002;16:491–7.
[19] Pecina M, Giltaij LR, Vukicevic S. Orthopaedic applications of osteogenic protein-1 (BMP-7). Int Orthop 2001;25:203–8.
[20] Hulth A. Current concepts of fracture healing. Clin Orthop 1989;249:265–84.
[21] Kay P, Freemont A, Edwards J, et al. Quantification of fracture repair by direct stiffness measurement and vibration analysis. J Bone Joint Surg [Br] 1992;74(Suppl 11):134.
[22] Reckling FW, Waters CH. Treatment of non-unions of fractures of the tibial diaphysis by posterolateral cortical cancellous bone-grafting. J Bone Joint Surg [Am] 1980;62:936–41.
[23] Owen MA. Use of the Ilizarov method to manage a septic tibial fracture nonunion with a large cortical defect. J Small Anim Pract 2000;41:124–7.
[24] Richardson JB, Cunningham JL, Goodship AE, et al. Measuring stiffness can define healing of tibial fractures. J Bone Joint Surg [Br] 1994;76:389–94.
[25] Shahcheraghi GH, Bayatpoor A. Infected tibial nonunion. Can J Surg 1994;37:209–13.
[26] Jenny G, Jenny JY, Mosser JJ. Ilizarov's method in infected tibial pseudo-arthrosis and for reconstruction of bone defects. Orthop Traumatol 1993;3:55–8.
[27] Aronson J. Limb-lengthening, skeletal reconstruction, and bone transport with the Ilizarov method. J Bone Joint Surg [Am] 1997;79:1243–58.
[28] Garg NK, Gaur S, Sharma S. Percutaneous autogenous bone marrow grafting in 29 cases of ununited fracture. Acta Orthop Scand 1993;64:671–2.
[29] Helfet DL, Jupiter JB, Gasser S. Indirect reduction and tension-band plating of tibial non-union with deformity. J Bone Joint Surg [Am] 1992;74:1286–97.
[30] Paley D, Herzenberg JE. Intramedullary infections treated with antibiotic cement rods: preliminary results in nine cases. J Orthop Trauma 2002;16:723–9.
[31] Schmitt JM, Hwang K, Winn SR, et al. Bone morphogenetic proteins: an update on basic biology and clinical relevance. J Orthop Res 1999;17:269–78.
[32] Schwartsman V, Choi SH, Schwartsman R. Tibial nonunions: treatment tactics with the Ilizarov method. Orthop Clin North Am 1990;21:639–53.
[33] Green SA. Ilizarov-type treatment of nonunions, malunions and post-traumatic shortening. In: Chapman MW, editor. Operative orthopaedics. Philadelphia: JB Lippincott; 1993. p. 949–64.
[34] Ilizarov GA. The transosseous osteosynthesis. Theoretical and clinical aspects of the regeneration and growth of tissue. New York: Springer-Verlag; 1992.

[35] Paley D, Chaudray M, Pirone AM, et al. Treatment of malunions and mal-nonunions of the femur and tibia by detailed preoperative planning and the Ilizarov techniques. Orthop Clin North Am 1990;21:667–91.

[36] Paley D. Problems, obstacles, and complications of limb lengthening by the Ilizarov technique. Clin Orthop 1990;250:81–104.

[37] Cattaneo R, Catagni M, Johnson EE. The treatment of infected nonunions and segmental defects of the tibia by the methods of Ilizarov. Clin Orthop 1992;280:143–52.

[38] Ilizarov GA. Clinical application of the tension-stress effect for limb lengthening. Clin Orthop 1990;250:8–26.

[39] Lane JM, Yasko AW, Tomin E, et al. Bone marrow and recombinant human bone morphogenetic protein-2 in osseous repair. Clin Orthop 1999;361:217–27.

[40] Milgram JV. Nonunion and pseudarthrosis of fracture healing: a histopathologic study of 95 humans specimens. Clin Orthop 1991;268:203–13.

[41] Marsh JL, Prokuski L, Biermann JS. Chronic infected tibial nonunions with bone loss: conventional techniques versus bone transport. Clin Orthop 1994;301:139–46.

[42] Ring D, Barrick WT, Jupiter JB. Recalcitrant nonunion. Clin Orthop 1997;340:181–9.

[43] Saleh M, Royston S. Management of nonunion of fractures by distraction with correction of angulation and shortening. J Bone Joint Surg [Br] 1996;78:105–9.

ELSEVIER
SAUNDERS

Clin Podiatr Med Surg
23 (2006) 455–465

CLINICS IN
PODIATRIC
MEDICINE AND
SURGERY

Current Concepts and Techniques in Posttraumatic Arthritis

Vasilios D. Polyzois, MD, PhD[a,*], Ioannis Papakostas, MD[a],
Thomas Zgonis, DPM[b], Demetrios G. Polyzois, MD[c],
Panayotis N. Soucacos, MD[d]

[a]KAT Hospital, 2 Nikis str, 14561, Kifisia, Athens, Greece
[b]Division of Podiatry, Department of Orthopaedics, University of Texas Health Science Center at
San Antonio, 7773 Floyd Curl Drive, San Antonio, TX 78229, USA
[c]Department of Orthopaedic Surgery, Metropolitan Hospital, Athens, Greece
[d]Department of Orthopaedics and Traumatology, University of Athens Medical School,
Athens, Greece

Posttraumatic arthritis is a commonly encountered clinical problem, but the pathoetiology of its development is not yet clarified. Many contributing mechanical biologic factors interplay with the traumatic event that necessarily precedes the posttraumatic syndrome. New biologic concepts involving the ability of the cartilage to repair and how such healing can be promoted are being realized in new modalities of treatment. The traumatic event as such and the resulting pathomechanical consequences require new ways of evaluation.

Currently, the tools necessary to evaluate the full spectrum of injuries to the various tissues involved in a traumatic event are lacking. Radiologic examination with limitations, defines, with limitations, the bony injury, but there are no available methods to assess the more important trauma to the cartilage tissue itself. The treatment of intra-articular injuries has focused on the anatomic restoration of joint congruity and early mobilization. Current research clarifies the predominant role of the primary chondral damage, which largely defines the final outcome irrespective of the method of treatment. Current concepts of minimal invasive surgery and indirect reduction techniques take precedence over perfect anatomic reduction at all costs.

* Corresponding author.
E-mail address: bpolyzois@yahoo.com (V.D. Polyzois).

0891-8422/06/$ – see front matter © 2006 Elsevier Inc. All rights reserved.
doi:10.1016/j.cpm.2006.01.006   *podiatric.theclinics.com*

The biologic events that follow after an intra-articular injury are matters of intense research [1–6]. The study of the structure of articular cartilage and the impact of the traumatic event on the normal potential of chondral self repair opens new biologic ways to promote healing and to prevent the progression of posttraumatic arthritis. The traumatic events that lead to the development of posttraumatic osteoarthritis include direct and indirect articular and periarticular injuries [7–11]. The nature of the injury largely defines the posttraumatic prognosis [12,13].

Types of chondral and osteochondral damage

There are three basic types of chondral and osteochondral injuries [14–16]. The first type consists of damage to the matrix and cellular elements with no visible injury to the chondral surface. The clinician lacks appropriate methods for evaluating this type of damage. MRI examination or even arthroscopy does not provide the necessary information. An impact load of lower magnitude than necessary to produce chondral disruption affects the pericellular elements, and the first consequence is a reduction in proteoglycan aggregation [17]. Chondrocytes respond to such injury with increased proteoglycan synthesis; providing that the fibrillar elements remain intact and the number of adapting cells is sufficient, there is a possibility for restoration. On the other hand, it has been shown that impact loading increases the apoptosis of chondrocytes [18–21]. If the injury exceeds the tissue's capability for restoration, the articular defect remains permanent, and there is increased risk for joint degeneration [22,23].

With the second type of injury there is a chondral fracture or disruption that does not extent to the subchondral bone. This type of injury can be evaluated with MRI or CT scan. Because the articular cartilage has no blood supply, it is aneural with no lymphatics and depends on the diffusion of the interstitial fluid and on anaerobic glycolysis to survive. As a result, after this type of injury, there are no signs of inflammation or fibrin clot formation. Chondrocytes increase their anabolic activity, producing new macromolecules and proliferating, but increased activity is not adequate to restore the defect [24]. This lesion may proceed to the development of posttraumatic arthritis depending on the extent and intra-articular location of the lesion. Cartilage responds to this type of injury, but the repair process usually is not sufficient to fill the defect.

The third type of injury is the osteochondral fracture. CT scan can usually be of help in evaluating this type of damage [25]. Cartilage and subchondral bone disruption leads to the formation of a fibrin clot and to inflammation. Besides the presence of the articular fracture, this type of damage usually includes areas of chondral damage or cartilage disruption.

When there is a gap between the intra-articular fragments, healing take place with the formation of fibrocartilage. This process involves various growth factors and the differentiation of mesenchymal cells. With this process in the chondral region of the defect, cells develop that assume the rounded form of chondrocytes, and in the bony portion cells begin to synthesize immature bone. The resulting fibrocartilage is not durable and usually (depending on mechanical and biologic factors) begins to show signs of degeneration. There is a depletion of proteoglycans and increased fragmentation; the end result is a matrix consisting primarily of closely packed collagen fibers. This tissue cannot support the necessary loads and usually fragments and exposes the underlying bone.

In intra-articular step-offs animal studies indicate there is potential for remodeling after trauma if there is no instability or mechanical malalignment [26,27]. Step-offs of the same height as the thickness of the involved cartilage have good potential for remodeling [28,29]. Another study showed that intra-articular gaps 3 mm wide with 2-mm step off in a rabbit femoral condylar surface can be restored to a congruent articular surface [30]. This study does not support the necessity of perfect anatomic reduction in intra-articular fractures [31].

Evaluation of joint injury

One important aspect in the pathogenesis of posttraumatic arthritis is the residual joint instability and its role in the progression of arthritis [32]. Joint instability may result from ligament rupture, injury to the menisci or joint capsule, or loss of the articular congruity. This instability results in abnormal translational and rotational movement that, in combination with the loss of articular congruity, leads to rapid joint degeneration.

Joint trauma may result from loss of protective innervation, which may further compromise the ability of the joint to withstand axial, shear, and rotational loads. Open reduction techniques using capsulotomy may result in partial joint denervation, further compromising the result [5]. One great advantage of techniques that do not use incisions (external fixation, the Ilizarov method) is that they respect the blood supply and the innervation of the capsule and the intra-articular fragments.

Different joints have different potential for remodeling. Every joint has different anatomic and mechanical characteristics that define the prognosis of an intra-articular injury. To a great extent, the thickness of the articular cartilage, the biomechanical characteristics of the particular cartilage, and the overall joint congruity define the potential for remodeling [33,34].

Posttraumatic arthritis is more common than primary arthritis in the ankle. The knee is less susceptible than the ankle to the development of posttraumatic arthritis.

The age of the individual influences the characteristics of the injury. The cartilage defect' potential for remodeling reduces with increasing age [35–37]. Cartilage cells have decreased ability for anabolic activity, and the older individual is more susceptible overall to the progression of posttraumatic arthritis. Therefore treatment of both primary intra-articular fracture and posttraumatic arthritis should be individualized according to the nature of the trauma, the particular joint involved, the age of the patient, and other factors.

Conservative treatment

There are many palliative conservative measures for managing posttraumatic arthritis. Pharmacologic intervention, physical therapy for muscle strengthening, and proprioceptive training can be of benefit. Various types of ankle foot orthoses (eg, custom-made molded-propylene, metal double upright, patella tendon-bearing ankle–foot orthoses, and others) may provide symptom relief.

Surgical treatment

There are six broad categories of surgical options for posttraumatic arthritis [38]:

- Osteotomy (mechanical realignment, bone reconstruction with internal fixation of malunited fractures)
- Joint débridement
- Arthroscopy (débridement, arthroscopic arthrodesis)
- Arthrodiastasis
- Arthrodesis
- Arthroplasty

Joint reconstruction

Malunited ankle fractures can become symptomatic as a result of inadequate reduction or loss of reduction after open or closed treatment. Because of the malalignment there is a shift of the talus in the mortise, resulting in loss of articular congruency and cartilage wear. The success of the reconstruction depends to a great extent on the timing of the operation, because late reconstruction has the added burden of increased cartilage wear. A malunited fibula can be osteotomized, lengthened, and internally rotated to restore Shenton's and the arcuate line. A medial malleolar malunion can be osteotomised and fixed with lag screws, tension band construct, a medial spring plate, or a buttress pate. A posterior malleolar malunion should be treated in symptomatic patients if it includes more than 25% of the articular surface when the fragment is significantly displaced or associated with joint instability. Overall these procedures involve realignment of articular surfaces with osteotomies and bone grafting, removal of debris, scar, and hypertrophic synovium, long bone osteotomies, and ligamentous repair. When arthritis is limited to one side of the joint, with medial joint-space narrowing and preservation of the lateral side, tibial medial-opening osteotomies can improve the symptoms and the ability of walking. Usually this type of intervention does not improve the range of movement of the joint.

Joint débridement

Joint débridement has a place in the treatment of arthritis of mild-to-moderate severity.

Anterior tibiotalar impingement caused by the presence of anterior bone spurs and the subsequent posterior opening in dorsiflexion responds well to open or arthroscopic methods. Débridement consists of removing the osteophytes from the leading edge of the tibia and talar neck, excision of hypertrophic synovium and scar tissue, and removal of loose bodies from the anterior ankle.

Arthroscopic débridement with rigid intraoperative distraction has been shown to improve function and range of motion. This method is worth considering as an alternative to arthrodesis in patients who have mild deformity and no instability. If symptoms are refractory, the surgeon can still perform arthrodesis. With this technique arthrodesis can be delayed or even avoided in more than half the patients.

Arthrodiastasis

Distraction using the Ilizarov apparatus (Fig. 1) has been studied by van Valburg and colleagues [39]. In this study a 5-mm distraction was applied across the ankle joint for 18 to 34 weeks (with hinges added 6 to 12 weeks after surgery). The results showed promise, with more than half of the subjects increasing their range of movement, all subjects experiencing some pain relief

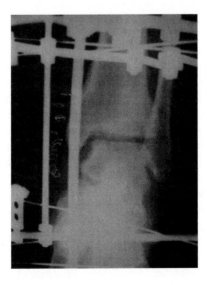

Fig. 1. Arthrodiastasis with Ilizarov technique.

(40% experiencing complete relief), and more than 50% showing joint widening on radiographs. Long-term sustained results are needed for complete evaluation of this method.

Arthrodesis

Arthrodesis is the criterion standard in the treatment of moderate and severe posttraumatic arthritis [40–42]. Currently there are many techniques for ankle arthrodesis, which can be grouped in five categories [38]:

- Compression arthrodesis with internal fixation
- Compression arthrodesis with external fixation
- Arthroscopic arthrodesis combined with internal fixation
- Arthrodesis using the fibula as a graft
- Arthrodesis using the tibia as a sliding graft

The preferred position of arthrodesis is in slight external rotation (5°–10°), neutral or slight valgus (5°–8°), and neutral plantar dorsiflexion [43]. When the lower fibula is preserved, some slight medial translation of the talus may be acceptable. Some authors stress the importance of positioning the center of the talar dome posterior to the midline of the tibia to improve the posterior lever arm of the calcaneus.

The surgical approaches can be classified as anterior, medial or lateral, and posterior. The anterior approach may lead to postoperative complications such as neuromas and tendon adhesions. Because of the improved cosmesis and the decreased risk of postoperative complications, the currently preferred approach is lateral or anterolateral with the addition of a medial incision if necessary.

For internal fixation of the arthrodesis site the bony configuration is the principal determinant factor for achieving union. The congruent apposition with compression of the two bone surfaces ensures rapid union if there is adequate blood supply. The apposed bone surfaces may be simply denuded of cartilage, or the surgeon may remove the subchondral bone, creating flat parallel surfaces or a chevron type cut [44]. The removal, transposition, or incorporation of the malleoli is the subject of many controversies. Malleoli may be removed if the surgeon thinks they may cause impingement postoperatively. Others believe that the medial malleolus stabilizes the talus postoperatively. Removal of the fibula is not detrimental to the function of the subtalar joint. Biomechanical studies have been shown that the malleoli can be reattached with lag screws to improve the strength of the arthrodesis.

Many authors advocate the use of lag screws for internal fixation of the arthrodesis site [45,46]. Lag screws attached in crossed fashion have increased biomechanical strength, but the parallel configuration provides improved compression. With crossed screws inadequate compression may inhibit fusion. A construct with two parallel lag screws from the tibia to the talus and a third posterior screw from the posterior malleolus to the neck and head of the talus provides improved stabilization at plantar and dorsiflexion stresses. Some authors have good results with the use of T plate fixation, which provides a more rigid construct at the expense of increased stripping of the soft tissues.

Retrograde intramedullary nailing for tibio-talo-calcaneal arthrodesis has been described recently [47,48]. This technique can be used in severely osteoporotic bone, providing adequate stability to allow weight bearing. Retrograde nailing is not without complications because of its insertion from the sole of the foot. Anatomic structures at risk at the sole of the foot are the origin of the short flexors, the lateral plantar nerve and artery, and the plantar fascia.

For minimal deformity but severe cartilage destruction, a new method is arthroscopic arthrodesis. Because of its minimal invasiveness, it allows earlier mobilization and reduced hospitalization. Poor blood supply, bleeding disorders, and the presence of flaps around the ankle are some of the conditions for which arthroscopic arthrodesis is more appropriate. It is a difficult technique even for advanced ankle arthroscopists. The cartilage is removed down to bone using curettes and power burs, and the site then is stabilized with cannulated screws. Postoperatively the ankle is immobilized in plaster, and then mobilization is encouraged using a brace.

Ilizarov ankle arthrodesis

The Ilizarov technique in ankle fusion remains a reliable and very successful method of treatment [49–51]. This method has many advantages:

- Full weight bearing
- Increased stabilization of fusion site
- Increased compression at fusion site
- Decreased trauma of the talus
- Ability to increase compression after surgery
- Ability to distract the subtalar joint while compressing the ankle joint

Before the application of the frame the authors advocate using a lateral approach for lateral dissection and splitting of the fibula, ankle joint resection with resection of the lateral aspect of the talus, and onlay fibular sliding grafting at the lateral aspect of the talus. Compression with the frame is achieved with the bent-wire technique (Fig. 2).

There are basically two frame configurations for ankle arthrodesis. The first construct (Fig. 3) includes one proximal tibial ring, one distal tibial ring, one talar ring, and a footplate. The second type (Fig. 4) includes one proximal tibial ring, one distal tibial ring, and a footplate without talar ring. With the latter configuration compression is exerted through the subtalar joint. Subtalar joint compression can be prevented with the use of raised wires from the footplate.

The Ilizarov method has diverse applications. It can be used in complex foot deformities, osteomyelitis, and limb-length discrepancies. The technique requires extensive experience and a dedicated team approach with continuous patient evaluations. The patient should be compliant and dedicated to achieving satis-

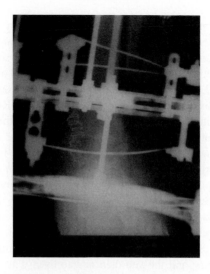

Fig. 2. Bent-wire technique.

factory results. In the authors' series using a ring fixator, union was achieved in 93% of the cases at 7 weeks.

Ankle arthroplasty

Because arthrodesis always imparts some disability and increases the load transmitted through the others joints of the hindfoot, efforts have been made to

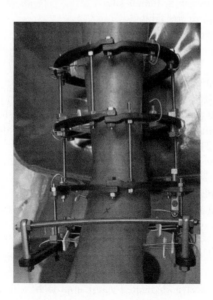

Fig. 3. First type of configuration.

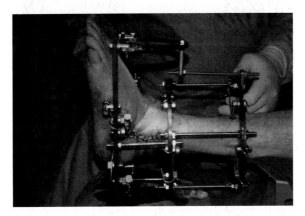

Fig. 4. Second type of configuration.

improve the results of ankle arthroplasty in the long term [52–55]. Earlier designs had an unacceptable rate of failure, often 10% per annum. Earlier designs were of the constrained type, which does not allow distal fibular rotation to optimize lateral ligamentous function. Also, constrained designs fail to accommodate rotational or shear loads, which are transmitted to the bone implant interface. These loads increase the rate of loosening of the prosthesis. Newer semiconstrained mobile bearing designs have improved biomechanical characteristics and with diligent surgical incision and wound management can achieve satisfactory results. Survivorship of 92% at 12 years has been reported with these newer implants.

References

[1] Borrelli Jr J, Torzilli PA, Grigiene R, et al. Effect of impact load on articular cartilage: development of an intra-articular fracture model. J Orthop Trauma 1997;11:319–26.

[2] D'Lima DD, Hashimoto S, Chen PC, et al. Impact of mechanical trauma on matrix and cells. Clin Orthop 2001;391(Suppl):S90–9.

[3] Haut RC. Contact pressures in the patellofemoral joint during impact loading on the human flexed knee. J Orthop Res 1989;7:272–80.

[4] O'Connor BL, Palmoski MJ, Brandt KD. Neurogenic acceleration of degenerative joint lesions. J Bone Joint Surg [Am] 1985;67:562–72.

[5] O'Connor BL, Visco DM, Brandt KD, et al. Neurogenic acceleration of osteoarthritis. J Bone Joint Surg [Am] 1992;74:367–76.

[6] Oloyede A, Flachsmann R, Broom ND. The dramatic influence of loading velocity on the compressive response of articular cartilage. Connect Tissue Res 1992;27:211–24.

[7] Aspden RM, Jeffrey JE, Burgin LV. Impact loading of articular cartilage. Osteoarthritis Cartilage 2002;10:588–90.

[8] Buckwalter JA. Osteoarthritis and articular cartilage use, disuse and abuse: experimental studies. J Rheumatol 1995;22(Suppl 43):13–5.

[9] Patwari P, Fay J, Cook MN, et al. In vitro models for investigation of the effects of acute mechanical injury on cartilage. Clin Orthop 2001;393(Suppl):S61–71.

[10] Torzilli PA, Grigiene R, Borrelli Jr J, et al. Effect of impact load on articular cartilage: cell metabolism and viability, and matrix water content. J Biomech Eng 1999;121:433–41.

[11] Zang H, Vrahas MS, Baratta RV, et al. Damage to rabbit femoral articular cartilage following direct impacts of uniform stresses: an in vitro study. Clin Biomech 1999;14:543–8.

[12] Buckwalter JA. Evaluating methods of restoring cartilaginous articular surfaces. Clin Orthop 1999;367(Suppl):224–38.

[13] Buckwalter JA, Stanish WD, Rosier RN, et al. The increasing need for nonoperative treatment of osteoarthritis. Clin Orthop 2001;385:36–45.

[14] Buckwalter JA. Articular cartilage injuries. Clin Orthop 2002;402:21–37.

[15] Buckwalter JA, Mankin HJ. Articular cartilage: I. Tissue design and chondrocyte-matrix interactions. J Bone Joint Surg [Am] 1997;79:600–11.

[16] Buckwalter JA, Mankin HJ. Articular cartilage: II. Degeneration and osteoarthrosis, repair, regeneration and transplantation. J Bone Joint Surg [Am] 1997;79:612–32.

[17] Patwari P, Cook MN, DiMicco MA, et al. Proteoglycan degradation after injurious compression of bovine and human articular cartilage in vitro: interaction with exogenous cytokines. Arthritis Rheum 2003;48:1292–301.

[18] Duda GN, Eilers M, Loh L, et al. Chondrocyte death precedes structural damage in blunt impact trauma. Clin Orthop 2001;393:302–9.

[19] Ewers BJ, Dvoracek-Driksna D, Orth MW, et al. The extent of matrix damage and chondrocyte death in mechanically traumatized articular cartilage explants depends on rate of loading. J Orthop Res 2001;19:779–84.

[20] Ewers BJ, Jayaraman VM, Banglmaier RF, et al. Rate of blunt impact loading affects changes in retropatellar cartilage and underlying bone in the rabbit patella. J Biomech 2002;35:747–55.

[21] Kim H, Lo M, Pillarisetty R. Chondrocyte apoptosis following intraarticular fracture in humans. Osteoarthritis Cartilage 2002;10:747–9.

[22] Ewers BJ, Weaver BT, Haut RC. Impact orientation can significantly affect the outcome of a blunt impact to the rabbit patello-femoral joint. J Biomech 2002;35:1591–8.

[23] Ewers BJ, Weaver BT, Sevensma ET, et al. Chronic changes in rabbit retro-patellar cartilage and subchondral bone after blunt impact loading of the patellofemoral joint. J Orthop Res 2002;20:545–50.

[24] Kafka V. Surface fissures in articular cartilage: new concepts, hypotheses and modeling. Clin Biomech (Bristol, Avon) 2002;17:73–80.

[25] Bohndorf K. Imaging of acute injuries of the articular surfaces (chondral, osteochondral and subchondral fractures). Skeletal Radiol 1999;28:545–60.

[26] Bai B, Kummer FJ, Sala DA, et al. Effect of articular step-off and meniscectomy on joint alignment and contact pressures for fractures of the lateral tibial plateau. J Orthop Trauma 2001;15:101–6.

[27] Lovasz G, Park SH, Ebramzadeh E, et al. Characteristics of degeneration in an unstable knee with a coronal surface step-off. J Bone Joint Surg [Br] 2001;83:428–36.

[28] Lefkoe TP, Walsh WR, Anastasatos J, et al. Remodeling of articular step offs: is osteoarthrosis dependent on defect size? Clin Orthop 1995;314:253–65.

[29] Llinas A, McKellop HA, Marshall JG, et al. Healing and remodeling of articular incongruities in a rabbit fracture model. J Bone Joint Surg [Am] 1993;75:1508–23.

[30] Lovasz G, Llinas A, Benya PD, et al. Cartilage changes caused by a coronal surface stepoff in a rabbit model. Clin Orthop 1998;354:224–34.

[31] Marsh JL, Buckwalter JA, Gelberman R, et al. American Orthopedic Association symposium: articular fractures: does an anatomic reduction really change the result? J Bone Joint Surg [Am] 2002;84A:1259–71.

[32] Blokker CP, Rorabeck CH, Bourne RB. Tibial plateau fractures: an analysis of the results of treatment in 60 patients. Clin Orthop 1984;182:193–9.

[33] Huber-Betzer H, Brown TD, Mattheck C. Some effects of global joint morphology on local stress aberrations near imprecisely reduced intra-articular fractures. J Biomech 1990;23:811–22.

[34] Stevens DG, Beharry R, McKee MD, et al. The long-term functional outcome of operatively treated tibial plateau fractures. J Orthop Trauma 2001;15:312–20.

[35] Martin JA, Buckwalter JA. Fibronectin and cell shape affect age related decline in chondrocyte synthetic response to IGF-I. Trans Orthop Res Soc 1996;21:306.

[36] Martin JA, Buckwalter JA. The role of chondrocyte senescence in the pathogenesis of osteoarthritis and in limiting cartilage repair. J Bone Joint Surg [Am] 2003;85(Suppl 2): 106–10.

[37] Martin JA, Ellerbroek SM, Buckwalter JA. The age-related decline in chondrocyte response to insulin-like growth factor-I: the role of growth factor binding proteins. J Orthop Res 1997; 15:491–8.

[38] Cooke PH. Ankle arthritis. In: Bulstrode C, Buckwalter J, Carr A, et al, editors. Oxford textbook of orthopaedics and trauma. 1st edition. Oxford (UK): Oxford University Press; 2002. p. 1217–24.

[39] van Valburg AA, van Roermund PM, Lammens J, et al. Can Ilizarov joint distraction delay the need for an arthrodesis of the ankle? A preliminary report. J Bone Joint Surg [Br] 1995; 77:720–5.

[40] Abdo RV, Wasilewski SA. Ankle arthrodesis: a long-term study. Foot Ankle 1992;13:307–12.

[41] Mann RA, Chou LB. Tibiocalcaneal arthrodesis. Foot Ankle 1995;16:401–5.

[42] Mann RA, Van Manen JW, Wapner K, et al. Ankle fusion. Clin Orthop 1991;268:49–55.

[43] Buck P, Morrey BF, Chao EYS. The optimum position of arthrodesis of the ankle. J Bone Joint Surg [Am] 1987;69:1052–62.

[44] Marcus RE, Balourdas GM, Heiple KG. Ankle arthrodesis by Chevron fusion with internal fixation and bone-grafting. Bone Joint Surg [Am] 1983;65:833–8.

[45] Dohm MP, Benjamin JB, Harrison J, et al. A biomechanical evaluation of three forms of internal fixation used in ankle arthrodesis. Foot Ankle 1994;15:297–300.

[46] Holt ES, Hansen ST, Mayo KA, et al. Ankle arthrodesis using internal screw fixation. Clin Orthop 1991;268:21–8.

[47] Kite TA, Donnelly RE, Gehrke JC, et al. Tibiotalocalcaneal arthrodesis with an intramedullary device. Foot Ankle 1994;15:669–73.

[48] Moore TJ, Prince R, Pochatko D, et al. Retrograde intramedullary nailing for ankle arthrodesis. Foot Ankle 1995;16:433–44.

[49] Hawkins III B, Langerman III R, Anger DM, et al. The Ilizarov technique in ankle fusion. Clin Orthop 1994;303:217–25.

[50] Johnson EE, Weltmer J, Lian GJ, et al. Ilizarov ankle arthrodesis. Clin Orthop 1992;280: 160–9.

[51] Moeckel BH, Patterson BM, Inglis AE, et al. Ankle arthrodesis: a comparison of internal and external fixation. Clin Orthop 1991;268:78–83.

[52] Boobbyer GN. The long-term results of ankle arthrodesis. Acta Orthop Scand 1981;52: 107–10.

[53] Hintermann B, Nigg BM. Influence of arthrodeses on kinematics of the axially loaded ankle complex during dorsiflexion/plantarflexion. Foot Ankle 1995;16:633–6.

[54] Morrey BF, Wiedeman GP. Complications and long-term results of ankle arthrodesis following trauma. J Bone Joint Surg [Am] 1980;62:777–84.

[55] Buckwalter JA, Einhorn TA, Marsh JL. Bone and joint healing. In: Rockwood CA, Green DP, Bucholz RW, et al, editors. Fractures. Philadelphia: Lippincott; 2001. p. 245–71.

ELSEVIER
SAUNDERS

Clin Podiatr Med Surg
23 (2006) 467–483

CLINICS IN
PODIATRIC
MEDICINE AND
SURGERY

The Management of Acute Charcot Fracture-Dislocations with the Taylor's Spatial External Fixation System

Thomas S. Roukis, DPM[a],*, Thomas Zgonis, DPM[b]

[a]Department of Vascular Surgery MCHJ-SOP, Madigan Army Medical Center,
9040-A Fitzsimmons Avenue, Tacoma, WA 98431, USA
[b]Division of Podiatry, Department of Orthopaedics,
The University of Texas Health Science Center at San Antonio, 7773 Floyd Curl Drive,
San Antonio, TX 78229, USA

Diabetic Charcot foot deformity (ie, neuropathic osteoarthropathy) is a progressive and disfiguring condition characterized by joint dislocation, pathologic fracture, and extensive destruction of the foot architecture secondary to severe peripheral neuropathy. This is a progressive disease process driven by repetitive trauma (ie, weight bearing, taut Achilles tendon, or equinus contracture) that goes unrecognized because of loss of sensation (ie, dense peripheral neuropathy) and reactive hyperemia (ie, osteopenia, reduced bone stiffness, reduced bone density). The end result is usually a severely deformed and disabling foot that is difficult to shoe and brace properly, recurrent ulceration and infection, and ultimately amputation [1].

The diabetic Charcot foot deformity is most commonly classified using the Eichenholtz classification, which is a temporal classification based on characteristic clinical and radiographic changes that occur over time [2]. This classification divides the diabetic Charcot foot deformity into a process with three stages: stage I or the developmental phase characterized by soft-tissue edema, joint fragmentation, and dislocation; stage II or the coalescent phase characterized by edema reduction, bone callus proliferation, and fracture consolidation; and stage III or the reconstructive phase characterized by osseous ankylosis and hypertrophic proliferation stages. In clinical practice, the first stage is considered active, and

---

* Corresponding author.
E-mail address: troukis@footankledeformity.com (T.S. Roukis).

the last two stages are considered the quiescent or reparative stages. The Sanders/ Frykberg classification of diabetic Charcot foot deformity is based upon the anatomic location of the neuroarthropathic process: (1) toes, metatarsophalangeal joints, metatarsals; (2) tarso-metatarsal joints; (3) naviculo-cuneiform, talonavicular, and calcaneo-cuboid joints; (4) ankle joint; and (5) calcaneus [3].

The goal of any treatment for the diabetic Charcot foot deformity is to create a plantigrade, stable and shoeable/braceable foot that will be free of significant risk for further breakdown, ulceration, or infection [1,4–6]. Conservative and surgical intervention has been discussed for all stages of disease and anatomic locations of deformity. The actual decision between conservative and surgical intervention depends on the assessment of the risks and advantages of each in terms of the deformity present, patient compliance, comorbidities, nutrition status, family support capabilities, and other factors. One must usually choose the "lesser of two evils" when deciding between conservative care with whole-limb immobilization and non–weight bearing (with the associated problems of reliance on casting/bracing to maintain reduction and the risk of skin breakdown and deep venous thrombosis) or surgical intervention (with the risks of incision breakdown, infection, hardware failure, and vascular compromise). Because these patients have dense peripheral neuropathy, and pain is not an issue to them, the worst-case scenario must be assumed, and the treatment plan must be made as "patient-proof" as possible.

Management of diabetic Charcot foot deformity: literature review

Eichenholtz stage I

The management of Eichenholtz stage I diabetic Charcot foot deformities has predominantly involved the use of immobilization (ie, using various types of over-the-counter or custom-made casts, splints, or braces, total-contact casts, fixed-ankle walkers, bivalved casts, total-contact prosthetic walkers, patellar tendon–bearing braces) and complete non–weight bearing (ie, complete bed rest, crutches, quad-walker, wheelchair) [1]. Although these are accepted forms of treatment, weight bearing on the contralateral limb (ie, a three-point gait) increases pressure to this foot, which is also at risk, predisposing it to repetitive stress, ulceration, or Charcot foot deformity during the 4-to-6–month period required for the original Charcot foot deformity to heal fully and stabilize [7]. A chronic degree of bone resorption has also been implicated in both the development and the maintained bone fragmentation and delayed healing seen in diabetic Charcot neuroarthropathy [8]. A recent immunohistochemical study of 20 bone specimens obtained from predominantly male patients with a mean age of 55 years who had an Eichenholtz stage II Charcot midfoot deformity revealed a significant number of large osteoclasts and cell mediators for increased bone resorption [9]. This finding suggests that therapy aimed at increasing osseous consolidation and limiting resorption, such as the use of bisphosphonate intravenous therapy [10] or bone-growth stimulation [11,12], would be beneficial in the early stages of treatment of the Charcot deformity. Although ancillary bone-growth stimulation seems promising, it has not been conclusively proven to be effective in this disease state [11–13].

Surgical intervention (ie, open reduction internal fixation [ORIF] and arthrodesis with plates and large-diameter screws) in the Eichenholtz stage I diabetic Charcot foot deformity has been discussed infrequently in the literature, but the few published studies seem to support this form of treatment in select patients.

Myerson and colleagues [14], in a retrospective review, treated eight unstable Eichenholtz stage I diabetic Charcot foot deformities using ORIF, immobilization in a non–weight-bearing cast for 8 to 10 weeks, and then a total-contact weight-bearing cast for 2 to 7 months. These feet remained stable, shoeable/braceable, and free of ulceration at a mean of 28 months [14].

Simon and colleagues [15], in a retrospective review, treated 14 unstable Eichenholtz stage I diabetic Charcot foot deformities with ORIF, immobilization in a non–weight-bearing cast for a mean of 10 to 16 weeks, followed by a total-contact weight-bearing cast for an additional 10 to 16 weeks. These feet remained stable, shoeable/braceable, and free of ulceration at a mean of 41 months.

Eichenholtz stage II and III

The management of Eichenholtz stage II and III diabetic Charcot foot deformities with osseous prominence, instability, or ulceration has predominantly involved the use of either immobilization using various types of over-the-counter or custom-made casts, splints, or braces (ie, total-contact casts, fixed-ankle walkers, bivalved casts, total-contact prosthetic walkers, patellar tendon–bearing braces) or limited surgical intervention in the form of resection of the osseous prominence and excision of the ulceration with or without soft tissue plastic surgery reconstruction [1].

Brodsky and Rouse [16], in a retrospective review of 12 patients who had Eichenholtz stage II and III diabetic Charcot foot deformities and persistent or recurrent ulceration, performed an exostectomy and cast immobilization (mean duration of 3 months) and followed the patients for a mean of 25 months. Complications arose in 25% of patients during the postoperative recovery, and one patient required a more proximal Syme's-type amputation.

Rosenblum and colleagues [17], in a retrospective review of 31 patients (32 feet) with Eichenholtz stage II and III diabetic Charcot foot deformities and persistent or recurrent ulceration, performed an exostectomy with primary closure following ulcer excision or soft tissue plastic surgery reconstruction. Twenty-one patients (66%) healed uneventfully or with minor complications (ie, superficial infection or wound dehiscence) after the initial procedure and remained stable and shoeable. The remaining 11 patients had serious complications (ie, deep wound dehiscence, infection, ulcer recurrence) and required revision surgery. Additional surgical intervention was unsuccessfully in three patients. At a mean follow-up of 21 months, functional limb salvage was attained in 29 of 32 feet (91%).

The use of realignment arthrodesis using ORIF for the management of Eichenholtz stage II and III diabetic Charcot foot deformities with osseous prominence, instability, or ulceration has been supported in the literature as well.

Papa and colleagues [18], in a retrospective review of 29 patients who had Eichenholtz stage II and III diabetic Charcot foot or ankle deformities and osseous prominences with instability, performed an arthrodesis with ORIF, non–weight-bearing casts progressing to weight-bearing total-contact casts, and finally custom ankle foot orthoses use indefinitely. Nineteen patients (66%) developed a solid arthrodesis at a mean of 5 months. Of the 10 patients who developed a pseudoarthrosis, 7 were deemed stable. In total, two feet were not plantigrade, two developed a malunion, one required a below-knee amputation, and one developed a recurrent ulceration. None of the patients treated with solid arthrodesis or stable pseudoarthrosis broke down during the follow-up period of 43 months.

Myerson and colleagues [14], in a retrospective review of 12 feet with Eichenholtz stage II and III diabetic Charcot foot deformities and osseous prominences with instability, performed an arthrodesis with ORIF, tendo-Achilles lengthening, and cast immobilization for a mean of 6.5 months. All 12 feet were deemed stable at a mean follow-up of 28 months.

Early and Hansen [19], in a retrospective review of 21 feet with Eichenholtz stage II and III diabetic Charcot foot deformities and osseous prominences with instability, performed an arthrodesis with ORIF, tendo-Achilles lengthening, and cast immobilization and wheelchair use for a mean of 5 months. At a mean follow-up of 28 months, 18 feet (86%) had been successfully treated with their surgical protocol; one patient died of a myocardial infarction on the third postoperative day, and two required below-knee amputations because of uncontrolled osteomyelitis.

Deresh and Cohen [20], in a retrospective case series of three patients who had Eichenholtz stage II and III diabetic Charcot foot deformities and osseous prominences with instability, performed an arthrodesis with ORIF and bone grafting, tendo-Achilles lengthening, and cast immobilization for a total of 4 to 6 months. One patient received an implantable bone growth stimulation device as well. Each patient developed a stable arthrodesis, plantigrade foot, and was free of ulceration at final follow-up, at 10 months, 3 years, and 6 years, respectively.

Johnson and colleagues [21], in a non–peer-reviewed, retrospective abstract of 27 feet from 25 patients who had Eichenholtz stage II and III diabetic Charcot foot or ankle deformities and osseous prominences with instability, performed arthrodesis with ORIF. Twenty-six feet (96%) were eventually rendered stable and braceable; one foot required a below-knee amputation secondary to a deep infection.

Horton and Schon [22], in a non–peer-reviewed, retrospective abstract of 27 feet with Eichenholtz stage II and III diabetic Charcot foot deformities and osseous prominences with instability, performed arthrodesis with ORIF using an extensile plantar approach and plantar plate application. There were two significant deep infections and eight minor wound complications; one reoperation was required.

Sammarco and colleagues [23], in a non–peer-reviewed, retrospective abstract of 12 patients who had Eichenholtz stage II and III diabetic Charcot foot deformities and osseous prominences with instability, performed arthrodesis with ORIF using multiple large-diameter, long intramedullary axial screws to bridge the apex of the deformity. Stable arthrodesis was achieved in 10 feet (83%) at a mean of 5.3 months, and full ambulation begun at a mean of 7 months. At a mean follow-up of 35 months, two feet developed an unstable pseudoarthrosis, and three feet required hardware removal because of loosening, but there were no recurrent ulcerations, and the successful feet retained alignment and stability.

Role of external fixation in the treatment of the diabetic Charcot foot deformity

The role of external fixation in the surgical treatment of acutely unstable or chronically malaligned or ulcerated diabetic Charcot foot deformity remains a matter for conjecture because of the paucity of peer-reviewed, scientifically sound and meaningful studies available.

Papa and colleagues [18] described the use of external fixation in four patients who had chronic ulceration and unstable diabetic Charcot foot or ankle deformities. None of the patients healed, and all required additional open surgery for salvage.

Johnson [24] simply stated that the use of external fixation in the management of diabetic Charcot foot deformities "provides adequate stability," but positioning the foot and ankle is extremely difficult, and early removal is frequently required because of serious pin-tract problems.

Myerson and Edwards [25] discussed the use of an external ring fixation system in the management of the infected diabetic Charcot foot deformity or as a supplemental means of protecting tenuous internal fixation following ORIF. No further information was provided.

Farber and colleagues [26], in a retrospective review of 11 patients who had Eichenholtz stage II and III diabetic Charcot foot deformities and osseous prominences with instability, performed a single-stage correction with complete ulcer excision, osteotomy, and realignment arthrodesis and external fixation stabilization for a mean of 57 days with minimal weight bearing. This treatment was followed by application of a total-contact cast for a mean of 131 days and progression into custom-molded diabetic shoes or patellar tendon–bearing braces. At a mean follow-up of 24 months, all feet were free of ulceration and stable in custom-molded diabetic-type shoes, although only four feet (36%) developed a solid arthrodesis. The remainder developed a stable pseudoarthrosis.

Wang and colleagues [27] performed a retrospective review of 28 feet from 28 patients who had nonspecified Eichenholtz stages of diabetic Charcot foot and ankle deformities and underwent a percutaneous tendo-Achilles lengthening, external ring fixation about the lower leg and hindfoot, application of mini external fixation about the forefoot and midfoot, and use of an external bone growth stimulator. The authors claim that osseous consolidation was achieved at a mean of 3.1 months (range, 2.1–5.0 months) and that no osseous collapse occurred over a follow-up period of up to 24 months.

Cooper [28], in a non–peer-reviewed, retrospective abstract of 77 feet from 77 patients who had Eichenholtz stage II and III diabetic Charcot foot deformities and osseous prominences with instability and ulceration, performed a single-stage correction with complete ulcer excision, osteotomy, and realignment arthrodesis plus external fixation stabilization for a mean of 91 days. At a mean follow-up of 20 months, two patients developed Charcot deformities at adjacent joints, but no recurrent ulcerations developed at the previous sites. No further data were provided; however, this same information was later published in a non–peer-reviewed study [29].

Wang [30], in a non–peer-reviewed "techniques" article on the use of external fixation in "over 75 patients" who had Eichenholtz stage I diabetic Charcot foot deformities, states that, "all of the patients experienced complete consolidation and arthrodesis ... and none of the patients experienced recurrence, breakdown, or reulceration, with the longest follow-up at 60 months." In a similar non–peer-reviewed "techniques" article, Jolly and colleagues [31] discuss the use of external fixation in the surgical treatment of Eichenholtz stage I diabetic Charcot foot deformities, but they presented no formal data of any kind.

Finally, Herbst [32], in a non–peer-reviewed "techniques" article on the use of external fixation in the surgical treatment of unbraceable diabetic Charcot foot and ankle deformities, described his approach to realignment arthrodesis but presented no formal data of any kind. Herbst cites unpublished data from Lew Schon, MD, involving a "large series of unpublished frame cases" for Charcot foot and ankle deformities as having a 92.5% limb salvage rate [32].

Surgical reconstruction of the acute Charcot midfoot fracture dislocation with the Taylor spatial external fixation system

Surgical reconstruction of the Eichenholtz stage I Charcot midfoot fracture dislocation (ie, Sanders/Frykberg classification types II and III) represents a difficult challenge, as evidenced by the paucity of literature available for review (Fig. 1). The authors' preferred technique involves the use of minimally invasive surgical incisions that respect the cutaneous and underlying osseous vasculature [33,34]. Because most diabetic Charcot neuropathic osteoarthropathy fracture-dislocation patterns in this stage involve collapse of the medial longitudinal arch and medial dislocation of the cuneiforms along with plantar dislocation of the cuboid, the authors prefer to perform midline (ie, junction of the dorsal and plantar skin edges) medial and lateral incisions directly overlying the deformities.

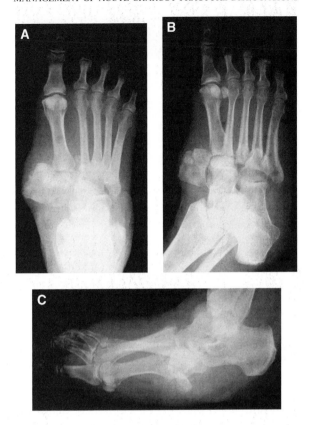

Fig. 1. Preoperative non–weight-bearing radiographs of an Eichenholtz stage I Charcot fracture dislocation about the midfoot demonstrating the typical fracture pattern seen. (*A*) Anterior-posterior. (*B*) Oblique. (*C*) Lateral.

These incisions also allow the use of either local cutaneous flaps or intrinsic muscle flaps covered with a split-thickness skin graft should wound healing problems develop about the incisions during the initial postoperative recovery period [35,36]. The incisions are carried down to the underlying osseous structures in a single full-thickness layer without excessive undermining, for the reasons described previously. The dislocated joints are debrided of articular cartilage, and the underlying cancellous surfaces are fenestrated with an osteotome to create slurry of bone while leaving the surrounding cortical surfaces intact (Fig. 2). The use of allogenic bone graft material impregnated with autogenous platelet-rich plasma is then packed within the arthrodesis site (Fig. 3) [37–39]. The midfoot is then manually molded until normal alignment is appreciated about the medial and lateral columns of the midfoot with the plantar surfaces of each metatarsal head lying at the same level. This series of maneuvers is most easily performed by first distracting the midfoot through longitudinal manual traction about the forefoot, followed by simultaneous dorsiflexion of all five toes

474ROUKIS & ZGONIS

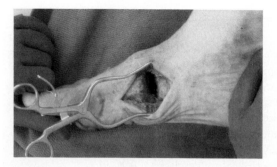

Fig. 2. Intraoperative photograph demonstrating the distraction technique used by the authors and the minimally invasive medial incision.

at the metatarso-phalangeal joints, and finally by compression of the midfoot through longitudinal compression. Large-diameter, smooth Kirschner wires are then driven across the arthrodesis sites, and osseous apposition and alignment are assessed under image intensification. These wires are removed once the external fixation system has been attached to the foot, ankle, and lower leg. Once proper alignment has been verified, the surgical sites are irrigated, and the incisions are closed as a single layer.

The authors prefer to apply the Taylor spatial external fixation system, which is a computer-assisted program that uses a six-axis coordinate system and a series of spatial relationships between the osseous structures and external fixation device to provide stability while allowing postoperative manipulation of the arthrodesis site in all three cardinal planes. The Ilizarov external fixation system

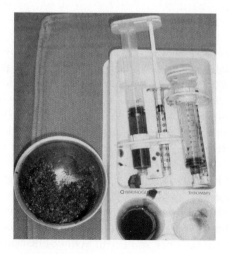

Fig. 3. Intraoperative photograph of allogenic bone-graft material impregnated with autogenous platelet-rich plasma.

uses a large number of components as well as hinges and translation mechanisms designed for a specific case, requires sequential correction for multiaxial deformities, and is associated with a steep learning curve [40–48]. The Taylor spatial external fixation system eliminates the challenges of calculating hinge placement, assembling translation and rotational constructs, and performing complex trigonometric calculations; also, the attachment to the limb undergoing deformity correction is simplified [40]. In addition, the Taylor spatial external fixation system has been shown to be equal to the Ilizarov external fixation system in axial compression, two times stronger in bending, and 2.3 times stronger in torsional resistance (data on file: Smith and Nephew, Inc., Memphis, Tennessee) [40]. Finally, the Taylor spatial external fixation system has been shown to have a mechanical accuracy within $0.7°$ and 2 mm and mathematical accuracy of 1/1,000,000 inches and 1/10,000° for correction of six-axis deformity (data on file: Smith and Nephew, Inc.) [40]. This system has been predominantly used for deformity correction (ie, malunion, non-union, limb-length discrepancy, triplane malalignment) and correction of traumatic injuries involving the tibia [40–48]. Although the Taylor spatial external fixation system has been used predominantly in the treatment of long bone deformities, the foot-specific Taylor spatial frame web software upgrade version 3.0 was released for general use on October 26, 2004. To date no reports of the step-by-step process have been published, and users must request an account to have access to the computer-based software and actually use the foot-specific frames available (www.spatialframe.com). After an account is set up, the initial step in the process involves determining the correction type that will be performed.

There are four correction types available: (1) long bone; (2) forefoot 6 × 6 miter; (3) forefoot 6 × 6 butt; and (4) forefoot 6 + 6. The long bone correction type is used when planning correction of tibia, femur, knee-spanning, and ankle-spanning deformities. The forefoot 6 × 6 miter correction type is used when planning a forefoot frame with a proximal two-thirds calcaneal ring at an oblique angle to the plane of the midfoot and employs the distal two-thirds forefoot ring as the reference fragment. The forefoot 6 × 6 butt correction type is used when planning a forefoot frame with a proximal U-shaped calcaneal ring orthogonal/perpendicular to the axis of the midfoot and employs either the distal two-thirds forefoot ring or the proximal U-shaped ring as the reference fragment. Finally, the forefoot 6 + 6 correction type is used whenever the specialized Lobe plate attachment is used to span the forefoot, which is connected to the distal U-shaped forefoot ring that is parallel to the plantar aspect of the forefoot and serves as the reference fragment.

The next step is to understand the quite specific terminology used for the Taylor spatial external fixation system. The icon for the left foot is lime colored and that for the right foot is rose colored to prevent inadvertent use of the wrong foot during the subsequent analysis and deformity correction. Once the proper foot is selected, anterior-posterior and lateral radiographs that are orthogonal to the rings must be obtained. The joint and intended level of attachment of the rings must be within the radiographs.

Once these parameters have been assured, the reference fragment is then assigned. The reference fragment is the piece(s) of bone that does not move (ie, remains stationary) during the correction. The reference fragment can be either the distal or the proximal fragment. By convention, the orthopedic literature usually characterizes the deformity of the distal fragment relative to the proximal fragment. Therefore, the proximal fragment is the reference fragment, and the distal fragment is the moving fragment. Ideally, the location of the reference ring should be as close as possible to the deformity to increase accuracy, because the further the reference ring is from the deformity, the greater is the likelihood of measurement error and the potential for the radiographs not to show properly the reference ring and reference fragment together [40]. Regardless of which foot is undergoing deformity correction, the forefoot is usually regarded as the distal reference fragment and the rearfoot as the proximal fragment. Once these parameters have been identified, the next step is to identify the origin and the corresponding point. The origin is the location on the reference fragment that matches exactly the location of the corresponding point on the moving fragment. The best points to select are ones that are coincident (ie, identical) in the anatomic or corrected state. The most common choice for the origin and corresponding points are the intersection of the reference and moving fragments along the mechanical axis or longitudinal bisection of the specific bone(s) being treated. For the tibia, selection of the origin and corresponding points are self-explanatory, but specific and rather unconventional bisections are used for the foot. On the anterior-posterior view the bisection of the center of the talar neck and second metatarsal should form one continuous line. On the lateral view the bisection of talar neck and the first metatarsal (ie, Meary's angle) should form one continuous line. Finally, on the axial view the plantar aspect of the metatarsal heads should be perpendicular to the bisection of the calcaneus.

Once these terms are selected, the next step is to identify the parameters. There are three frame, four mounting, and six deformity parameters that are used to allow the Internet-based computer software to produce the deformity correction program. The three frame parameters are the internal diameters of the proximal and distal rings and the neutral strut length (ie, length of the six struts used that would create a symmetrical frame). The frame parameters are obviously based on the components selected for the patient's specific anatomy. For the foot-specific program, the frame components are a full ring, U-plate, two-thirds ring, Lobe plate, or combination of these; the strut family type is either the standard or the Fast-Fx; and strut sizes are extra-short, short, medium, or long. The four mounting parameters or dimensions are

1. Anterior-posterior view frame offset (ie, medial or lateral translation of the center of the reference ring with respect to the origin)
2. Lateral view frame offset (ie, anterior or posterior translation of the center of the reference ring with respect to the origin)
3. Axial frame offset (ie, proximal or distal translation of the reference ring with respect to the origin)

4. Rotary frame offset (ie, rotation in the sagittal plane of the reference ring from the sagittal plane of the reference fragment).

The center of the rings (ie, center line) relative to the underlying osseous anatomy is usually offset because of the constraints of the soft tissue envelope. Therefore, origin and corresponding points usually are offset to some degree from the center of the rings, and this deviation needs to be incorporated into the entire coordinate system to avoid major errors. Next, the master tab needs to be selected. The master tab is always located on the reference ring and is located directly anterior (ie, dorsal). The master tab is the place where the universal joints for struts number 1 and number 2 attach (with each strut attachment progressing in a counterclockwise direction when viewed proximally). The six deformity parameters or dimensions are

1. Anterior-posterior view translation (ie, medial or lateral translation from the origin to the corresponding point)
2. Lateral view translation (ie, anterior or posterior translation from the origin to the corresponding point)
3. Anterior-posterior view angulation (ie, angle between the fragment center lines)
4. Lateral view angulation (ie, angle between the center lines)
5. Axial translation (ie, proximal or distal translation from the origin to the corresponding point)
6. Axial view angulation (ie, the angle between the reference fragment and moving fragment).

For the foot-specific program the following definitions are employed. On the anterior-posterior view the transverse plane angulation is defined as the degree of varus or valgus malalignment as well as the distance in millimeters of medial or lateral translation of the forefoot relative to the rearfoot. On the lateral view the sagittal plane angulation is defined as the degree of apex plantar (ie, rocker-bottom deformity) or apex dorsal (ie, cavus foot posture), as well as the distance in millimeters of plantar or dorsal translation of the forefoot relative to the rear-foot. Finally, on the axial view the degree of forefoot supination or pronation is defined, as well as the distance in millimeters of either excessive length or foreshortening of the forefoot relative to the rearfoot.

Once these parameters have been entered, the screen is refreshed to create regenerated views. The regenerated views are reviewed to make certain that the computer icons match the deformity present clinically and that the correct foot has been chosen. The final step is to define the structures at risk during the correction (ie, the important biologic structure—nerve, vessel, bone, muscle, skin—that will undergo the greatest or most critical elongation or compression during the deformity correction. The coordinates of the structures at risk relative to the reference fragment are used to determine the actual rate of deformity correction.

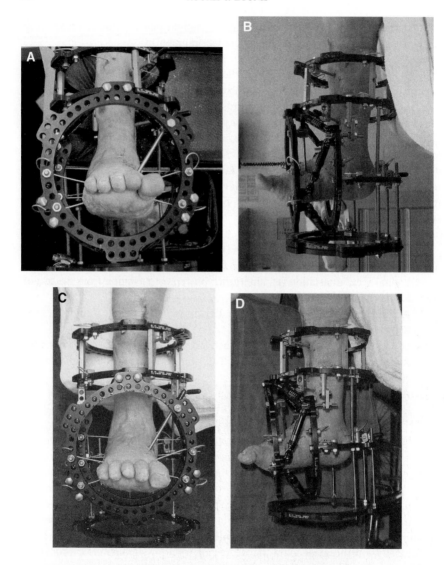

Fig. 4. (*A*) End-on and (*B*) medial views of the foot shown in the previous figures after the technique described within the text and application of a Taylor spatial external fixation system. Note (*A*) the excessive plantarflexion of the first metatarsal head and forefoot valgus and (*B*) the over-corrected medial longitudinal arch. (*C*) End-on and (*D*) medial views of the same foot 10 days after total residual correction to the deformities until each metatarsal head rests at (C) the same level with a rectus forefoot and (*D*) theappropriate medial longitudinal arch height.

The next screen gives the prescription that shows each of the starting strut lengths (ie, day zero) and the daily progression necessary to achieve full correction of the deformity over the specific time necessary, as based upon the structures at risk (Fig. 4). Any necessary strut changes (ie, from an extra-short to a long) are stated in bold so that the patient can be seen during these change-out times to avoid jamming of the struts throughout the correction phase.

Throughout the deformity-correction phase, repeat radiographs are obtained, as defined previously, and the parameters are reviewed with any changes requiring repeat measurement and data input to create a new prescription. Once the deformity has been fully corrected, no further alterations are performed, and the consolidation phase is entered, which allows the osseous components to solidify. The authors have found it useful to compress and distract the reference and moving fragments (ie, "accordion" the axial length) slowly to stimulate osseous regeneration and also to keep the patient involved in their care, because patients have a tendency to grow tired of the constant presence of the external fixation device unless some are daily modifications employed (ie, "cage rage"). In addition, the authors have found it helpful to use a specialized postoperative shoe that is attached to an extra "dummy-ring" about the undersurface of the external fixation system to allow the patient to perform weight sharing on the involved limb with the appropriate gait aide [40,49]. This technique allows some limited mobility while suspending the foot and transmitting the weight-sharing forces to the more proximal rings.

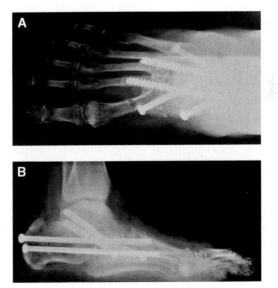

Fig. 5. Weight-bearing (*A*) anterior-posterior and (*B*) lateral radiographs of the same foot 1 year after surgical correction demonstrating complete osseous incorporation of the allogenic bone graft impregnated with autogenous platelet-rich plasma with a stable midfoot arthrodesis and well-aligned foot. Note the presence of multiple large-diameter internal screws that were placed through percutaneous incisions at the time of external fixation removal to afford osseous stability (ie, internal splitage).

After osseous consolidation, the external fixation system is removed, most commonly under local anesthesia, and the osseous consolidation is assessed under image intensification. If any motion whatever is detected, the authors insert multiple large cannulated screws in multiple planes to provide internal splintage (ie, rebar). This technique allows continued osseous apposition and limits the potential for delayed collapse of the corrected deformity (Fig. 5). This assessment is followed by the application of a well-padded, short-leg, partial–weight-bearing cast with gradual transition into a removable over-the-counter or customized walking brace as determined by serial radiographs that demonstrate continued osseous consolidation and maintained correction of the deformity. A useful technique for the potentially or frankly noncompliant patient is to apply the initial cast with the foot held in a plantarflexed and inverted position relative to the lower leg, because this position is not conducive to formal weight bearing as is possible in a cast applied with the foot at a right angle to the lower leg. A formal fixed-ankle gauntlet-type brace or posterior ankle-foot orthosis is used for approximately 12 months, after which a proper extra-depth shoe and customized in-shoe orthoses are used indefinitely.

Discussion

Because external fixation technology allows minimally invasive acute or gradual reduction and stabilization of deformity and early assisted partial weight bearing (or rather, weight sharing), it would seem to be the obvious first choice for surgical treatment of the acutely unstable or chronically malaligned and ulcerated diabetic foot with Charcot neuropathic osteoarthropathy deformity. Few prospective studies exist for any form of treatment, and despite numerous lectures at both podiatric and orthopedic meetings regarding the use of external fixation in the surgical management of the unstable diabetic Charcot neuropathic osteoarthropathy foot deformity, no studies beyond unpublished abstracts, poorly controlled case series, or descriptive "how-to" technique guides have been presented to support its use. There is a significant need for a well-designed, prospective, randomized, controlled study on the use of external fixation for the surgical treatment of the unstable diabetic Charcot foot deformity. The use of the Taylor spatial external fixation system has been shown to increase the accuracy of correction of long bone deformity and trauma repair, and similar improvement should be attainable with the foot-specific program once it has been fully embraced by the foot and ankle community.

Summary

The surgical repair of acute diabetic Charcot neuropathic osteoarthropathy about the midfoot remains a formidable challenge with little guidance offered in the medical literature. The use of external fixation systems to reduce the deformity and afford a stable, plantigrade foot that can be fitted with proper brace/shoe gear to support the repeat shear and vertical forces associated with ambulation is currently popular but has not been supported by well-controlled, prospective studies involving a large patient population followed for a long period of time. The gradual correction of the deformity with the use of the foot-specific Taylor spatial external fixation system shows great promise and overcomes some of the problems associated with the use of the traditional Ilizarov external fixation system. Like the external fixation for foot deformity correction, however, the Taylor spatial external fixation system is a complicated process with multiple opportunities for patient and physician error and requires proper research to define fully its role in the reconstructive foot and ankle surgeons' armamentarium.

References

[1] Frykberg RG, Armstrong DA, Edwards A, et al, American College of Foot and Ankle Surgeons. Diabetic foot disorders: a clinical practice guideline. J Foot Ankle Surg 2000;39:S1–60.

[2] Eichenholtz SN. In: Wilson P, editor. Charcot joints. Springfield (IL): CC Thomas; 1966.

[3] Sanders LJ, Frykberg RG. Diabetic neuropathic osteoarthropathy. The Charcot foot. In: Frykberg RG, editor. The high risk foot in diabetes mellitus. New York: Churchill Livingston; 1991. p. 297.

[4] Larsen K, Fabrin J, Holstein PE. Incidence and management of ulcers in diabetic Charcot feet. J Wound Care 2001;10:323–8.

[5] Bowering CK. Diabetic foot ulcers: pathophysiology, assessment, and therapy. Can Fam Physician 2001;47:1007–16.

[6] Brem H, Sheehan P, Boulton AJM. Protocol for treatment of diabetic foot ulcers. Am J Surg 2004;187:1S–10S.

[7] Lesko P, Maurer RC. Talonavicular dislocations and midfoot arthropathy in neuropathic diabetic feet: natural course and principles of treatment. Clin Orthop 1989;240:226.

[8] Gough A, Abraha H, Purewal TS, et al. Measurement of markers of osteoclast and osteoblast activity in patients with acute and chronic diabetic Charcot neuroarthropathy. Diabet Med 1997; 14:527.

[9] Baumhauer JF, O'Keefe R, Schon LC, et al. Free cytokine induced osteoclastic bone resorption in Charcot arthropathy: an immunohistochemical study. Presented at the 20th Annual Summer Meeting of the American Orthopaedic Foot and Ankle Society. Seattle, WA, July 29–31, 2004.

[10] Anderson JJ, Woelffer KE, Holtzman JJ, et al. Bisphosphonates for the treatment of Charcot neuroarthropathy. J Foot Ankle Surg 2004;43:285.

[11] Hanft JR, Goggin JP, Landsman A, et al. The role of combined magnetic field bone growth stimulation as an adjunct in the treatment of neuroarthropathy/Charcot joint: an expanded pilot study. J Foot Ankle Surg 1998;37:510–5.

[12] Grady JF, O'Connor KJ, Axe TM, et al. Use of electrostimulation in the treatment of diabetic neuroarthropathy. J Am Podiatr Med Assoc 2000;90:287.

[13] Rubin C, Bolander M, Ryaby JP, et al. The use of low-intensity ultrasound to accelerate the healing of fractures. J Bone Joint Surg [Am] 2001;83:259–70.

[14] Myerson MS, Henderson MR, Saxby T, et al. Management of midfoot diabetic neuroarthropathy. Foot Ankle Int 1994;15:233–41.

[15] Simon SR, Tejwani S, Wilson D, et al. Arthrodesis as an early alternative to non-operative management of Charcot arthropathy of the diabetic foot. J Bone Joint Surg [Am] 2000;82: 939–50.

[16] Brodsky JW, Rouse AM. Exostectomy for symptomatic bony prominences in diabetic Charcot feet. Clin Orthop Rel Res 1993;296:21–6.

[17] Rosenblum BI, Giurini JM, Miller LB, et al. Neuropathic ulcerations plantar to the lateral column

in patients with Charcot foot deformity: a flexible approach to limb salvage. J Foot Ankle Surg 1997;36:360–3.

[18] Papa J, Myerson M, Girard P. Salvage, with arthrodesis, in intractable diabetic neuropathic arthropathy of the foot and ankle. J Bone Joint Surg [Am] 1993;75:1056–66.

[19] Early JS, Hansen ST. Surgical reconstruction of the diabetic foot: a salvage approach for midfoot collapse. Foot Ankle Int 1996;17:325–30.

[20] Deresh GM, Cohen M. Reconstruction of the diabetic Charcot foot incorporating bone grafts. J Foot Ankle Surg 1996;35:474–88.

[21] Johnson JE, O'Brien TS, Hart TS, et al. Reconstruction of the Charcot foot and ankle: an outcome study of long-term results. Presented at the Annual Meeting of the American Orthopaedic Foot and Ankle Society. Hilton Head, South Carolina. June 30, 1996.

[22] Horton GA, Schon L. An extensile plantar exposure of the midfoot for treatment of the severe rocker bottom deformity. American Association of Orthopaedic Surgeons Specialty Day. San Francisco, March 23, 2001.

[23] Sammarco VJ, Guiao RP, Sammarco GJ, et al. Surgical treatment of severe Charcot midfoot collapse with transverse midtarsal arthrodesis fixed with multiple long intramedullary screws. Presented at the American Orthopaedic Foot and Ankle Society Summer Meeting. Traverse City, Michigan, July 13, 2002.

[24] Johnson JE. Surgical reconstruction of the diabetic Charcot foot and ankle. Foot Ankle Clin 1997;2:37–55.

[25] Myerson MS, Edwards WH. Management of neuropathic fractures in the foot and ankle. J Am Acad Orthop Surg 1997;7:8–18.

[26] Farber DC, Juliano PJ, Cavanagh PR, et al. Single stage correction with external fixation of the ulcerated foot in individuals with Charcot neuroarthropathy. Foot Ankle Int 2002;23:130–4.

[27] Wang JC, Le AW, Tsukuda RK. A new technique for Charcot's foot reconstruction. J Am Podiatr Med Assoc 2002;92:429–36.

[28] Cooper P, et al. Fine wire external fixation for the management of chronic ulcerations associated with Charcot arthropathy. American Orthopaedic Foot and Ankle Society Summer Meeting 2002.

[29] Cooper PS. Application of external fixations for management of Charcot deformities of the foot and ankle. Foot Ankle Clin 2002;7:207–54.

[30] Wang JC. Use of external fixation in the reconstruction of the Charcot foot and ankle. Clin Podiatr Med Surg 2003;20:97–117.

[31] Jolly GP, Zgonis T, Polyzois V. External fixation in the management of Charcot neuro-arthropathy. Clin Podiatr Med Surg 2003;20:741–56.

[32] Herbst SA. External fixation of Charcot arthropathy. Foot Ankle Clin 2004;9:595–609.

[33] Attinger C, Cooper P, Blume P. Vascular anatomy of the foot and ankle. Operative Techniques in Plastic and Reconstructive Surgery 1997;4:183–98.

[34] Attinger C, Cooper P, Blume P, et al. The safest surgical incisions and amputations applying the angiosome principles and using the Doppler to assess the arterial-arterial connections of the foot and ankle. Foot Ankle Clin 2001;6:745–99.

[35] Attinger CE, Ducic I, Cooper P, et al. The role of intrinsic muscle flaps of the foot for bone coverage in foot and ankle defects in diabetic and nondiabetic patients. Plast Reconstr Surg 2002;110:1047–54.

[36] Papp CT, Hasenohrl C. Small toe muscles for defect coverage. Plast Reconstr Surg 1990;86:941–5.

[37] Slater M, Patava J, Kingham K, et al. Involvement of platelets in stimulating osteogenic activity. J Orthop Res 1995;13:655–63.

[38] Marx RE, Carlson ER, Eichstaedt RM, et al. Platelet-rich plasma: growth factor enhancement for bone grafts. Oral Surg Oral Med Oral Pathol Oral Radiol Endod 1998;85:638–46.

[39] Dugrillon A, Eichler H, Kern S, et al. Autologous concentrated platelet-rich plasma (cPRP) for local application in bone regeneration. Int J Oral Maxillofac Surg 2002;31:615–9.

[40] Taylor JC. Six-axis deformity analysis and correction. In: Paley D, editor. Principles of deformity correction. Berlin: Springer-Verlag; 2002. p. 411–36.

[41] Rozbruch SR, Helfet DL, Blyakher A. Distraction of hypertrophic nonunion of tibia with deformity using Ilizarov/Taylor spatial frame. Arch Orthop Trauma Surg 2002;122:295–8.

[42] Schatz KD, Nehrer S, Dorotka R, et al. 3D-navigated high energy shock wave therapy and axis correction after failed distraction treatment of congenital tibial pseudarthrosis. Orthopade 2002; 31:663–6.

[43] Feldman DS, Shin SS, Madan S, et al. Correction of tibial malunion and nonunion with six-axis analysis deformity correction using the Taylor spatial frame. J Orthop Trauma 2003;17:549–54.

[44] Sluga M, Pfeiffer M, Kotz R, et al. Lower limb deformities in children: two-stage correction using the Taylor spatial frame. J Pediatr Orthop 2003;12:123–8.

[45] Feldman DS, Madan SS, Koval KJ, et al. Correction of tibia vara with six-axis deformity analysis and the Taylor spatial frame. J Pediatr Orthop 2003;23:387–91.

[46] Rödl R, Leidinger B, Böhm A, et al. Correction of deformities with conventional and hexapod frames: comparison of methods. Z Orthop Ihre Grenzgeb 2003;141:92–8.

[47] Höll S, Stoll V. Application of the Taylor spatial frame with unilateral implantation of a medial sledge prosthesis after post-traumatic dislocation of the femur: a complicated progression. Unfallchirurg 2004;107:433–66.

[48] McFadyen I, Atkins RM. The Taylor spatial frame in limb reconstruction surgery: review of 100 cases. Presented at the annual congress of the British Orthopaedic Association. Manchester (UK), September 15, 2004.

[49] Roukis TS, Zgonis T. Post-operative shoe modifications for weightbearing with the Ilizarov external fixation system. J Foot Ankle Surg 2004;43:433–5.

Further readings

Cooper PS. Orthopedic considerations in wound healing of the lower extremity. Foot Ankle Clin 2001;6:715–44.

Daniels TR. Ankle and hindfoot Charcot arthropathy. In: Nunley JA, Pfeffer GB, Sanders RW, et al, editors. Advanced reconstruction: foot and ankle. Rosemont (IL): American Academy of Orthopaedic Surgeons; 2004. p. 419–26.

Early JS. Surgical intervention in diabetic neuroarthropathy of the foot. Foot Ankle Clin 1997;2:23.

Schon L. Chronic midfoot Charcot rocker-bottom reconstruction. In: Nunley JA, Pfeffer GB, Sanders RW, et al, editors. Advanced reconstruction: foot and ankle. Rosemont (IL): American Academy of Orthopaedic Surgeons; 2004. p. 411—8.

Schon LC, Marks RM. The management of neuropathic fracture-dislocations in the diabetic patient. Orthop Clin North Am 1995;26:375.

Trepman E. Reconstruction of acute midfoot Charcot arthropathy. In: Nunley JA, Pfeffer GB, Sanders RW, et al, editors. Advanced reconstruction: foot and ankle. Rosemont (IL): American Academy of Orthopaedic Surgeons; 2004. p. 405–10.

ELSEVIER
SAUNDERS

Clin Podiatr Med Surg
23 (2006) 485–486

CLINICS IN
PODIATRIC
MEDICINE AND
SURGERY

Erratum

Erratum to "External Fixation for the Foot and Ankle in Children" [Clin Podiatr Med Surg 23 (1) (2006) 137–166]

Bradley M. Lamm, DPM*, Shawn C. Standard, MD,
Ian J. Galley, MD, John E. Herzenberg, MD, Dror Paley, MD

*Rubin Institute for Advanced Orthopedics, Sinai Hospital of Baltimore, 2401 West Belvedere Avenue,
Baltimore, MD 21215, USA*

In the January 2006 issue "Pediatric Foot and Ankle Disorders," in the article "External Fixation for the Foot and Ankle in Children" by Bradley M. Lamm and colleagues, an error in the file for Fig. 3E published incorrectly. We apologize for this error and have printed the correct Fig. 3E and its legend below.

DOI of original article title 10.1016/j.cpm.2005.10.007.
* Corresponding author.
E-mail address: blamm@lifebridgehealth.org (B.M. Lamm).

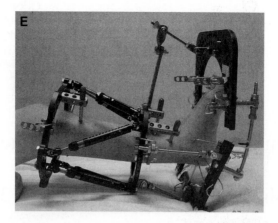

Fig. 3. (*E*) After the equinus deformity is corrected, the foot ring is cut (medial and lateral) to allow for correction of the cavus deformity. The gradual distraction is accomplished by adding pusher and puller Ilizarov rods.

ELSEVIER
SAUNDERS

Clin Podiatr Med Surg
23 (2006) 487–495

CLINICS IN
PODIATRIC
MEDICINE AND
SURGERY

Index

Note: Page numbers of article titles are in **boldface** type.

Changing Your Address?

Make sure your subscription changes too! When you notify us of your new address, you can help make our job easier by including an exact copy of your Clinics label number with your old address (see illustration below.) This number identifies you to our computer system and will speed the processing of your address change. Please be sure this label number accompanies your old address and your corrected address—you can send an old Clinics label with your number on it or just copy it exactly and send it to the address listed below.

We appreciate your help in our attempt to give you continuous coverage. Thank you.

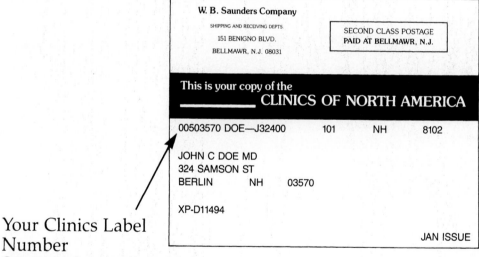

W. B. Saunders Company

SHIPPING AND RECEIVING DEPTS.
151 BENIGNO BLVD.
BELLMAWR, N.J. 08031

SECOND CLASS POSTAGE
PAID AT BELLMAWR, N.J.

This is your copy of the
_____ CLINICS OF NORTH AMERICA

00503570 DOE—J32400   101   NH   8102

JOHN C DOE MD
324 SAMSON ST
BERLIN   NH   03570

XP-D11494

JAN ISSUE

Your Clinics Label Number
Copy it exactly or send your label
along with your address to:
W.B. Saunders Company, Customer Service
Orlando, FL 32887-4800
Call Toll Free 1-800-654-2452

Please allow four to six weeks for delivery of new subscriptions and for processing address changes.